T0259416

Adult Behavioral Sleep Medicine

Guest Editor

KENNETH L. LICHSTEIN, PhD

SLEEP MEDICINE CLINICS

www.sleep.theclinics.com

December 2009 • Volume 4 • Number 4

SAUNDERS an imprint of ELSEVIER, Inc.

W.B. SAUNDERS COMPANY
A Division of Elsevier Inc.

1600 John F. Kennedy Boulevard ● Suite 1800 ● Philadelphia, PA 19103-2899

http://www.sleep.theclinics.com

SLEEP MEDICINE CLINICS Volume 4, Number 4
December 2009, ISSN 1556-407X, ISBN-13: 978-1-4377-1274-2, ISBN-10: 1-4377-1274-6

Editor: Sarah E. Barth
Developmental Editor: Donald Mumford

Sleep Medicine Clinics (ISSN 1556-407X) is published quarterly by Elsevier, 360 Park Avenue South, New York, NY 10010. Months of issue are March, June, September and December. Application to mail at periodicals postage rates is pending at New York, NY and at additional mailing offices. Subscription prices are $150.00 per year (US individuals), $76.00 (US residents), $346.00 (US institutions), $185.00 (foreign individuals), $106.00 (foreign residents), and $381.00 (foreign institutions). Foreign air speed delivery is included in all *Clinics* subscription prices. All prices are subject to change without notice. **POSTMASTER:** Send change of address to *Sleep Medicine Clinics*, Elsevier Health Sciences Division, Subscription Customer Service, 3251 Riverport Lane, Maryland Heights, MO 63043 Customer Service, (orders, claims, online, change of address): **Elsevier Health Sciences Division, Subscription Customer Service, 3251 Riverport Lane, Maryland Heights, MO 63043 Tel: 1-800-654-2452 (U.S. and Canada); 314-447-8871 (outside U.S. and Canada). Fax: 314-447-8029. E-mail: journalscustomerservice-usa@elsevier.com (for print support); journalsonlinesupport-usa@elsevier.com (for online support).**

Reprints. For copies of 100 or more of articles in this publication, please contact the Commercial Reprints Department, Elsevier Inc., 360 Park Avenue South, New York, NY 10010-1710. Tel.: 212-633-3812; Fax: 212-462-1935; E-mail: reprints@elsevier.com.

Printed and bound in the United Kingdom

Transferred to Digital Print 2011

Sleep Medicine Clinics

FORTHCOMING ISSUES

March 2010

Dental Sleep Medicine
Dennis R. Bailey, DDS,
Guest Editor

June 2010

Dreaming
James F. Pagel, MD,
Guest Editor

September 2010

Positive Airway Pressure Therapy
Richard Berry, MD,
Guest Editor

RECENT ISSUES

September 2009

Polysomnography
Lawrence J. Epstein, MD,
and Douglas B. Kirsch, MD,
Guest Editors

June 2009

Circadian Rhythm Sleep Disorders
Kenneth P. Wright, Jr, PhD,
Guest Editor

March 2009

**Epidemiology of Sleep Disorders: Clinical
Implications**
Edward O. Bixler, PhD,
Guest Editor

THE CLINICS ARE NOW AVAILABLE ONLINE!

Access your subscription at:
www.theclinics.com

Contributors

CONSULTING EDITOR

TEOFILO LEE-CHIONG, Jr., MD
Head, Division of Sleep Medicine, National Jewish
Health; and Associate Professor of Medicine,
University of Colorado Denver School of Medicine,
Denver, Colorado

GUEST EDITOR

KENNETH L. LICHSTEIN, PhD, CBSM
Professor of Psychology; Director, Sleep
Research Project, Department of Psychology,
The University of Alabama, Tuscaloosa, Alabama

AUTHORS

MARK S. ALOIA, PhD, CBSM
Associate Professor of Medicine, National Jewish
Health, Department of Medicine, Denver,
Colorado

LYNDA BÉLANGER, PhD
Université Laval, École de Psychologie; Centre de
Recherche Université Laval/Robert-Giffard,
Québec, Canada

GENEVIÈVE BELLEVILLE, PhD
Département de Psychologie, Université du
Québecà Montréal; Centre de Recherche
Fernand-Seguin, Hôpital Louis-H.-Lafontaine,
Montréal, Québec, Canada

IAN ALPS CHEN, MD, MPH
Associate Professor of Internal Medicine,
Department of Internal Medicine, Eastern Virginia
Medical School, Norfolk, Virginia

JAMIE A. CVENGROS, PhD
Instructor of Behavioral Sciences, Rush Medical
College; Fellow in Behavioral Sleep Medicine,
Sleep Disorders Service and Research Center,
Rush University Medical Center, Chicago, Illinois

SEAN DRUMMOND, PhD
Laboratory of Sleep and Behavioral Neuroscience,
UCSD and VA San Diego Healthcare System,
San Diego, California

JOSEPH M. DZIERZEWSKI, MS
Department of Clinical and Health Psychology,
University of Florida, Gainesville, Florida

**COLIN A. ESPIE, MAppSci, PhD, CPsychol,
FBPsS, FCS, FRSM**
Professor, University of Glasgow Sleep Centre,
Sackler Institute of Psychobiological Research,
Faculty of Medicine, Southern General Hospital,
Glasgow, Scotland, United Kingdom

JAMES FINDLEY, PhD
Behavioral Sleep Medicine Program, Department
of Psychiatry, University of Pennsylvania,
Philadelphia, Pennsylvania

PHILLIP GEHRMAN, PhD
Behavioral Sleep Medicine Program, Department
of Psychiatry, University of Pennsylvania,
Philadelphia, Pennsylvania

ANNE GERMAIN, PhD
Assistant Professor of Psychiatry, Department of
Psychiatry, University of Pittsburgh School of
Medicine, Pittsburgh, Pennsylvania

LAURA E. GIBBONS, PhD
Senior Research Scientist, Department of General
Internal Medicine, University of Washington,
Seattle, Washington

ALLISON G. HARVEY, PhD
Associate Professor, Department of Psychology,
University of California, Berkeley, Berkeley,
California

BRANT P. HASLER, PhD
Postdoctoral Fellow, Department of Psychiatry,
University of Pittsburgh School of Medicine,
Pittsburgh, Pennsylvania

KATHERINE A. KAPLAN, MA
Department of Psychology, University of
California, Berkeley, Berkeley, California

DANIEL B. KAY, MS
Department of Clinical and Health Psychology,
University of Florida, Gainesville, Florida

SIMON D. KYLE, MA
University of Glasgow Sleep Centre, Sackler
Institute of Psychobiological Research, Faculty of
Medicine, Southern General Hospital, Glasgow,
Scotland, United Kingdom

REBECCA G. LOGSDON, PhD
Research Professor, Department of Psychosocial
and Community Health, University of Washington,
Seattle, Washington

HANNAH G. LUND, BA
Department of Psychology, Virginia
Commonwealth University, Richmond, Virginia

LAURIN MACK, MS
Department of Psychology, Virginia
Commonwealth University, Richmond, Virginia

ELLYN E. MATTHEWS, PhD, RN, AOCN
Assistant Professor of Nursing, University of
Colorado, College of Nursing, Aurora, Colorado

CHRISTINA S. McCRAE, PhD
Associate Professor, Department of Clinical and
Health Psychology, University of Florida,
Gainesville, Florida

SUSAN M. McCURRY, PhD
Research Professor, Department of Psychosocial
and Community Health, University of Washington,
Seattle, Washington

CHARLES M. MORIN, PhD
Université Laval, École de Psychologie; Centre de
Recherche Université Laval/Robert-Giffard,
Québec, Québec, Canada

MICHAEL PERLIS, PhD
Behavioral Sleep Medicine Program, Department
of Psychiatry, University of Pennsylvania,
Philadelphia, Pennsylvania

WILFRED R. PIGEON, PhD, CBSM
Assistant Professor, Department of Psychiatry,
Sleep and Neurophysiology Research Laboratory,
University of Rochester Medical Center,
Rochester, New York

BRUCE RYBARCZYK, PhD
Department of Psychology, Virginia
Commonwealth University, Richmond, Virginia

EDWARD STEPANSKI, PhD
Clinical Assistant Professor, Department of
Internal Medicine, University of Tennessee Health
Science Center; Chief Operating Officer,
Accelerated Community Oncology Research
Network, Inc (ACORN), Memphis, Tennessee

LISA S. TALBOT, MA
Department of Psychology, University of
California, Berkeley, Berkeley, California

LINDA TERI, PhD
Professor, Department of Psychosocial and
Community Health, University of Washington,
Seattle, Washington

MICHAEL V. VITIELLO, PhD
Professor, Department of Psychiatry and
Behavioral Sciences, University of Washington,
Seattle, Washington

ROBERT DANIEL VORONA, MD
Associate Professor of Internal Medicine, Department of Internal Medicine, Eastern Virginia Medical School; Medical Director, Eastern Virginia Medical School/Sentara Norfolk General Hospital Sleep Disorders Center, Norfolk, Virginia

J. CATESBY WARE, PhD
Professor of Internal Medicine, Division of Sleep Medicine, Department of Internal Medicine, Eastern Virginia Medical School; Professor of Psychiatry and Behavioral Medicine, Department of Psychiatry and Behavioral Medicine, Eastern Virginia Medical School, Norfolk, Virginia

JAMES K. WYATT, PhD
Associate Professor of Behavioral Sciences, Rush Medical College; Director, Sleep Disorders Service and Research Center, Rush University Medical Center, Chicago, Illinois

MICHAEL YURCHESHEN, MD
Assistant Professor, Department of Neurology and Strong Sleep Disorders Center, University of Rochester Medical Center, Rochester, New York

Contents

> Although continuous positive airway pressure (CPAP) is highly efficacious in the elimination of nocturnal apneas and hypopneas of obstructive sleep apnea (OSA), suboptimal adherence to treatment is common. Investigations of CPAP adherence reveal frequent adverse effects, and weak relationships between personality factors, OSA severity, symptoms, and CPAP use. Several well-conducted studies of mechanical interventions to overcome CPAP disadvantages have reported success; however, corresponding increase in adherence is not proportional to the reduction in adverse effects. Psychoeducational approaches provide promise for improving adherence, but are currently less rigorously evaluated. As appreciation for behavioral factors and technology increases, additional research is needed to identify which factors, in combination with mechanical interventions, provide the best prescription for CPAP adherence.

> Restless legs syndrome (RLS) and periodic limb movement disorder (PLMD) are sleep disorders that are commonly seen in clinical practice. The standard treatment recommendations for these disorders are pharmacologic; both conditions are typically managed with pramipexole or ropinirole, which are approved by the Food and Drug Administration for the treatment of RLS. A mix of behavioral suggestions is included in treatment algorithms for providers and in patient education materials. Although these suggestions have considerable merit, they are typically not delivered as an intervention, but instead provided as a series of helpful tips. There is emerging evidence for providing such suggestions as part of a cognitive-behavioral package to be delivered as active treatments for RLS or PLMD.

> Sleep and wakefulness are regulated by two modulatory processes: a homeostatic drive for sleep and a circadian timekeeping system. This article reviews the etiology, diagnosis, and treatment of the circadian rhythm sleep disorders that result from misalignment or dysfunction of these two processes. A review of the homeostatic and circadian regulation of sleep and wakefulness including measurement and modulation of circadian phase is also provided. This article concludes with a brief summary of the literature examining role of circadian factors in insomnia.

This article discusses the notion that insomnia is too often described in solely psychological terms. It is proposed that a comprehensive perspective on insomnia requires one that takes into account the neurobiologic abnormalities that may also function as predisposing, precipitating, and perpetuating factors for chronic Insomnia. To justify this claim, the reader is provided with a review of the neurobiology of sleep and wakefulness as it pertains to sleep initiation and maintenance problems, sleep state misperception, and such psychological factors as worry and attention bias. Following the review it is suggested that the temptation to define insomnia solely in neurobiological terms ("of the brain and by the brain") is also likely to be unproductive. Ultimately both sides of the equation must be taken into consideration and in a way that doesn't pander to dualism.

Primary insomnia is a prevalent disorder of sleep disturbance, impairing daytime functioning and health-related quality of life, leading to increased health care use. This article gives a brief overview of cognitive behavioral therapy as the treatment modality of choice for effectively ameliorating chronic sleep difficulties. Recommended and endorsed cognitive behavioral components are briefly described, and future research directions, focusing on improving the psychological management of insomnia, are outlined.

This article reviews the theoretical and empirical foundation for the new understanding of comorbid insomnia (CI) as a functional equivalent to primary insomnia. In both cases cognitive behavioral therapy for insomnia (CBT-I) should be considered as a highly efficacious first line of treatment. This article reviews the growing body of evidence supporting CBT-I interventions for CI and new research on methods to reduce barriers to access. Lower cost and more accessible interventions are needed to serve as a first step in a stepped-care model of CI treatment. The article also examines the specific advances in the domains of cancer, depression, and pain disorders.

The management of hypnotic discontinuation after regular and prolonged use may be a challenging task for patients and clinicians alike. Evidence suggests that a stepped-care approach may be a cost-effective approach to assist patients in tapering hypnotics. This approach may involve simple information about the need to discontinue medication; implementation of a supervised and systematic tapering schedule, with or without professional guidance; and cognitive behavioral therapy. Research evidence shows that this approach appears to be promising; further research is, however, necessary to identify treatment and individual characteristics associated with better outcomes.

A variety of factors contribute to the high prevalence of insomnia in later life. Although insomnia can occur as an acute disorder (7 days or less), older adults are often afflicted with chronic insomnia (12 months or more). This article focuses on the conceptualization, assessment, and treatment of late-life insomnia from a behavioral sleep medicine perspective. Evidence for both behavioral and pharmacologic treatment approaches is presented. As is shown, however, late-life insomnia's chronic and comorbid nature make behavioral techniques the preferable treatment approach.

Foreword

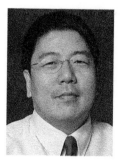

Teofilo Lee-Chiong, Jr., MD
Consulting Editor

Chico Marx one stated, "Who are you gonna believe—me or your own eyes?" This lighthearted statement captures one of the key elements of behavioral sleep medicine: that to modify behavior, one often has to challenge certain long-held precepts that have functioned so well in the past; the notion that many of the things we believe in, although reasonably plausible, are, unfortunately, either wrong or at least not always true.

Who can argue with a person's past experiences that staying in bed longer can offer immense relief whenever one is tired or sleep deprived; or that certain habits (eg, watching television in bed) that have never disturbed sleep in the past could possibly do so now? These discussions form the basis of many sleep medicine patient encounters.

There are other questions that behavioral sleep medicine specialists have to grapple. Does one encourage positive airway pressure use, or is penalizing non-adherence to therapy more effective in altering use of the device? Is behavioral change sustainable, and, if not, how rapidly does a person revert to old habits without episodic reinforcements?

How does one type of intervention compare with another? How does one go about choosing the best technique to address the specific needs and character of an individual? Many behavioral sleep medicine therapies are well known to primary care clinicians; these include avoiding alcohol use at bedtime ("you might feel good, but you will feel worse"), cognitive therapy ("many of the things you think you know about your sleep are wrong"), paradoxical intention ("I dare you to try to stay awake"), sleep restriction ("less bedtime for more sleep time"), stimulus control ("do not multitask in bed"), and multi-component cognitive behavioral therapy ("let's try everything"). Nevertheless, it takes an astute behavioral sleep medicine specialist to transform these concepts into a coherent, individualized, and synergistic process.

Other sleep behavioral medicine techniques will certainly emerge in the future. Similar to other medical disciplines, these novel techniques should ideally be (1) physiologically relevant (ie, address true neurobiologic changes in the sleep process that need to be altered); (2) applicable to a diverse group of sleep disorders presenting in a similar fashion, such as sleep initiation insomnia; (3) use the full potential of nonconventional treatment approaches, including self-help programs (books or audiovisual presentations), therapist-guided individual sessions, group therapy, and web portal based interventions; and (4) allow more widespread applications, including management of sleep-related breathing disorders, parasomnias, and hypersomnia.

Teofilo Lee-Chiong, Jr., MD
Division of Sleep Medicine
National Jewish Health
University of Colorado Denver School of Medicine
1400 Jackson Street
Room J221, Denver, CO 60206, USA

E-mail address:
Lee-ChiongT@NJC.ORG (T. Lee-Chiong)

Sleep Med Clin 4 (2009) xiii
doi:10.1016/j.jsmc.2009.07.014

Preface

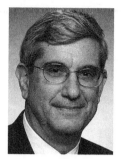

Kenneth L. Lichstein, PhD, CBSM
Guest Editor

By 2000, owing to its roots in psychosomatic medicine, behavioral medicine, and behavior therapy, behavioral/cognitive science and its therapeutic application, cognitive behavioral therapy (CBT), had established a strong footing in sleep medicine, particularly in the clinical management of the insomnias, continuous positive airway pressure (CPAP) adherence, parasomnias (particularly nocturnal enuresis and nightmares), and circadian rhythm disorders. Comprehensive reviews of the history of behavioral sleep medicine (BSM) are available elsewhere.[1]

BSM was invented in 2000 when Daniel Buysse, then president of the American Academy of Sleep Medicine, created an ad hoc presidential committee to broaden the role and stimulate the growth of psychology and related disciplines within sleep medicine. In its early deliberations, the committee took on the task of describing the boundaries of BSM and adopted the following definition that is now seen in the training accreditation standards:

"BSM comprises the behavioral dimension of normal and abnormal sleep mechanisms, and the prevention, assessment, and treatment of sleep disorders and associated behavioral and emotional problems through the application of established principles of behavior change."

In the decade that has followed the creation of the BSM committee, the predictable conclusion that much has been accomplished and much remains undone is applicable. The field of BSM has stabilized, and the foundation for steady growth has been laid. At the time of this writing, about 130 individuals have earned certification in BSM, and nine BSM training sites have been accredited. Practical matters of insurance reimbursement and growing the number of certified BSM practitioners, to achieve adequate dissemination, are enduring challenges.

The scientific underpinnings of BSM have grown rapidly and are, by now, prodigious. This issue summarizes the state of adult BSM science. The issue is organized in two clusters of articles. The first cluster, varied BSM targets, is a series of articles on disorders, strategies, and critical issues. The first article, by Matthews and Aloia, is on the topic of CPAP adherence. Adherence to medical regimens is one of the enduring, paramount obstacles to effective healthcare, and the article examines this obstacle with respect to the most important treatment for sleep apnea. The second article, by Pigeon and Yurcheshen, explores periodic limb movement disorder/restless leg syndrome. These disorders are typically managed pharmacologically, but this article is a call to action to expand the range and power of behavioral interventions for these disorders. The third article, by Cvengros and Wyatt, addresses circadian rhythm disorders. This article elucidates this complex web of processes and available strategies for taming these disorders when circadian rhythm drifts off. The fourth article, by Hasler and Germain, targets nightmares. This area has made great progress in recent years, and this article highlights effective interventions for nightmares, whether or not they are associated with posttraumatic stress disorder. The fifth article by McCurry, Gibbons, Logsdon, Vitiello, and Teri investigates sleep disturbance in caregivers. Home-based caregivers of dementia patients, often older adults themselves, are a special group of individuals whose sleep needs are significant and often overlooked. The sixth article by Vorona, Chen, and

Sleep Med Clin 4 (2009) xv–xvi
doi:10.1016/j.jsmc.2009.07.013

Ware examines sleep deprived physicians. It demonstrates with startling clarity the serious hazards to physicians and their patients when healthcare providers do not obtain adequate sleep.

The second cluster, the insomnias, is comprised of articles on varied aspects of the premier topic in BSM. The first two articles by Kaplan, Talbot, and Harvey and by Perlis, Gehrman, Pigeon, Findley, and Drummond investigate the two main theories of insomnia mechanisms: cognitive and neurobiologic. The third article, by Espie and Kyle, is on the major topic of primary insomnia. This article presents a broad survey of the research and clinical procedures of insomnia unaccompanied by overt medical and psychiatric comorbidities. The fourth article by Rybarczyk, Lund, Mack, and Stepanski is on comorbid insomnia. Having shed its untouchable status when it was referred to as secondary insomnia, this article documents significant progress in directly treating comorbid insomnia emphasizing the most prevalent types of comorbidity—depression, cancer, and pain. The fifth article by Bélanger, Belleville, and Morin tackles dependence in long-term hypnotic use. This article describes the hazards of hypnotic use and effective rescue with CBT for insomnia when hypnotic use becomes problematic. The sixth article by McCrae, Dzierzewski, and Kay discusses late-life insomnia.

Insomnia in older adults is more frequent, severe, and disabling than in younger adults. This article presents a comprehensive approach to understanding and managing late-life insomnia.

Last, I express my deep appreciation to my colleagues, who invented time to prepare these articles amidst densely packed schedules that yield time grudgingly. I am proud to be associated with these high quality scholarly pieces that may serve the dual purpose of advancing BSM a bit further and expanding the availability of effective, safe treatments for people experiencing sleep disorders.

Kenneth L. Lichstein, PhD, CBSM
Sleep Research Project
Department of Psychology
The University of Alabama
Box 870348
Tuscaloosa, AL 35487-0348, USA

E-mail address:
Lichstein@ua.edu (K.L. Lichstein)

REFERENCE

1. Stepanski EJ. Behavioral sleep medicine: a historical perspective. Behav Sleep Med 2003;1(1):4–21.

Continuous Positive Airway Pressure Treatment and Adherence in Obstructive Sleep Apnea

Ellyn E. Matthews, PhD, RN, AOCN[a], Mark S. Aloia, PhD, CBSM[b],*

KEYWORDS

- Obstructive sleep apnea
- Continuous positive airway pressure
- Treatment adherence • Health psychology
- Behavioral medicine

Obstructive sleep apnea (OSA) is a serious and prevalent sleep breathing disorder, characterized by repeated episodes of obstructed (apnea) or reduced (hypopnea) flow in the upper airway. Episodes of apnea and hypopnea result in intermittent hypoxemia, arousal from sleep, and sympathetic nervous system activation.[1,2] Nocturnal apnea and hypoxemia are associated with increase risk of cognitive deficits,[3] hypertension, cardiovascular disease, metabolic syndrome, stoke,[4] and type II diabetes.[5] There are significant, high mortality risks with untreated OSA, independent of age, gender, and body mass index (BMI).[6] The importance of adherence to standard treatment for OSA (ie, positive airway pressure) is underscored by a higher 5-year survival rate from adherent users compared with nonusers.[7]

The severity of sleep apnea is defined by the apnea-hypopnea index (AHI; total number of apneas plus hypopneas divided by the hours of sleep) or the respiratory disturbance index (RDI; total of apneas, hypopneas, and respiratory event-related arousals). Mild sleep apnea is defined as an AHI or RDI of 5 to less than 15, moderate is 15 to 30, and severe is greater than 30.[8] AHI and RDI are frequently outcome measures of OSA treatment efficacy. Positive airway pressure (PAP) is highly efficacious in the elimination of nocturnal apneas and hypopneas, and is the gold standard for moderate to severe OSA.

POSITIVE AIRWAY PRESSURE TREATMENT

PAP devices act like a pneumatic pump supplying positive pressure to the upper airway, preventing collapse and occlusion during sleep. Several randomized controlled trials have demonstrated that continuous positive airway pressure (CPAP) reduces the AHI or RDI and improves subjective and objective sleepiness.[9–11] In addition, sleep quality and quality-of-life improvements have been reported for OSA patients and their bed partners.[12–14] Unfortunately, patients often experience discomfort related to their interface or CPAP pressure among other factors, which may make them want to abandon treatment that has proved to be beneficial.

NONADHERENCE STATISTICS

Despite its effectiveness, overall treatment adherence remains suboptimal. It is estimated that 15%

[a] University of Colorado, College of Nursing, 13120 East 19th Avenue, Aurora, CO 80045, USA
[b] National Jewish Health, Department of Medicine, 1400 Jackson Street, Denver, CO 80206, USA
* Corresponding author.
E-mail address: aloiam@njhealth.org (M.S. Aloia).

Sleep Med Clin 4 (2009) 473–485
doi:10.1016/j.jsmc.2009.07.004
1556-407X/09/$ – see front matter © 2009 Elsevier Inc. All rights reserved.

to 30% of patients do not accept CPAP treatment from the onset[15] and approximately 25% of patients discontinue PAP within the first year.[16] Although sleep medicine experts disagree over the minimal amount of nightly PAP that is necessary for therapeutic effect for OSA patients, several investigators suggest the benefits of CPAP are directly related to the average duration of nightly use.[17–19] Symptom improvement may occur with just a few hours of nightly use; however, daytime alertness is impaired even with a single night of missed treatment.[20] Estimates of long-term CPAP use are as low as 50%.[21–23] Poor adherence rates and patterns are not unique to CPAP. In the past 50 years of research, average adherence ranged from 65% for sleep disorder treatments to 88.3% for HIV medication regimens.[24] In a study comparing adherence across different medical interventions, OSA patients who declined or discontinued CPAP had similar adherence to three medication treatments (for cardiovascular disease) as patients who were CPAP adherent. This suggests that patients are selective in choosing which interventions they will adhere to, and challenges the notion of "healthy user" bias.[25,26]

Adherence to treatment is important for satisfactory health outcomes. CPAP treatment remains a significant therapeutic challenge, requiring considerable change in patients' lifestyle and behavior. Recent investigations of methods to improve PAP adherence have centered around (1) predictors of adherence and nonadherence, (2) benefits of mechanical and physical interventions and titration methods, and (3) efficacy of behavioral and educational approaches. This article reviews the evidence regarding predictors of CPAP adherence, describes mechanical and behavioral-educational interventions that have been tested, and discusses theoretical models that can be adapted into clinical practice.

ADHERENCE FACTORS

There has been much speculation, but inconsistent findings, relating demographic and disease-specific factors to CPAP adherence. In some studies, CPAP adherence has been found to be associated with male gender,[27] older age,[16,28] race,[29] obesity,[30] and short sleep duration.[31] Others, however, have found these relations not to hold true. Some studies have found that women are less adherent.[27,32,33] One study found that women are more adherent to CPAP,[34] whereas other studies have reported no differences between men and women.[29,35–38] With regard to age, a few studies have reported patterns of adherence in older individuals is consistent with that of middle-aged adults,[37,39] whereas several others demonstrated greater adherence associated with older age.[29,34,36] In two studies, younger OSA patients were found to be more adherent.[16,33] Race has not been consistently associated with CPAP adherence. Among African Americans, lower adherence rates have been reported[29,32] and no racial differences in adhering to CPAP therapy have been found[40] (despite more severe OSA among African Americans). Another predictor with mixed results is BMI.[21,33,38]

Disease Severity and Improvements in Disease Variables

It is logical to think that those with more severe disease and symptoms would more readily use therapy. There is little evidence to support a relation between CPAP adherence and nocturnal hypoxemia,[29,41–44] however, although some studies have noted moderate correlations between AHI and adherence.[21,28,45–47] When comparing patients who maintained CPAP use with those who abandoned CPAP treatment early, two studies demonstrated adherence was related to severe AHI levels.[48,49] The association between baseline subjective sleepiness, measured by the Epworth Sleepiness Scale (ESS) score, has shown a modest association with eventual CPAP adherence[16,21,50] and self-referral,[51] although other studies have failed to demonstrate such a relationship.[52–54] Subjective improvement in sleep quality and sleepiness, however, seems to be associated with greater adherence to treatment.[45,46,55] The overall lack of association between adherence and demographic or disease measures has been disappointing and points to the need to focus on other factors that might improve adherence.

Patient-Reported Barriers

Initial patient satisfaction with CPAP and early management of problems seems to be associated with long-term adherence.[42,46,52] The pattern of adherence is established in the early weeks of treatment and predicts long-term use.[16,38,56] Reasons for discontinuing CPAP therapy have been primarily related to issues of mask discomfort, skin irritation, nasal dryness, congestion, air leaks, and difficulty adapting to the positive pressure.[28,57] Nasal stuffiness, dry nose and throat, and sore throat affect approximately 40% of patients using nasal CPAP.[58] Less common symptoms associated with adherence are feeling closed in by the device or mask (eg, claustrophobia) and noise of the machine.[28,52,59]

Anatomic characteristics, such as mouth breathing and nasal resistance, can also be a barrier to treatment. Mouth breathers with moderate-to-severe sleep-disordered breathing have been shown to be less adherent to CPAP compared with nose breathers.[60] Initial acceptance of CPAP treatment may be affected by increased nasal resistance and poor nasal airflow. In a study of OSA patients, CPAP use in patients with smaller nasal passages and reduced volume was lower than in those with larger passages and greater volume.[61] In another study, nasal resistance was lower in patients with primary OSA who accepted CPAP than in those who did not accept CPAP.[62] To evaluate the impact of conventional nasal surgery to treat nasal obstruction, 12 male patients who were refractory to treatment by CPAP were studied.[63] Surgery resulted in a significant decrease in nasal resistance and subjective sleepiness, but the AHI did not change significantly. Nasal airflow and resistance may be predictive of the initial acceptance of CPAP. Surgery may improve acceptance, but this has not yet been fully explored.

Psychologic and Personality Factors

Studies of patient-reported barriers, anatomic characteristics, OSA severity, and symptoms do not fully explain the problem of CPAP nonadherence. Recent studies examining the association between psychologic variables and CPAP adherence have produced equivocal findings.[32,64] Lower levels of pretreatment anxiety and depression predicted subsequent CPAP adherence in some studies[21,65,66] but not others.[27,67] For instance, lower pretreatment depression and hypochodriasis predicted subjective nightly CPAP use at 6-month follow-up,[26] whereas others found that anxiety and depression did not correlate with CPAP adherence at 1 week posttreatment.[54] In a study of Alzheimer patients, greater depressive symptoms were associated with poorer adherence, and patients who chose to continue using CPAP after the study had fewer depressive symptoms.[65] It is unclear if CPAP improves depressive symptoms, which in turn predicts better adherence, or whether symptoms of depression (eg, fatigue, poor concentration, hopelessness, cognitive distortions, and increased sensitivity to side effects) interfere with adherence to CPAP.[68] With a high prevalence of depression in OSA patients, sorting out the role of depression remains a worthy avenue of investigation. In addition to anxiety and depression, a type D personality (negative affectivity and social inhibition) may be associated with poor adherence. In 247 patients with OSA (average CPAP use of 55 months), objective adherence was significantly lower in type D compared with non–type D patients with regard to mean CPAP use per night and self-rated sleep.[64] The impact of psychologic factors in acceptance may be advanced by considering these factors in the social environment.

Potential Social Factors and Adherence

Most research on predictors of adherence has focused on the individual, with few studies examining the influence of relationship support or conflict with their partner. OSA patients who lived alone have been shown to use CPAP less (3.2 hours) compared with 4.5 hours for those with live-in partners ($P = .04$).[27] Others found that patients within 2 weeks of CPAP initiation were more likely to use CPAP when sleeping with their spouse compared with nights sleeping alone.[69] In studies testing spousal and relationship influences, one study reported objective CPAP adherence was predicted by marital conflict but not marital support,[70] whereas another reported no association with marital functioning.[71] Additionally, patients whose spouses were instrumental in their seeking treatment demonstrated lower adherence over the first 3 months of treatment, with adherence continuing to decline with time.[51] The importance of psychologic and social variables remains unclear and most studies have not taken a theoretical approach to the study of social factors influence on adherence.

THEORETICAL APPROACHES

Recently, investigators have begun to emphasize the importance of psychologic constructs and learning theories in predicting CPAP adherence. Such investigations might reduce the inconsistencies noted in previous studies. Four primary theories have been applied to CPAP adherence: (1) the health belief model (HBM),[72] (2) transtheoretical model (TTM),[73] (3) social cognitive theory (SCT),[74,75] and (4) Wallston's health locus of control and social learning theory.[76] Studies of CPAP adherence have incorporated constructs from these models.[53,77]

Health Belief Model

The HBM explains and predicts health behaviors by focusing on individual attitudes and beliefs.[72] The HBM is based on the notion that health-related actions occur when an individual (1) believes that a negative health condition can be avoided, (2) has a positive expectation that their actions can avoid negative health consequences, and (3) holds the belief that they themselves can successfully take the recommended action. Related constructs include perceived susceptibility, severity, benefits, barriers, and self-efficacy.

Studies using the HBM constructs in predicting CPAP use found the constructs of perceived benefits and barriers were predictive of CPAP adherence (average daily hours of CPAP use).[53,77] Perceived benefits of CPAP were inversely associated with percentage of daily CPAP nonadherence.[77] The model may be of use in the early prediction of CPAP acceptance and adherence, which is critical in establishing long-term CPAP usage patterns.[38,42,78] Another study reported CPAP adherence at 4 months was best explained by higher outcome expectancies with treatment and lower risk perception.[53] Health belief model constructs alone explained 21.8% of the variance in CPAP adherence, whereas constructs of the HBM and biomedical indices together explained 31.8% of the variance in CPAP adherence. These findings support the use of HBM constructs in the prediction of CPAP adherence and provide focus for future studies.[53]

Wallston's Health Locus of Control and Social Learning Theory

Wallston's[76] modified SLT posits that a patient's perception about the level of control over their illness determines health-related behavior change. Health locus of control is a concept that incorporates internality, chance, and powerful others. Internality (or internal locus of control) is the extent to which an individual believes that they are responsible for their own health and illness. Chance measures the extent to which health and illness are believed to be a matter of fate or luck. Powerful others (or external locus of control) relates to beliefs that health is determined by influential others (eg, health care providers). Individuals with a higher internal locus of control are more likely to adhere to treatment compared with those with an external locus of control. The value one places on maintaining good physical health (health value) is a moderator of the relationship between internal locus of control and health behavior. Only if an individual values their health does internal locus of control predict adherence. Locus of control, self-efficacy, and health value were examined in 119 CPAP-naive participants. Self-efficacy was not predictive of adherence 3 months after CPAP initiation; however, disease-specific variables (AHI, subjective sleepiness, CPAP pressure, and BMI) predicted 18% of the variance in CPAP adherence. Internal locus of control, lower belief in powerful others, and greater health value

independently predicted adherence.[79] Self-efficacy has been shown to predict adherence in other CPAP studies.[77,80] Its lack of association with adherence in this study may be caused by the use of general measures of self-efficacy, rather than CPAP-specific measure.

Social Cognitive Theory and Transtheoretical Model

According to Bandura's SCT, behavior change is influenced by (1) self-efficacy; (2) proper goal setting; and (3) an individual's expectations for favorable or unfavorable outcomes if a health behavior is performed (outcome expectancies).[74,75,81] SCT emphasizes the importance of knowledge and social support in adherence. The TTM model posits that an individual's readiness to engage in the required actions of change is an important predictor of treatment participation, dropout, efficacy, and long-term maintenance of improvement.[82–85] Individuals move through five stages of increasing readiness to change: (1) precontemplation, (2) contemplation, (3) preparation, (4) action, and (5) maintenance. A key assumption is that interventions need to be matched to a specific change stage to be effective.[85,86]

The relationship between objective CPAP adherence and variables from SCT and the TTM (eg, self-efficacy, outcome expectations, and decisional balance) was studied in 51 new CPAP users.[54] SCT and TTM variables were measured at CPAP fitting, 1 week postfitting, and 1 month postfitting. SCT and TTM variables measured 1 week post–CPAP fitting accounted for a significant amount of variance in objective CPAP adherence measured at 1 month. Decisional balance accounted for a significant amount of variance in objective CPAP compliance even when CPAP pressure was controlled, as did self-efficacy and outcome expectancies. Although SCT constructs measured at 1 week explained an additional 26% of variance in adherence, they did not individually predict adherence, suggesting intercorrelations between the predictors, and the use of future model building and testing.[87] This same author later examined the relationship between behavior change factors based on SCT and TTM and objectively measured CPAP adherence in experienced CPAP users (mean use = 2.1 years).[88] SCT and TM variables each accounted for a significant variance in CPAP adherence suggesting a relationship between social-cognitive factors and adherence in experienced CPAP users.

In a group of moderate to severe treatment-naive OSA participants, TTM and SCT constructs of readiness to change, perceived self-efficacy, and decisional balance measures were all predictive of adherence at 6 months.[80] Contrary to findings by others,[54] decisional balance was only predictive of adherence at 6 months when measured at 1 week, but not baseline.[80] These constructs did not predict adherence when measured before using CPAP, indicating the TTM and SCT constructs became more predictive with increasing exposure to the therapy.

MECHANICAL INTERVENTIONS TO IMPROVE ADHERENCE

Several mechanical interventions have been investigated to determine their impact on adherence. Approaches aimed at overcoming PAP disadvantages have had some successes, including different types of interfaces, such as nasal, oral, or full-face masks; heated humidification; and pressure delivery modes. Mask types and autotitration devices have not shown a corresponding increase in adherence proportional to the reduction in side effects.[89,90]

Mask Types

Many patients have difficulty tolerating CPAP because of the interface-related symptoms (eg, nasal airway problems, mouth leak, and general discomfort from the headgear). Several investigations have examined adherence, efficacy, patient preference, and mask comfort comparing masks that cover the nose, the mouth, both the nose and mouth, and the entire face. When a nasal mask was compared with an oral mask[91,92] no difference was found between the interfaces in mean hours of use per night at 1 month, polysomnography (PSG) variables, mask preference, ESS, or the total side effect score. The nature of the side effects differed slightly. For example, the nasal mask produced nasal congestion, air leaks, mask and strap pressure, and mask dislodgement. Mask users reported dry mouth or throat, excess salivation, and sore lips or gums.[92,93] Three interfaces were studied in 98 CPAP-naive patients who self-selected a nasal, oranasal, or oral mask.[91] The oral mask was selected by 27% of the patients, compared with 66% who chose a nasal mask, and 7% who chose an oronasal mask. After 3 weeks, efficacy and mask comfort were similar between groups of the three mask users, although the oronasal group had a disproportionately greater number of dropouts from therapy than the nasal group.[91] The nasal mask is a useful alternative interface, despite more complaints of upper airway dryness and "rain-out" by nasal mask.

In a study comparing nasal pillows with nasal masks in 39 middle-aged patients during the first 3 weeks of CPAP therapy,[94] the use of nasal pillows was associated with greater adherence in percentage of days used. There were no differences in mean daily use between nasal pillows and masks. Fewer adverse effects, less trouble getting to sleep and staying asleep, and less air leak were reported with nasal pillows. There was no difference in ESS or quality of life between nasal pillows and nasal mask users.

In a study comparing face mask and nose mask therapy in 20 newly diagnosed OSA patients, nightly adherence was significantly higher with use of the nasal mask (mean difference 1 hour per night; 95% confidence interval, 0.3–1.8; $P<.01$).[95] The nasal mask was rated significantly more comfortable than the face mask, despite more mouth leak symptoms and reports of dry throat, mouth, and nose with the nasal mask. The face mask was associated with more complaints of air leaks, red or sore eyes, claustrophobia, and difficulty exhaling, suggesting the face mask is best used when nasal obstruction or dryness limits the use of nasal mask. The ESS score was significantly lower with the use of a nasal mask compared with a face mask.

In a study assessing the efficacy of humidified air through a nasal cannula, a reduction was found in the AHI to less than 10 events per hour in 8 of 11 subjects, and less than five events per hour in four subjects.[96] These findings provide preliminary evidence of the efficacy, but not adherence, for a minimally invasive interface to treat a diverse group of patients with OSA.

Despite the wide range of options continually being introduced into the market, there are few studies addressing adherence in relation to various interfaces for CPAP. Small sample sizes and lack of standardized measures for the reporting of outcomes, such as symptoms, quality of life, and adverse effects of treatment, have limited statistical comparisons and the ability to draw conclusions about which interfaces are the best. Most studies evaluating the effectiveness of CPAP to treat OSA have used nasal masks; thus, nasal masks have emerged as the first choice during CPAP titration. Recent studies are comprised of primarily newly diagnosed OSA patients, and no data are available that examine interfaces in patients who have tried but are not able to tolerate conventional masks. Most patients in the reported studies had AHI indicative of severe OSA. The impact of CPAP interfaces on adherence in patients with milder forms of OSA is not well understood. Long-term outcomes and adherence rates associated with different interface types have not been adequately explored.

Humidification

The use heated humidification has been suggested to improve tolerance, acceptance, and adherence to nasal CPAP therapy by decreasing nasopharyngeal symptoms. Nasal stuffiness is commonly associated with CPAP treatment, and the resultant nasal resistance could be attenuated using heated humidification. Nasal mask leak significantly reduces nasal humidity and CPAP. Heated humidification compensates for dehydration effects by increasing the humidity levels at the anterior turbinate area. A study of 38 OSA patients compared heated humidity, cold pass over humidity, and a washout period without humidity. CPAP adherence with heated humidity was greater than CPAP use without humidity, but not with cold pass over humidity.[97] Patients were more satisfied with CPAP with either type of humidity compared with absence of humidification; however, only heated humidity resulted in feeling more refreshed on awakening. Side effects, such as dry mouth or throat and dry nose, were reported less frequently with heated humidity compared with CPAP use without humidity. Others have found no added benefit of heated humidification.[98]

Positive Airway Pressure Delivery Modes

In addition to heated humidification, pressure delivery modes are thought to provide greater comfort and result in improved therapeutic adherence. Delivery modes include autoadjusting PAP (APAP), bi-level PAP (Bi-PAP), and flexible PAP (C-Flex). The most frequently studied mechanical intervention is APAP.

Autoadjusting positive airway pressure

The advantage of APAP devices is the ability simultaneously to detect and prevent upper airway obstruction using the lowest possible pressure during sleep. APAP was developed to improve adherence by decreasing average pressure levels; however, there is little evidence that APAP results in greater acceptance or increased hours of use. A number of studies have compared APAP with standard, fixed pressure CPAP. There have been no significant differences in the mean number of hours per night of CPAP usage in studies of APAP versus CPAP.[99–103] There is one report of greater average nightly use, better quality, more restful sleep, less discomfort from pressure, and decreased trouble falling asleep in the APAP compared with the CPAP group.[104] Participants in this study may have benefited more from APAP because they had more severe apnea, requiring greater pressure to treat OSA compared with other study samples.[90]

No difference has been observed for percentage of days PAP was used in APAP versus CPAP users.[104–107] In three studies, patients preferred APAP over either CPAP or neither treatment.[102,106,108] Others report participants (N = 29) prefer neither APAP nor CPAP.[106] No significant differences were observed between APAP and CPAP on subjective sleepiness as measured by the ESS score.[99,101,103,104]

In a recent meta-analysis of randomized trials comparing APAP with CPAP, APAP was associated with a reduction in mean pressure, but it was similar to standard CPAP in adherence, the ability to eliminate respiratory events, and improvements in subjective sleepiness.[109] Interpreting the dissimilar results in APAP versus CPAP trials is difficult because of the clinically diverse populations, various machines, and operating principles used,[90] and because the dose of CPAP includes both the pressure level and time exposed.[110]

Bi-level positive airway pressure

Bi-PAP deliver two independently adjusted levels of pressure: high pressure during inhalation and a low pressure during exhalation. To date, few published studies have compared Bi-PAP with other modes of PAP delivery. Studies have not demonstrated differences between Bi-PAP and fixed CPAP with regard to treatment adherence.[111,112] In a study comparing standard CPAP with Bi-PAP in 27 adults newly referred for suspected OSA, both groups reduced AHI during the laboratory titration and improved scores on the ESS and Functional Outcomes of Sleep Questionnaire.[111] At 1 month, there were no group differences in adherence as determined by percentage of nights with at least 4 hours of use, and hours of use per night.

In a study of 62 OSA patients receiving either CPAP or Bi-PAP, both were similar in the percentage of time that the machine was running and the prescribed pressure delivered.[44] Both groups had equal complaints about mask discomfort, machine noise, and nasal stuffiness. Of note, five patients in the study stopped CPAP as a result of mask discomfort or treatment intolerance, but none of the withdrawals from the Bi-PAP group were related to treatment intolerance. These two studies suggest that Bi-PAP is as effective as CPAP for the treatment of OSA but offers no advantages in patients receiving therapy for OSA.[111]

C-Flex

C-Flex lowers the pressure level at the beginning of exhalation, returning to set pressure before exhalation ends. The flexible amount of pressure relief is thought to increase comfort and result in better therapeutic adherence. In a trial of CPAP therapy compared with C-Flex in 89 participants experiencing moderate-to-severe OSA, greater adherence was found in C-flex users over a 3-month follow-up period.[113] There were no significant differences in the subjective sleepiness or functional outcomes associated with sleep. Self-efficacy showed a trend toward being higher in the C-Flex users suggesting greater confidence in their ability to adhere to treatment.[113] In a multisite study comparing C-Flex and CPAP on adherence and subjective measures of comfort in 148 middle-aged participants (average AHI of 51.9 ± 27.7), C-Flex users had comparable average hours of use per night and total nights of use across the study, but had a trend (P<.07) toward achieving greater total hours of use.[114] Both groups had comparable decreases in sleepiness, comparable AHI on titration, and PAP pressure requirements. Understanding the impact of C-flex devices on adherence and comfort is needed.

Titration Methods

The current standard of practice for manual titration of CPAP and Bi-PAP to treat OSA consists of attended PSG, during which PAP is adjusted to eliminate apneas, hypopneas, respiratory effort–related arousals, and snoring (or the maximum recommended CPAP pressure is reached). According to American Academy of Sleep Medicine practice guidelines, full-night titration is the preferred method to determine optimal PAP, but split-night studies are considered both common and sufficient.[115,116] Split-night trials consist of PSG in the first half of the night followed by CPAP titration for the remainder of the night if there is an abnormal frequency of apneas and hypopneas. Several studies[116–120] have supported the adequacy of prescribing PAP therapy based on split night titration, but have not found significant differences in patient acceptance or adherence of CPAP (long-term or median nightly use).[117–120]

Advances in autoadjusting PAP technology permit treatment to be initiated outside of the sleep laboratory environment or at home. Little research has addressed how home versus sleep laboratory initiation affects adherence. One study found that patients' sleep laboratory experience with CPAP and the support and education provided by sleep technologists are important factors in facilitating CPAP compliance.[121]

In a study of home APAP with care supervised by an experienced nurse, and another group undergoing standard attended PSG, change in ESS after 3 months of CPAP for the nurse-led management was no worse than standard attended PSG. There were also no differences between both groups in CPAP adherence at 3 months.[122] Additional research is needed to ensure adequate use of therapy under these new models of care delivery.

PSYCHOEDUCATIONAL APPROACHES

The problem of CPAP adherence is not fully explained by the reduction of side effects mode of pressure delivery, or manner of titration. This has led to greater interest in studying psychologic, motivational, and educational approaches toward improving adherence. A variety of psychoeducational interventions have been aimed at improving adherence CPAP. These approaches are consistent with a recent American Academy of Sleep Medicine report emphasizing the importance of close follow-up and support.[115] Interventions have included systematic desensitization, self-management, motivational enhancement, cognitive behavioral therapy, and educational support.

Systematic Desensitization

In vivo desensitization has been used in a male apnea patient who initially failed CPAP therapy because of his claustrophobia.[121] The patient became able to tolerate CPAP use throughout his nocturnal sleep periods, which continued 6.5 years after desensitization. In another study, desensitization and sensory awareness training provided sufficient protection from anxiety and discomfort to proceed with treatment successfully, suggesting the process of desensitization and sensory awareness training can be useful in increasing the adherence rate in nasal CPAP.[123]

Sleep Apnea Self-Management Program

The sleep apnea self-management program[124] is based on the premise that OSA is a chronic illness requiring self-management. Distinct from "traditional" patient education, "self management" is a systematic behavioral approach to help patients with chronic conditions participate actively in self-monitoring, decision making, and problem solving. The sleep apnea self-management program is run in group format using a variety of activities. The sleep apnea self-management program pilot study offers evidence that the program has the potential to be efficacious, resulting in relatively high adherence levels postintervention, lower sleepiness scores, and less depressive symptoms. Self-efficacy and outcome expectation scores were high at postintervention.[88]

Motivational Enhancement Therapy for Continuous Positive Airway Pressure

Based on the theories of the transtheoretical model and social cognitive theory, motivational enhancement therapy for CPAP was developed. Motivational enhancement therapy is a patient-centered counseling approach adapted for medical settings that often have time-limited patient encounters.[125] A pilot study demonstrated efficacy of two 45-minute sessions of an motivational enhancement therapy intervention delivered to older adults before their starting CPAP versus a control with simple education. Motivational enhancement therapy CPAP increased CPAP adherence by over 3 hours per night on average.[126] In a larger study with 142 CPAP-naive OSA patients, the same group compared standard care with traditional education and a motivational enhancement therapy.[127] Both brief therapies decreased PAP discontinuation compared with standard care. The motivational enhancement therapy performed best under the condition of flexible delivery of PAP, although differences were not statistically significant.

Cognitive Behavioral Therapy

In a study of cognitive-behavioral therapy and CPAP, 100 subjects were randomized to either two 1-hour cognitive-behavioral therapy interventions plus treatment as usual (mask fitting and information) or only treatment as usual. Higher self-efficacy and adherence to CPAP therapy was found in the cognitive-behavioral therapy group, suggesting some relation to social cognitive theory.[128]

A theory-based music intervention was used to improve initial CPAP adherence in 97 moderate-to-severe OSA patients.[129] Materials included directions for CPAP nightly use, a diary for recording nightly use, and writing about CPAP benefits or problems. An audiotape with softly spoken instructions for placing the CPAP mask comfortably, using deep breathing and muscle relaxation along with the slowly decreasing music tempo, was provided to listen to at bedtime each night. Compared with placebo controls, a greater proportion of experimental patients were adhering at the end of the first month of CPAP onset. There were no differences in CPAP adherence at 3 and 6 months.

Psychoeducation

Educational interventions have ranged from simple telephone call follow-up and provision of patient literature[130] to intensive patient education and support protocols.[51,131,132] Proposing that increased knowledge about the risks of OSA and the consequences of nonadherence would result in greater CPAP use, several studies demonstrated some short-term improvement in adherence.[130,132,133] Additional studies examined the efficacy of intensive interventions for adherence compared with standard care with equivocal results.[51,131] Fewer patients in the didactic education and motivational enhancement therapy groups discontinued PAP at some point early in treatment.[127] Group differences were more pronounced under conditions of flexible PAP, with motivational enhancement therapy showing a clinically but not statistically significant advantage.[127]

SUMMARY

OSA is a serious health concern. Treatment with PAP is effective, but adherence to PAP has been limited by several factors. Among these factors are those related to the efficacy of the treatment and its comfort, and psychologic and social factors that more likely reflect a person's overall approach to health management and behavior change. Interventions to improve adherence to CPAP have provided some insight as to the limited effects of comfort management on adherence and have generally raised more questions than they have answered. Recent approaches, however, to the psychosocial aspects that contribute to behavior change provide promise for improving adherence. Some of these approaches have begun to be studied with mixed results. Others, however, such as social support, relationship-based approaches, and other theory-driven interventions, have yet to be studied. These interventions provide promise for an integrated, stepped-care approach to the management of the OSA patient. As the appreciation of these behavioral factors and new technologies increases, additional research is needed to identify which factors, in combination with which technologic factors, provide the best recipe for CPAP adherence on an individual case.

REFERENCES

1. Dyken ME, Yamada T, Glenn CL, et al. Obstructive sleep apnea associated with cerebral hypoxemia and death. Neurology 2004;62:491–3.
2. Meadows GE, Kotajima F, Vazir A, et al. Overnight changes in the cerebral vascular response to iso-capnic hypoxia and hypercapnia in healthy humans: protection against stroke. Stroke 2005;36: 2367–72.

3. Aloia MS, Ilniczky N, Di DP, et al. Neuropsychological changes and treatment compliance in older adults with sleep apnea. J Psychosom Res 2003; 54:71–6.

4. Coughlin SR, Mawdsley L, Mugarza JA, et al. Cardiovascular and metabolic effects of CPAP in obese males with OSA. Eur Respir J 2007;29: 720–7.

5. Malhotra A, White DP. Obstructive sleep apnoea. Lancet 2002;360:237–45.

6. Young T, Finn L, Peppard PE, et al. Sleep disordered breathing and mortality: eighteen-year follow-up of the Wisconsin sleep cohort. Sleep 2008;31:1071–8.

7. Campos-Rodriguez F, Pena-Grinan N, Reyes-Nunez N, et al. Mortality in obstructive sleep apnea-hypopnea patients treated with positive airway pressure. Chest 2005;128:624–33.

8. American Academy of Sleep Medicine Task Force. Sleep-related breathing disorders in adults: recommendations for syndrome definition and measurement techniques in clinical research. Sleep 1999;22:667–89.

9. George CF, Boudreau AC, Smiley A. Effects of nasal CPAP on simulated driving performance in patients with obstructive sleep apnoea. Thorax 1997;52:648–53.

10. Kiely JL, Murphy M, McNicholas WT. Subjective efficacy of nasal CPAP therapy in obstructive sleep apnoea syndrome: a prospective controlled study. Eur Respir J 1999;13:1086–90.

11. Meurice JC, Paquereau J, Neau JP, et al. Long-term evolution of daytime somnolence in patients with sleep apnea/hypopnea syndrome treated by continuous positive airway pressure. Sleep 1997; 20:1162–6.

12. Kingshott RN, Vennelle M, Hoy CJ, et al. Predictors of improvements in daytime function outcomes with CPAP therapy. Am J Respir Crit Care Med 2000; 161:866–71.

13. McMahon JP, Foresman BH, Chisholm RC. The influence of CPAP on the neurobehavioral performance of patients with obstructive sleep apnea hypopnea syndrome: a systematic review. WMJ 2003; 102:36–43.

14. Weaver TE, Maislin G, Dinges DF, et al. Relationship between hours of CPAP use and achieving normal levels of sleepiness and daily functioning. Sleep 2007;30:711–9.

15. Collard P, Pieters T, Aubert G, et al. Compliance with nasal CPAP in obstructive sleep apnea patients. Sleep Med Rev 1997;1:33–44.

16. McArdle N, Devereux G, Heidarnejad H, et al. Long-term use of CPAP therapy for sleep apnea/hypopnea syndrome. Am J Respir Crit Care Med 1999;159:1108–14.

17. Kaneko Y, Floras JS, Usui K, et al. Cardiovascular effects of continuous positive airway pressure in patients with heart failure and obstructive sleep apnea. N Engl J Med 2003;348:1233–41.

18. Pepperell JC, Ramdassingh-Dow S, Crosthwaite N, et al. Ambulatory blood pressure after therapeutic and subtherapeutic nasal continuous positive airway pressure for obstructive sleep apnoea: a randomised parallel trial. Lancet 2002;359: 204–10.

19. Weaver T, Maislin G, Venditti L, et al. CPAP dose duration for effective outcome response. Am J Respir Crit Care Med 2003;167:A324.

20. Kribbs NB, Pack AI, Kline LR, et al. Effects of one night without nasal CPAP treatment on sleep and sleepiness in patients with obstructive sleep apnea. Am Rev Respir Dis 1993;147:1162–8.

21. Edinger JD, Carwile S, Miller P, et al. Psychological status, syndromatic measures, and compliance with nasal CPAP therapy for sleep apnea. Percept Mot Skills 1994;78:1116–8.

22. Marquez-Baez C, Paniagua-Soto J, Castilla-Garrido JM. [Treatment of sleep apnea syndrome with CPAP: compliance with treatment, its efficacy and secondary effects]. Rev Neurol 1998;26: 375–80 [in Spanish].

23. Pepin JL, Krieger J, Rodenstein D, et al. Effective compliance during the first 3 months of continuous positive airway pressure: a European prospective study of 121 patients. Am J Respir Crit Care Med 1999;160:1124–9.

24. DiMatteo MR. Variations in patients' adherence to medical recommendations: a quantitative review of 50 years of research. Med Care 2004;42:200–9.

25. Platt AB, Kuna ST. To adhere or not to adhere-patients selectively decide. Sleep 2009;32:583–4.

26. Villar P, Isuel M, Carrizo S, et al. Medication adherence and persistence in severe obstructive sleep apnea. Sleep 2009;32:623–8.

27. Lewis KE, Seale L, Bartle IE, et al. Early predictors of CPAP use for the treatment of obstructive sleep apnea. Sleep 2004;27:134–8.

28. Zozula R, Rosen R. Compliance with continuous positive airway pressure therapy: assessing and improving treatment outcomes. Curr Opin Pulm Med 2001;7:391–8.

29. Budhiraja R, Parthasarathy S, Drake CL, et al. Early CPAP use identifies subsequent adherence to CPAP therapy. Sleep 2007;30:320–4.

30. Shigeta Y, Enciso R, Ogawa T, et al. Correlation between retroglossal airway size and body mass index in OSA and non-OSA patients using cone beam CT imaging. Sleep Breath 2008;12:347–52.

31. Bartlett DJ, Marshall NS, Williams A, et al. Predictors of primary medical care consultation for sleep disorders. Sleep Med 2008;9:857–64.

32. Joo MJ, Herdegen JJ. Sleep apnea in an urban public hospital: assessment of severity and treatment adherence. J Clin Sleep Med 2007;3: 285–8.

33. Pelletier-Fleury N, Rakotonanahary D, Fleury B. The age and other factors in the evaluation of compliance with nasal continuous positive airway pressure for obstructive sleep apnea syndrome: a Cox's proportional hazard analysis. Sleep Med 2001;2:225–32.

34. Sin DD, Mayers I, Man GC, et al. Long-term compliance rates to continuous positive airway pressure in obstructive sleep apnea: a population-based study. Chest 2002;121:430–5.

35. Anttalainen U, Saaresranta T, Kalleinen N, et al. CPAP adherence and partial upper airway obstruction during sleep. Sleep Breath 2007;11:171–6.

36. Ball EM, Banks MB. Determinants of compliance with nasal continuous positive airway pressure treatment applied in a community setting. Sleep Med 2001;2:195–205.

37. Nino-Murcia G, McCann CC, Bliwise DL, et al. Compliance and side effects in sleep apnea patients treated with nasal continuous positive airway pressure. West J Med 1989;150:165–9.

38. Weaver TE, Kribbs NB, Pack AI,, et al. Night-to-night variability in CPAP use over the first three months of treatment. Sleep 1997;20:278–83.

39. Weaver TE, Chasens ER. Continuous positive airway pressure treatment for sleep apnea in older adults. Sleep Med Rev 2007;11:99–111.

40. Scharf SM, Seiden L, DeMore J, et al. Racial differences in clinical presentation of patients with sleep-disordered breathing. Sleep Breath 2004;8:173–83.

41. Gay P, Weaver T, Loube D, et al. Evaluation of positive airway pressure treatment for sleep related breathing disorders in adults. Sleep 2006;29: 381–401.

42. Kribbs NB, Pack AI, Kline LR, et al. Objective measurement of patterns of nasal CPAP use by patients with obstructive sleep apnea. Am Rev Respir Dis 1993;147:887–95.

43. Krieger J. Long-term compliance with nasal continuous positive airway pressure (CPAP) in obstructive sleep apnea patients and nonapneic snorers. Sleep 1992;15:S42–6.

44. Reeves-Hoche MK, Meck R, Zwillich CW. Nasal CPAP: an objective evaluation of patient compliance. Am J Respir Crit Care Med 1994;149:149–54.

45. Drake CL, Day R, Hudgel D, et al. Sleep during titration predicts continuous positive airway pressure compliance. Sleep 2003;26:308–11.

46. Popescu G, Latham M, Allgar V, et al. Continuous positive airway pressure for sleep apnoea/hypopnoea syndrome: usefulness of a 2 week trial to identify factors associated with long term use. Thorax 2001;56:727–33.

47. Yetkin O, Kunter E, Gunen H. CPAP compliance in patients with obstructive sleep apnea syndrome. Sleep Breath 2008;12:365–7.

48. Janson C, Noges E, Svedberg-Randt S, et al. What characterizes patients who are unable to tolerate continuous positive airway pressure (CPAP) treatment? Respir Med 2000;94:145–9.

49. Rauscher H, Popp W, Wanke T, et al. Acceptance of CPAP therapy for sleep apnea. Chest 1991; 100:1019–23.

50. Engleman HM, Wild MR. Improving CPAP use by patients with the sleep apnoea/hypopnoea syndrome (SAHS). Sleep Med Rev 2003;7:81–99.

51. Hoy CJ, Vennelle M, Kingshott RN, et al. Can intensive support improve continuous positive airway pressure use in patients with the sleep apnea/hypopnea syndrome? Am J Respir Crit Care Med 1999;159:1096–100.

52. Hui DS, Choy DK, Li TS, et al. Determinants of continuous positive airway pressure compliance in a group of Chinese patients with obstructive sleep apnea. Chest 2001;120:170–6.

53. Olsen S, Smith S, Oei T, et al. Health belief model predicts adherence to CPAP before experience with CPAP. Eur Respir J 2008;32:710–7.

54. Stepnowsky CJ Jr, Marler MR, Ancoli-Israel S. Determinants of nasal CPAP compliance. Sleep Med 2002;3:239–47.

55. Wolkove N, Baltzan M, Kamel H, et al. Long-term compliance with continuous positive airway pressure in patients with obstructive sleep apnea. Can Respir J 2008;15:365–9.

56. Bhadriraju S, Kemp CR Jr, Cheruvu M, et al. Sleep apnea syndrome: implications on cardiovascular diseases. Crit Pathw Cardiol 2008;7:248–53.

57. Shadan FF, Dawson A, Kline LE. CPAP therapy may evoke a local nasal inflammation in patients. Rhinology 2008;46:347 [author reply].

58. Richards GN, Cistulli PA, Ungar RG, et al. Mouth leak with nasal continuous positive airway pressure increases nasal airway resistance. Am J Respir Crit Care Med 1996;154:182–6.

59. Chasens ER, Pack AI, Maislin G, et al. Claustrophobia and adherence to CPAP treatment. West J Nurs Res 2005;27:307–21.

60. Bachour A, Maasilta P. Mouth breathing compromises adherence to nasal continuous positive airway pressure therapy. Chest 2004;126:1248–54.

61. Li HY, Engleman H, Hsu CY, et al. Acoustic reflection for nasal airway measurement in patients with obstructive sleep apnea-hypopnea syndrome. Sleep 2005;28:1554–9.

62. Sugiura T, Noda A, Nakata S, et al. Influence of nasal resistance on initial acceptance of continuous positive airway pressure in treatment for obstructive sleep apnea syndrome. Respiration 2007;74:56–60.

63. Nakata S, Noda A, Yagi H, et al. Nasal resistance for determinant factor of nasal surgery in CPAP failure patients with obstructive sleep apnea syndrome. Rhinology 2005;43:296–9.

64. Brostrom A, Stromberg A, Martensson J, et al. Association of type D personality to perceived side effects and adherence in CPAP-treated patients with OSAS. J Sleep Res 2007;16:439–47.

65. Ayalon L, Ancoli-Israel S, Stepnowsky C, et al. Adherence to continuous positive airway pressure treatment in patients with Alzheimer's disease and obstructive sleep apnea. Am J Geriatr Psychiatry 2006;14:176–80.

66. Sandberg O, Franklin KA, Bucht G, et al. Nasal continuous positive airway pressure in stroke patients with sleep apnoea: a randomized treatment study. Eur Respir J 2001;18:630–4.

67. Wells RD, Freedland KE, Carney RM, et al. Adherence, reports of benefits, and depression among patients treated with continuous positive airway pressure. Psychosom Med 2007;69:449–54.

68. Wells RD, Day RC, Carney RM, et al. Depression predicts self-reported sleep quality in patients with obstructive sleep apnea. Psychosom Med 2004;66:692–7.

69. Cartwright R. Sleeping together: a pilot study of the effects of shared sleeping on adherence to CPAP treatment in obstructive sleep apnea. J Clin Sleep Med 2008;4:123–7.

70. Baron KG, Smith TW, Czajkowski LA, et al. Relationship quality and CPAP adherence in patients with obstructive sleep apnea. Behav Sleep Med 2009; 7:22–36.

71. McFadyen TA, Espie CA, McArdle N, et al. Controlled, prospective trial of psychosocial function before and after continuous positive airway pressure therapy. Eur Respir J 2001;18:996–1002.

72. Connor M, Norman P. Predicting health behaviour: research and practice with social cognition models. Buckingham: Open University Press; 1996.

73. Grimley D, Prochaska J, Velicer W, et al. The transtheoretical model of change. In: Brinthaupt T, Lipka R, editors. Changing the self: philosophies, techniques, and experiences. New York: State University of New York; 1994: 201–27.

74. Bandura A. Social foundations of thought and action: a social cognitive theory. Englewood Cliffs (NJ): Prentice Hall; 1986.

75. Bandura A. Human agency in social cognitive theory. Am Psychol 1989;44:1175–84.

76. Wallston K. Hocus-pocus, the focus isn't strictly on locus: Rotter's social learning theory modified for health. Cognit Ther Res 1992;16:183–99.

77. Sage CE, Southcott AM, Brown SL. The health belief model and compliance with CPAP treatment for obstructive sleep apnoea. Behav Change 2001;18:177–85.

78. Aloia MS, Arnedt JT, Stanchina M, et al. How early in treatment is PAP adherence established? Revisiting night-to-night variability. Behav Sleep Med 2007;5(3):229–40.

79. Wild MR, Engleman HM, Douglas NJ, et al. Can psychological factors help us to determine adherence to CPAP? A prospective study. Eur Respir J 2004;24:461–5.

80. Aloia MS, Arnedt JT, Stepnowsky C, et al. Predicting treatment adherence in obstructive sleep apnea using principles of behavior change. J Clin Sleep Med 2005;1:346–53.

81. Bandura A. Self-efficacy: toward a unifying theory of behavioral change. Psychol Rev 1977;84:191–215.

82. Prochaska JO, Diclemente CC. Stages and processes of self-change of smoking: toward an integrative model of change. J Consult Clin Psychol 1983;51:390–5.

83. Prochaska JO, Diclemente CC. Self change processes, self efficacy and decisional balance across five stages of smoking cessation. Prog Clin Biol Res 1984;156:131–40.

84. Prochaska JO, Velicer WF. The transtheoretical model of health behavior change. Am J Health Promot 1997;12:38–48.

85. Prochaska JO, Redding CA, Evers KE. The transtheoretical model and stages of change. In: Glanz K, Rimer BK, Viswanath K, editors. Health behavior and health education: theory, research, and practice. 4th edition. San Francisco (CA): Jossey-Bass; 2008. p. 97–121.

86. Weinstein ND, Rothman AJ, Sutton SR. Stage theories of health behavior: conceptual and methodological issues. Health Psychol 1998;17: 290–9.

87. Olsen S, Smith S, Oei TP. Adherence to continuous positive airway pressure therapy in obstructive sleep apnoea sufferers: a theoretical approach to treatment adherence and intervention. Clin Psychol Rev 2008;28:1355–71.

88. Stepnowsky CJ, Marler MR, Palau J, et al. Social-cognitive correlates of CPAP adherence in experienced users. Sleep Med 2006;7:350–6.

89. Chai CL, Pathinathan A, Smith B. Continuous positive airway pressure delivery interfaces for obstructive sleep apnoea. Cochrane Database Syst Rev 2006;4:CD005308.

90. Smith I, Lasserson TJ, Haniffa M. Interventions to improve compliance with continuous positive airway pressure for obstructive sleep apnea. Cochrane Database Syst Rev 2004;4:CD003531.

91. Beecroft J, Zanon S, Lukic D, et al. Oral continuous positive airway pressure for sleep apnea: effectiveness, patient preference, and adherence. Chest 2003;124:2200–8.

92. Khanna R, Kline LR. A prospective 8 week trial of nasal interfaces vs. a novel oral interface (Oracle)

for treatment of obstructive sleep apnea hypopnea syndrome. Sleep Med 2003;4:333–8.

93. Anderson FE, Kingshott RN, Taylor DR, et al. A randomized crossover efficacy trial of oral CPAP (Oracle) compared with nasal CPAP in the management of obstructive sleep apnea. Sleep 2003;26:721–6.

94. Massie CA, Hart RW. Clinical outcomes related to interface type in patients with obstructive sleep apnea/hypopnea syndrome who are using continuous positive airway pressure. Chest 2003;123: 1112–8.

95. Mortimore IL, Whittle AT, Douglas NJ. Comparison of nose and face mask CPAP therapy for sleep apnoea. Thorax 1998;53:290–2.

96. McGinley BM, Patil SP, Kirkness JP, et al. A nasal cannula can be used to treat obstructive sleep apnea. Am J Respir Crit Care Med 2007;176:194–200.

97. Massie CA, Hart RW, Peralez K, et al. Effects of humidification on nasal symptoms and compliance in sleep apnea patients using continuous positive airway pressure. Chest 1999;116:403–8.

98. Duong M, Jayaram L, Camfferman D, et al. Use of heated humidification during nasal CPAP titration in obstructive sleep apnoea syndrome. Eur Respir J 2005;26:679–85.

99. Ficker JH, Clarenbach CF, Neukirchner C, et al. Auto-CPAP therapy based on the forced oscillation technique. Biomed Tech (Berl) 2003;48:68–72.

100. Konermann M, Sanner BM, Vyleta M, et al. Use of conventional and self-adjusting nasal continuous positive airway pressure for treatment of severe obstructive sleep apnea syndrome: a comparative study. Chest 1998;113:714–8.

101. Meurice JC, Marc I, Series F. Efficacy of auto-CPAP in the treatment of obstructive sleep apnea/hypopnea syndrome. Am J Respir Crit Care Med 1996;153:794–8.

102. Randerath WJ, Schraeder O, Galetke W, et al. Autoadjusting CPAP therapy based on impedance efficacy, compliance and acceptance. Am J Respir Crit Care Med 2001;163:652–7.

103. Series F, Marc I. Efficacy of automatic continuous positive airway pressure therapy that uses an estimated required pressure in the treatment of the obstructive sleep apnea syndrome. Ann Intern Med 1997;127:588–95.

104. Massie CA, McArdle N, Hart RW, et al. Comparison between automatic and fixed positive airway pressure therapy in the home. Am J Respir Crit Care Med 2003;167:20–3.

105. Hudgel DW, Fung C. A long-term randomized, cross-over comparison of auto-titrating and standard nasal continuous airway pressure. Sleep 2000;23:645–8.

106. Senn O, Brack T, Matthews F, et al. Randomized short-term trial of two autoCPAP devices versus fixed continuous positive airway pressure for the treatment of sleep apnea. Am J Respir Crit Care Med 2003;168:1506–11.

107. Teschler H, Wessendorf TE, Farhat AA, et al. Two months auto-adjusting versus conventional nCPAP for obstructive sleep apnea syndrome. Eur Respir J 2000;15:990–5.

108. d'Ortho MP. Auto-titrating continuous positive airway pressure for treating adult patients with sleep apnea syndrome. Curr Opin Pulm Med 2004;10:495–9.

109. Ayas NT, Patel SR, Malhotra A, et al. Auto-titrating versus standard continuous positive airway pressure for the treatment of obstructive sleep apnea: results of a meta-analysis. Sleep 2004;27:249–53.

110. Stepnowsky CJ Jr, Moore PJ. Nasal CPAP treatment for obstructive sleep apnea: developing a new perspective on dosing strategies and compliance. J Psychosom Res 2003;54:599–605.

111. Gay PC, Herold DL, Olson EJ. A randomized, double-blind clinical trial comparing continuous positive airway pressure with a novel bilevel pressure system for treatment of obstructive sleep apnea syndrome. Sleep 2003;26:864–9.

112. Reeves-Hoche MK, Hudgel DW, Meck R, et al. Continuous versus bilevel positive airway pressure for obstructive sleep apnea. Am J Respir Crit Care Med 1995;151:443–9.

113. Aloia MS, Stanchina M, Arnedt JT, et al. Treatment adherence and outcomes in flexible vs standard continuous positive airway pressure therapy. Chest 2005;127:2085–93.

114. Dolan DC, Okonkwo R, Gfullner F, et al. Longitudinal comparison study of pressure relief (C-Flex-trade mark) vs. CPAP in OSA patients. Sleep Breath 2009;13:73–7.

115. Kushida CA, Morgenthaler TI, Littner MR, et al. Practice parameters for the treatment of snoring and obstructive sleep apnea with oral appliances: an update for 2005. Sleep 2006;29:240–3.

116. Kushida CA, Chediak A, Berry RB, et al. Clinical guidelines for the manual titration of positive airway pressure in patients with obstructive sleep apnea. J Clin Sleep Med 2008;4:157–71.

117. McArdle N, Grove A, Devereux G, et al. Split-night versus full-night studies for sleep apnea/hypopnoea syndrome. Eur Respir J 2000;15:670–5.

118. Sanders MH, Kern NB, Costantino JP, et al. Prescription of positive airway pressure for sleep apnea on the basis of a partial-night trial. Sleep 1993;16:S106–7.

119. Sanders MH, Kern NB, Costantino JP, et al. Adequacy of prescribing positive airway pressure therapy by mask for sleep apnea on the basis of a partial-night trial. Am Rev Respir Dis 1993;147: 1169–74.

120. Strollo PJ Jr, Sanders MH, Costantino JP, et al. Split-night studies for the diagnosis and treatment of sleep-disordered breathing. Sleep 1996;19:S255–9.

121. Means MK, Edinger JD. Graded exposure therapy for addressing claustrophobic reactions to continuous positive airway pressure: a case series report. Behav Sleep Med 2007;5:105–16.

122. Antic NA, Buchan C, Esterman A, et al. A randomised controlled trial of nurse led care for symptomatic moderate-severe obstructive sleep apnea. Am J Respir Crit Care Med 2009;179(6):501–8.

123. Speer TK, Fayle RW. The effect of systematic desensitization and sensory awareness training on adherence to CPAP treatment [abstract]. J Sleep Res 1997;26:216.

124. Stepnowsky CJ, Palau JJ, Gifford AL, et al. A self-management approach to improving continuous positive airway pressure adherence and outcomes. Behav Sleep Med 2007;5:131–46.

125. Aloia MS, Arnedt JT, Riggs RL, et al. Clinical management of poor adherence to CPAP: motivational enhancement. Behav Sleep Med 2004;2:205–22.

126. Aloia MS, Di DL, Ilniczky N, et al. Improving compliance with nasal CPAP and vigilance in older adults with OAHS. Sleep Breath 2001;5:13–21.

127. Aloia MS, Smith K, Arnedt JT, et al. Brief behavioral therapies reduce early positive airway pressure discontinuation rates in sleep apnea syndrome: preliminary findings. Behav Sleep Med 2007;5:89–104.

128. Richards D, Bartlett DJ, Wong K, et al. Increased adherence to CPAP with a group cognitive behavioral treatment intervention: a randomized trial. Sleep 2007;30:635–40.

129. Smith CE, Dauz E, Clements F, et al. Patient education combined in a music and habit-forming intervention for adherence to continuous positive airway (CPAP) prescribed for sleep apnea. Patient Educ Couns 2009;74:184–90.

130. Chervin RD, Theut S, Bassetti C, et al. Compliance with nasal CPAP can be improved by simple interventions. Sleep 1997;20:284–9.

131. Hui DS, Chan JK, Choy DK, et al. Effects of augmented continuous positive airway pressure education and support on compliance and outcome in a Chinese population. Chest 2000;117:1410–6.

132. Likar LL, Panciera TM, Erickson AD, et al. Group education sessions and compliance with nasal CPAP therapy. Chest 1997;111:1273–7.

133. Fletcher EC, Luckett RA. The effect of positive reinforcement on hourly compliance in nasal continuous positive airway pressure users with obstructive sleep apnea. Am Rev Respir Dis 1991;143:936–41.

Behavioral Sleep Medicine Interventions for Restless Legs Syndrome and Periodic Limb Movement Disorder

Wilfred R. Pigeon, PhD, CBSM[a],*, Michael Yurcheshen, MD[b]

KEYWORDS

- Restless legs syndrome
- Periodic limb movement disorder
- Behavioral • Cognitive-behavioral
- Behavioral medicine • Relaxation

BEHAVIORAL SLEEP MEDICINE INTERVENTIONS FOR RESTLESS LEGS SYNDROME AND PERIODIC LIMB MOVEMENT DISORDER

Restless legs syndrome (RLS) and periodic limb movement disorder (PLMD) are sleep disorders that are commonly seen in clinical practice, both by primary care providers and by sleep specialists. Unlike the vast majority of movement disorders, these conditions do not improve with sleep. The standard treatment recommendations for these disorders are pharmacologic, although behavioral interventions for these conditions are increasingly recognized, albeit underused.

RESTLESS LEGS SYNDROME AND ITS PHARMACOLOGIC MANAGEMENT

Although the first descriptions of RLS were recorded as early as 1672, Stephen Eckbolm is largely credited with the first modern report of the condition, identifying eight patients who had the condition in 1945.[1,2] Since these earliest accounts, diagnostic criteria for the condition have been established and refined.[3,4] In the most recent version of the *International Classification of Sleep Disorders*, RLS is grouped with other sleep-related movement disorders. Although this syndrome does not necessarily involve stereotyped movement, RLS is included among the movement disorders of sleep because of its close association with PLMD and periodic leg movements of wake. RLS has four features,[5] which include (1) a strong, "nearly irresistible" urge to move the legs; (2) sensations that are worsened with inactivity; (3) sensations that are improved or relieved with movement; and (4) symptoms that are exacerbated at night.

In clinical practice, not all of these features are necessary to make a diagnosis of RLS; there is also some variability in how frequently symptoms occur. In children younger than 12 years of

W.R.P. received funding support from NIH NR010408; Rochester Center for Mind-Body Research (NIH AG023956); VA Center of Excellence at Canandaigua, Canandaigua, NY; and Sanofi-Aventis.

The views and opinions expressed by the authors do not represent the views or opinions of the NIH or the VA.

[a] Department of Psychiatry, Sleep and Neurophysiology Research Laboratory, University of Rochester Medical Center, 300 Crittenden Boulevard, Box PSYCH, Rochester, NY 14642-8409, USA

[b] Department of Neurology and Strong Sleep Disorders Center, 919 Westfall Road, Building A, Suite 100, University of Rochester Medical Center, Rochester, NY 14618, USA

* Corresponding author.

E-mail address: wilfred_pigeon@urmc.rochester.edu (W.R. Pigeon).

Sleep Med Clin 4 (2009) 487–494

doi:10.1016/j.jsmc.2009.07.008

age, the condition can include probable or definite RLS, and diagnostic criteria are slightly different.[4,5]

This utilitarian description, however, in some ways minimizes the degree of sleep disruption that many of these patients experience. In some cases, the discomfort is so disruptive that afflicted patients wander nightly, sometimes for hours, until they finally collapse with exhaustion. The sensation has been described variably, and some descriptors of the sensation include "tingling," "stinging," or a "creepy-crawly" feeling. In up to 50% of cases, symptoms are severe enough to involve the upper extremities in addition to (or in rarer circumstances, instead of) the lower extremities.[6]

It is estimated that RLS has an incidence of about 5% to 15% in the general population, and most studies suggest it is up to twice as common in women.[7,8] RLS is commonly idiopathic, but many secondary causes of this condition have been identified. These secondary causes include, but are not limited to, neuropathy, diabetes, renal dysfunction, spinal stenosis, pregnancy, side effects from drugs/medications (such as antipsychotics or antiemetics), and iron or vitamin deficiency. A discussion of the secondary causes of RLS is beyond the scope of this article; however, a recent online review of RLS includes an extensive discussion.[9] Other less common causes of RLS have also been described. For instance, in a recent case series, five patients who had Chiari-I malformation were found to have RLS.[10] Some familial cases of RLS have also been identified, suggesting a genetic component. Indeed, a handful of genetic loci and polymorphisms of susceptible genes (including the BTBD9 gene) associated with RLS have been discovered.[11,12] Depending on the cause, symptoms may fluctuate. Pregnancy is a common example, with many women describing symptoms only during the term of pregnancy, but never before or after.

There has been some evidence that idiopathic RLS may actually be a harbinger of neurodegenerative conditions, such as Parkinson disease.[13] Confirmatory evidence of a definitive relationship between these conditions is lacking. A recent epidemiologic study also links RLS and vascular disease.[14] Causality and directionality in this association has not been firmly established.

The typical workup for RLS includes a diligent clinical encounter with close attention paid to sleep and past medical history. The physical examination should include a neurologic examination, particularly of the lower extremities. A comprehensive laboratory workup is of variable usefulness. Serum ferritin levels are often drawn, and some practitioners advocate for supplementing iron if the level is less than 50 ug/mL, although currently there are no clinical trials or even guidelines to support this practice. Although cerebrospinal fluid iron studies seem more sensitive for RLS, a lumbar puncture for such an evaluation is not recommended.[15] Neuroimaging of the lumbosacral spine and electromyography (EMG)/nerve conduction studies are not indicated in every patient. Polysomnography (PSG) is not routinely required in most cases of RLS, and an estimated 10% to 20% of patients who have RLS have a PSG free of any remarkable surface EMG finding.[16] Information from a nocturnal PSG can be useful in questionable cases of RLS or to identify the degree of sleep disruption from associated nighttime movements. The Suggested Immobilization Test (SIT) is a procedure wherein a patient rates their level of leg discomfort while surface EMG tracings of leg movements are recorded.[17] This test is used infrequently in clinical practice.

If a specific cause of RLS is identified, treating the underlying condition can be helpful in alleviating symptoms. Some examples include addressing any reversible causes of renal dysfunction, or delivery when pregnancy is the proximal cause.[18] The relationship between glucose control and RLS is just beginning to be explored.[19]

Treatment of the idiopathic form of RLS is most commonly pharmacologic. Standards of practice and algorithms for pharmacologic treatment have been developed, but the treatment landscape has changed since 2004 when these guidelines were published.[20,21] Specifically, dopamine D2 agonists have become first-line treatment of this condition.[22] According to the American Academy of Sleep Medicine (AASM) 2004 Practice Parameters, levodopa/carbidopa and pergolide are considered standards for treatment.[20] Since that time, pramipexole and ropinirole have been approved by the Food and Drug Administration for treating RLS, and many practitioners use these agents first. Evening administration at doses that are generally significantly less than what would be required for treatment of Parkinson Disease are usually effective. The most common side effects of these dopamine agonists include nausea and sleepiness. Dopamine dysregulation syndrome is uncommon, but should be considered when using dopamine agonists. Other agents that show significant efficacy include, but are not limited to, gabapentin and clonazepam.[23,24] Side effects to gabapentin include nonspecific drowsiness, nausea, and dizziness, among others. Clonazepam has a longer half-life than many benzodiazepines and therefore seems to carry a lower risk for abuse; however, clonazepam abuse does occur and this possibility remains at least a possible concern.[25] Opiates can also be effective; some (although not all) opiates are among the few RLS agents that are considered to be pregnancy risk category B. Dependency is a consideration with the use of any opiate. Supplemental iron (oral or intravenous) is sometimes effective in cases of iron deficiency (ferritin <50 mcg/L), but the evidence for this approach to date is based on case series, and controlled clinical trials are forthcoming.[26,27] Finally, magnesium may be a useful treatment in some cases.[28,29] There are few, if any, head-to-head clinical trials comparing these agents. A complete discussion of the specific therapeutic management of RLS is beyond the scope of this article, but considerations of comorbidities, tolerance, and augmentation, among others, will dictate which agents to use and when.

PERIODIC LIMB MOVEMENT DISORDER AND ITS PHARMACOLOGIC MANAGEMENT

This condition, initially referred to as nocturnal myoclonus, is characterized by nighttime limb movements during sleep. Sydmonds[30] first described the condition in 1953. Unlike RLS, no discomfort in the limbs is necessary for the diagnosis of PLMD. Patients might be completely unaware of the presence of these movements, were it not for a bed partner's complaints. Of course, many patients who have limb discomfort (of any kind) may also have comorbid PLMD. These patients may or may not meet diagnostic criteria for RLS. Most patients who have RLS also have PLMD.[16] PLMD is closely related to periodic limb movements of sleep, with one significant difference: patients who have PLMD have a sleep complaint, such as insomnia or daytime sleepiness.

PLMD is a relatively uncommon disorder. One study estimated that 3.9% of the adult population has PLMD, but these cases were identified by self-report and were not confirmed with polysomnography.[31] PLMD can also occur in children. A 2004 case series suggested that 23% of prepubertal children presenting to a sleep disorders clinic had periodic limb movements on polysomnography.[32] As with sleep-disordered breathing, the consequence of nighttime sleep disruption in a pediatric patient may not result in sleepiness, but rather in behavioral concerns. Specifically, symptoms of attention deficit hyperactivity disorder seem to be common in pediatric patients who have nocturnal sleep disruption from PLMD.[33]

PLMD is diagnosed through a combination of history along with polysomnographic data. Again, it is most often a bed partner's observation that a patient moves during the night. Particularly astute bed partners may notice that the movements are more likely to occur in the first half of the night. Non–rapid eye movement (REM) sleep, when leg movements are far more common than in REM sleep, predominates in the first half of the night. There is variability in the timing of these movements, however, and many patients' movements may continue throughout the entire sleep period.

On polysomnography, surface EMG activity from limb leads is recorded during the night. Using criteria recently established by the AASM, a limb movement can be scored if it has a duration of 0.5 to 10 seconds and has at least an 8 microvolt increase over the baseline resting EMG amplitude.[34] If four of these movements occur within 5 to 90 seconds, the movements can be scored as a periodic leg movement series (PLMS). A PLMS index of greater than 15 movements per hour in adults and greater than 5 in children should arouse suspicion for PLMD.[35] By strict criteria, movements that are precipitated by respiratory disturbances (such as apnea) should not be scored, and movements in this setting should not be considered periodic leg movement disorder. There is ongoing and considerable debate about whether disease severity, as assessed by PLMS index, has any correlation to patient complaints.

Correlative movements to this EMG activity can sometimes be witnessed using video monitoring. Classic clinical reports have characterized these movements as a partial or complete triple flexion response, with extension of the great toe, dorsiflexion of the ankle, and occasional flexion of the knee and hip.[36] The movements, however, can often be more vigorous, causing significant disruption to a bed partner's sleep.

Much has been written about clinical significance criteria for PLMD and how many if not most of these cases do not rise to this level and do not require treatment.[37] Clinical judgment is often a guide in these cases. If these limb movements are uncovered on polysomnography that is otherwise devoid of other obvious causes for daytime sleepiness, then they should certainly be addressed. Many times, however, limb movements on PSG are simply incidental and do not require treatment.

Because it can be difficult to determine if the limb movements noted on polysomnography are incidental to sleep complaints, or if they are germane, treatment of PLMD can be more complicated than for RLS. If there is an identified cause of the PLMD (ie, arthritis, RLS), then treatment of the primary condition is recommended. The 2004 AASM guidelines consider treatment of RLS and periodic limb movements of sleep to be one and the same.[20] The recommendations discuss a host of treatments, but ropinirole and pramipexole have since become leading agents in treatment of PLMD. Occasionally, several agents might be tried before an effective one is identified. In the absence of limb discomfort, judging treatment efficacy can be somewhat challenging. Again, a bed partner's reports are important to judge efficacy, as are patient reports of any improvements in sleep continuity or daytime sleepiness or fatigue.

BEHAVIORAL SLEEP MEDICINE INTERVENTIONS FOR RESTLESS LEGS SYNDROME AND PERIODIC LIMB MOVEMENT DISORDER

Behavioral sleep medicine (BSM) approaches to RLS and PLMD do exist, but the level of empiric support for their use is less complete than the body of evidence that exists for the use of BSM interventions in chronic insomnia, pediatric sleep disorders, and even continuous positive airways pressure adherence. Nonetheless, some BSM principles are already embedded in the existing treatment guidelines for RLS and PLMD. As conditions that tend to be chronic, RLS and PLMD are also appropriate targets for chronic disease management interventions with which practitioners in general behavioral medicine are familiar. There are also some data that support the direct and targeted treatment of RLS/PLMD with cognitive and behavioral interventions, some being specific to BSM and others coming from general behavioral medicine.

Although pharmacologic management is the standard of care for both RLS and PLMD, treatment guidelines and algorithms and patient information pamphlets highlight several nonpharmacologic suggestions. These are most well developed for RLS, but most of the suggestions apply to PLMD also. The list of such approaches/suggestions can be extensive and detailed.[21] They include eliminating medications that may cause or exacerbate RLS symptoms, especially dopamine-blocking agents (eg, neuroleptics), but also antiemetics and antihistamines (found in many over-the-counter allergy and sleep aids), and avoiding antidepressants that may cause or exacerbate periodic limb movements, especially the selective serotonin reuptake inhibitors. Other suggestions include maintaining a healthy weight and diet, getting moderate exercise, using support groups, and taking a hot bath, cold shower, or brief walk before bedtime. With the exception of exercise (see later discussion), none of these suggestions is based on anything other than anecdotal reports. The suggestions also usually mention some version of using good sleep hygiene.

Concerning sleep hygiene for RLS/PLMD, there are a two main points that bear highlighting. First, the avoidance of alcohol, caffeine, and nicotine should be underscored because of their potential contributions to RLS symptoms or PLMD. Second, other sleep hygiene practices may or may not have any usefulness for patients who have RLS/PLMD. Particularly when sleep hygiene is provided to patients as a handout or pamphlet, there is no indication that this helps promote sleep in any patient group. It is important for providers not familiar with delivering BSM interventions to know that sleep hygiene has little to no demonstrated efficacy as a monotherapy for insomnia. Moreover, even when it is delivered as part of a multipronged intervention, sleep hygiene as a psychoeducational therapy is an active process with patient–provider interaction, goal-setting, between-session homework assignments, and follow-up. In addition, it is equally important to note that some sleep hygiene or tips for good sleep include in them a suggestion that is not considered a sleep hygiene instruction, but a stimulus control instruction. In particular the suggestion to use the bedroom only for sleep and sex is a stimulus control instruction (without providing rationale for and complete instructions for stimulus control) and is in direct conflict with the suggestion to maintain a regular bed and wake time that is often an item on the same list. This suggestion is confusing to patients who may consistently go to bed at a regular time to abide by the latter instruction, regardless of whether they are sleepy, and get up at the same time each morning, despite waking much earlier than their rise time. In such cases, following good sleep hygiene may actually contribute to the development or maintenance of insomnia. A thorough BSM approach to sleep scheduling for patients who have RLS/PLMD is a much preferred approach than the standard sleep suggestions provide.

The treatment of comorbid insomnia or insomnia-like presentations in RLS/PLMD can be directly targeted with the cognitive-behavioral therapies for insomnia (CBT-I) that are the focus elsewhere in this issue.[38] As with many medical and psychiatric conditions, RLS/PLMD may directly precipitate insomnia or directly exacerbate pre-existing insomnia. One manner by which this may occur is that when nocturnal RLS symptoms or periodic limb movements lead to repeated full awakenings, one or more such awakenings may lead to lengthy wake times and difficulty reinitiating sleep. As is the case with going to bed before being sleepy and remaining in bed for more than

15 to 20 minutes following final awakening in the morning, these can set the stage for excessive time in bed relative to total sleep time, and potentially to conditioned arousal as seen in psychophysiologic insomnia. In one study, patients who had PLMD did not differ from primary insomnia patients in sleep hygiene factors (reading in bed), stimulus control behaviors (lying awake in bed), cognitive arousal, and physical arousal, whereas both groups differed significantly from normal sleepers on each of these domains.[36] For patients who have PLMD there can thus be an insomnia-like presentation. In such cases, or when comorbid insomnia is diagnosed in RLS or PLMD, CBT-I should be considered.

To date, there has been only one controlled trail of CBT-I in RLS/PLMD. In this study by Edinger and colleagues,[39] 16 patients who had PLMD were randomly assigned to receive four weekly sessions of CBT-I or 4 weeks of clonazepam at 0.5 to 1.0 mg. Both groups had significant improvements in self-reported sleep variables with no between-group differences, except that the CBT-I group had significantly more reductions in daytime napping and the clonazepam group had significantly more reductions in periodic limb movement arousals. One consideration when delivering CBT-I is the possibility that sleep deprivation can worsen RLS. If this is a concern, then the sleep restriction component of CBT-I may be modified to limit this possibility by replacing it with sleep compression.[40] On the other hand, in the seminal study of sleep restriction therapy for insomnia,[41] two study participants who had both RLS and PLMD demonstrated significant improvements in sleep with no reports of increased RLS symptoms. Overall, CBT-I, with some potential modifications on a patient-specific basis, can be considered a potentially promising approach to both RLS and PLMD with further empiric work clearly needed.

The role of exercise remains a somewhat confusing topic with respect to RSL/PLMD. Moderate exercise is often suggested for RLS. This suggestion is based on several factors. First, RLS symptoms tend to increase with prolonged inactivity and to be alleviated with physical activity. On the other hand, some individuals report exacerbation of symptoms with exercise. Specific findings on the topic have been mixed with one study showing an increased risk for RLS associated with physical activity before bedtime[31] and another showing an increased risk for RLS associated with lack of exercise.[42] The discussion is aided by the existence of two randomized controlled trials of exercise therapy. The first such study was a crossover trial conducted in 13

patients who had PLMD subsequent to spinal cord injury in which participants received 200 mg L-DOPA and 50 mg benserazide for 30 days or exercise on an ergometer three times a week for 45 days.[43] Despite the limitations of this design and the small sample size, both treatments resulted in significant reductions in PLM index from 35.1 to 19.9 for L-DOPA and from 35.1 to 18.5 for the exercise program. Such studies bear replication in other RLS/PLMD populations.

The second exercise study was conducted in 23 patients who had RLS who were randomized to receive a 12-week trial of exercise therapy or a control condition.[44] Both groups received basic instructions in lifestyle management that included cigarette and alcohol cessation, avoidance of excessive caffeine, and proper sleep hygiene, with no specific goals being set and no follow-up on these suggestions. The exercise intervention consisted of lower body resistance training exercises and 30 minutes of treadmill walking, which took place three times per week for 12 weeks at a local community center (participants were free to do more or less than instructed). Compared to the control group, the exercise group achieved significant reductions in RLS symptom severity at a 6-week assessment, which was maintained at the 12-week assessment. Notably, the control group had no improvements from baseline at either time point, an indirect test of the usefulness of lifestyle instructions for RLS. Although these are small trials, they begin to clear up some confusion with respect to exercise and suggest that an exercise program (as opposed to a suggestion to exercise), may be a promising approach to managing RLS/PLMD.

Although spontaneous, episodic, or treatment-specific remission of RLS/PLMD does occur, for many patients these are chronic conditions. Comprehensive nonpharmacologic approaches to other chronic diseases, either independent from or in concert with pharmacologic interventions, share some similarities with treatments for RLS/PLMD. For instance, one such approach, albeit untested in any controlled fashion, exists for RLS in the form of a patient guide that greatly expands the standard suggestions for RLS.[45] In addition, Hornyak and colleagues[46] have recently published results of an uncontrolled trial of CBT for RLS. In this preliminary study, 25 participants who had RLS (15 medicated and 10 unmedicated) took part in a weekly 90-minute group therapy sessions for 8 weeks. The intervention included modules on psychoeducation about RLS symptoms and treatments, mindfulness-based breathing relaxation, cognitive therapy for sleep disturbances, stress-reduction and coping strategies, cognitive therapy for depression, and identifying and managing individual triggers for RLS. Overall, participants reported significant improvements on subjective scales of RLS severity and quality of life (including satisfaction with sleep) at posttreatment and these gains were maintained at a 3-month follow-up assessment. Although further work is needed in this area, this study provides the first evidence that a comprehensive behavioral medicine approach can be implemented with positive outcomes for patients who have RLS.

SUMMARY

RLS and PLMD are most often treated pharmacologically as is suggested by standards of practice. Although treatment algorithms and patient materials do highlight the use of nonpharmacologic approaches, these are seldom delivered in any systematic or rigorous manner. Nonetheless, several behavioral sleep medicine approaches are available to assist in the management of RLS/PLMD. The first and perhaps most obvious use of a BSM approach in these conditions is in the case of diagnosed comorbid insomnia or the presence of several insomnia-like symptoms, wherein CBT-I would be indicated. Due caution is noted in using the all-too-pervasive lists of sleep hygiene and sleep tips as "hand-out" therapies. Except when such services are not available, there is little rationale for providing sleep hygiene instructions alone apart from multicomponent CBT-I. Second, the recent evidence supporting exercise therapy for PLMD and RLS and comprehensive CBT for RLS highlight their potential usefulness. Third, BSM and general behavioral medicine strategies can target lifestyle factors contributing to pathophysiology. Fourth, similar behavioral medicine approaches can be undertaken to help patients cope with their conditions using a model of chronic disease management. In addition, any or all BSM approaches may be useful for patients experiencing augmentation or tolerance to medications, and accordingly during a drug holiday.

The use of BSM approaches in RLS and PLMD represent not only an underused set of strategies that can be delivered to patients but also an area with several empiric questions to be addressed. Most, if not all, of the BSM interventions reviewed require additional support before being considered evidence-based treatments. Exercise therapy and comprehensive CBT, in particular, deserve some further assessment in randomized, controlled trial designs. There is also ample opportunity to assess various combinations of therapies, including modifying CBT-I to include exercise therapy or components of CBT for RLS. Similarly, research designs that could evaluate these BSM approaches as adjuvants to standard medication management would be informative.

In sum, it is incumbent on the sleep medicine field to more fully include BSM approaches in the management of RLS and PLMD. The emerging findings suggest that patients may benefit from a more multidisciplinary approach than is typically the norm, while underscoring the importance of conducting additional clinical research in this area.

REFERENCES

1. Willis T. De anima brutorum quæ hominis vitalis ac sensitiva est, excertitationes duæ; prior physiologica ejusdem naturam, partes, potentias et affectiones tradit; altera pathologica morbos qui ipsam, et sedem ejus primarium, nempe ceerebrum et nervosum genus atticiunt, explicat, eorumque therapeias instituit [in Latin]. London, R. Davis, 1672. English translation by Samuel Pordage, London, 1683: Two Discourses concerning The Soul of Brutes, Which is that of the Vital and Sensitive of Man.
2. Ekbom KA. Restless legs: a clinical study. Acta Med Scand 1945;158(l):1–122.
3. Allen R, Earley C. Restless legs syndrome: a review of clinical and pathophysiologic features. J Clin Neurophysiol 2001;18:128–47.
4. Allen R, Piccietti D, Hening W, et al. Restless legs syndrome: diagnostic criteria, special considerations, and epidemiology. A report from the restless legs syndrome diagnosis and epidemiology workshop at the National Institutes of Health. Sleep Med 2003;4:101–19.
5. Sleep related movement disorders-restless legs syndrome. In: The international classification of sleep disorders. 2nd edition. Westchester (IL): American Academy of Sleep Medicine; 2005. p. 178–81.
6. Michaud M, Chabli A, Lavigne G, et al. Arm restlessness in patients with restless legs syndrome. Mov Disord 2000;15:289–93.
7. Hening W, Walters AS, Allen RP, et al. Impact, diagnosis and treatment of restless legs syndrome (RLS) in a primary care population: the REST (RLS epidemiology, symptoms, and treatment) primary care study. Sleep Med 2004;5:237–46.
8. Winkelman JW, Finn L, Young T. Prevalence and correlates of restless legs syndrome symptoms in the Wisconsin Sleep Cohort. Sleep Med 2006;7: 545–52.
9. Latorre J, Irr WG. Restless legs syndrome. EMedicine. Available at: http://emedicine.medscape.com/article/1188327-overview. Accessed January 26, 2008.

10. Kaplan Y, Oksuz E. Association between restless legs syndrome and Chiari type 1 malformation. Clin Neurol Neurosurg 2008;110:408–10.

11. Trotti LM, Bhadriraju S, Rye D. An update on the pathophysiology and genetics of restless legs syndrome. Curr Neurol Neurosci Rep 2008;8:281–7.

12. Winkelmann J, Schormair B, Lichtner P, et al. Genome-wide association study of restless legs syndrome identifies common variants in three genomic regions. Nat Genet 2007;39:1000–6.

13. Iranzo A, Comella C, Santamaria J, et al. Restless legs syndrome in Parkinson's disease and other neurodegenerative diseases of the central nervous system. Mov Disord 2007;22(Suppl):S424–30.

14. Winkelman JW, Shahar E, Sharief I, et al. Association of restless legs syndrome and cardiovascular disease in the Sleep Heart Health Study. Neurology 2008;70:35–42.

15. Mizuno S, Mihara T, Miyaoka T, et al. CSF iron, ferritin and transferring levels in restless legs syndrome. J Sleep Res 2005;14:43–7.

16. Montplaisir J, Boucher S, Poirier G, et al. Clinical, polysomnographic, and genetic characteristics of restless legs syndrome: a study of 133 patients diagnosed with new standard criteria. Mov Disord 1997;12:61–5.

17. Michaud M, Paquet J, Lavigne G, et al. Sleep laboratory diagnosis of restless legs syndrome. Eur Neurol 2002;48:108–13.

18. Manconi M, Govoni V, De Vito A, et al. Restless legs syndrome and pregnancy. Neurology 2004;63:1065–9.

19. Cuellar NG, Ratcliffe SJ. A comparison of glycemic control, sleep, fatigue, and depression in type 2 diabetes with and without restless legs syndrome. J Clin Sleep Med 2008;4:50–6.

20. Littner R, Kushida A, Anderson WM, et al. Practice parameters for the dopaminergic treatment of restless legs syndrome and periodic limb movement disorder. Sleep 2004;27:557–9.

21. Silber MH, Ehrenberg BL, Allen RP, et al. An algorithm for the management of restless legs syndrome. Mayo Clin Proc 2004;79:916–22.

22. Montplaisir J, Nicolas A, Denesle R, et al. Restless legs syndrome improved by pramipexole: a double-blind randomized trial. Neurology 1999;52:938–43.

23. Garcia-Borreguero D, Larrosa D, de la Llave O, et al. Treatment of restless legs syndrome with gabapentin: a double-blind, crossover study. Neurology 2002;59:1571–9.

24. Matthews W. Treatment of restless legs syndrome with clonazepam [letter]. BMJ 1979;1:751.

25. Roache JD, Meisch RA. Findings from self-administration research on the addition potential of benzodiazepines. Psychiatr Ann 1995;25:153–7.

26. Earley CJ, Heckler D, Allen RP. Repeated IV doses of iron provides effective supplemental treatment of restless legs syndrome. Sleep Med 2005;6:301–5.

27. O'Keeffe ST, Gavin K, Lavan JN. Iron status and restless legs syndrome in the elderly. Age Ageing 1994;23:200–3.

28. Hronyak M, Voderhozer U, Hohagen F, et al. Magnesium therapy for periodic leg movements-related insomnia and restless legs syndrome: an open pilot study. Sleep 1998;21:501–5.

29. Bartell S, Zallek S. Intravenous magnesium sulfate may relieve restless legs syndrome in pregnancy. J Clin Sleep Med 2006;2:187–8.

30. Symonds CP. Nocturnal myoclonus. J Neurosurg Psychiatry 1953;16:166–71.

31. Ohayon MM, Roth T. Prevalence of restless legs syndrome and periodic limb movement disorder in the general population. J Psychosom Res 2002;53:547–54.

32. Martinez S, Guilleminault C. Periodic leg movements in prepubertal children with sleep disturbance. Dev Med Child Neurol 2004;46:765–70.

33. Picchietti DL, Underwood DJ, Farris WA, et al. Further studies on periodic limb movement disorder and restless legs syndrome in children with attention-deficit hyperactivity disorder. Mov Disord 1999;14:1000–7.

34. Iber C, Ancoli-Israel S, Chesson A, et al. Movement rules. In: The AASM manual for the scoring of sleep and associated events. Westchester (IL): American Academy of Sleep Medicine; 2007. p. 41.

35. Sleep related movement disorders-periodic limb movement disorder. In: The international classification of sleep disorders. 2nd edition. Westchester (IL): American Academy of Sleep Medicine; 2005. p. 182–6.

36. Smith RC. Relationship of periodic limb movements in sleep (nocturnal myoclonus) and the Babinski's sign. Sleep 1985;8:239–43.

37. Montplaisir J, Michaud M, Denesle R, et al. Periodic leg movements are not more prevalent in insomnia or hypersomnia but are specifically associated with sleep disorders involving a dopaminergic mechanism. Sleep Med 2000;1:163–7.

38. Edinger JD. Periodic limb movements: assessment and management strategies. In: Perlis M, Lichstein KL, editors. Treating sleep disorders: principles and practice of behavioral sleep medicine. New York: John Wiley & Sons, Inc; 2003. p. 286–304.

39. Edinger JD, Fins AI, Sullivan RJ, et al. Comparison of cognitive-behavioral therapy and clonazepam for treating periodic limb movement disorder. Sleep 1996;19(5):442–4.

40. Lichstein KL, Riedel BW, Wilson NM, et al. Relaxation and sleep compression for late-life insomnia: a placebo-controlled trial. J Consult Clin Psychol 2001;69(2):227–39.

41. Spielman AJ, Saskin P, Thorpy MJ. Treatment of chronic insomnia by restriction of time in bed. Sleep 1987;10:45–56.

42. Phillips B, Young T, Finn L, et al. Epidemiology of restless legs syndrome in adults. Arch Intern Med 2000;160:2137–41.

43. deMello MT, Esteves AM, Tufik S. Comparison between dopaminergic agents and physical exercise as treatment for periodic limb movements in patients with spinal cord injury. Spinal Cord 2004; 42(4):218–21.

44. Aukerman MM, Aukerman D, Bayard M, et al. Exercise and restless legs syndrome: a randomized controlled trial. J Am Board Fam Med 2006;19(5): 487–93.

45. Gunzel J. Restless legs syndrome: the RLS Rebel's survival guide. Tucson (AZ): Wheatmark, Inc; 2006.

46. Hornyak M, Grossmann C, Kohnen R, et al. Cognitive behavioural group therapy to improve patients' strategies for coping with restless legs syndrome: a proof-of-concept trial. J Neurol Neurosurg Psychiatr 2008;79:823–5.

Circadian Rhythm Disorders

Jamie A. Cvengros, PhD*, James K. Wyatt, PhD

KEYWORDS

- Circadian rhythms • Jet lag • Shift work
- Delayed sleep phase • Advanced sleep phase
- Free running

There are two primary modulatory processes that govern timing, duration, and depth of sleep, and timing, duration, and degree of wakefulness. Borbély[1] first introduced this concept as the "two process model" of sleep-wake regulation. The first process is referred to as the "homeostatic drive for sleep." With each hour of sustained wakefulness, homeostatic drive for sleep builds. Remaining awake for 14 to 18 hours builds sufficient homeostatic sleep pressure to initiate the major nocturnal sleep episode. This homeostatic system is very efficient, however, and most sleep drive from it is satiated approximately halfway through the nocturnal sleep episode. This raises the question: how do humans remain asleep for the second half of the night? A similar question is how do humans maintain a relatively stable level of alertness during a 16-hour daytime, wake episode in the face of homeostatic sleep drive building each and every hour?

The second modulatory process affecting sleep and wake is the intrinsic circadian system. The circadian timekeeping system allows for the synchronization of multiple physiologic processes to the desired sleep-wake schedule. As a diurnal species, humans typically sleep during darkness at night and are active during daylight. The circadian system receives its primary zeitgeber (literally "time giver") from the environmental light-dark cycle. Transduction of this time cue occurs in special retinal ganglion cells.[2] Light-dark information is passed through the retinohypothalamic tract to the suprachiasmatic nucleus (SCN) of the hypothalamus, the primary circadian oscillator or clock.[3,4] The SCN has myriad output pathways, allowing it to exert a modulatory influence on such physiologic functions as core body temperature, endogenous melatonin, cortisol, and even the sleep-wake cycle. The circadian modulation of core body temperature and endogenous melatonin are so robust that these physiologic parameters are typically used in research as markers of circadian phase. Although the SCN exerts a circadian modulation of other physiologic parameters (eg, urine concentration, cortisol), core body temperature and endogenous melatonin have emerged as the gold standard markers of circadian phase.

Research has demonstrated that the circadian system exerts an active promotion of wakefulness during the daytime. This drive for wake building across the 16-hour wake episode counteracts the mounting homeostatic drive for sleep, resulting in a relatively stable level of alertness across the waking day. The circadian system reaches its maximal wake drive a few hours before bedtime, at a time referred to as the "forbidden zone for sleep"[5] or the "wake maintenance zone."[6] Nearer to bedtime, the circadian system lowers its drive for wakefulness, permitting the homeostatic system to initiate and consolidate sleep. The circadian system begins actively driving sleep during the night, reaching its maximal promotion of sleep near and just after the normal wake time, in the "circadian sleep maintenance zone."[7,8] The circadian system allows humans to maintain sleep during the second half of the night when homeostatic sleep drive is insufficient to accomplish this task.

EFFECT OF LIGHT ON THE CIRCADIAN SYSTEM

The circadian timing system uses the environmental light-dark cycle as its primary

Sleep Disorders Service and Research Center, Department of Behavioral Sciences, Rush University Medical Center, 1653 West Congress Parkway, Chicago, IL 60612-3833, USA
* Corresponding author.
E-mail address: jamie_cvengros@rush.edu (J. A. Cvengros).

Sleep Med Clin 4 (2009) 495–505
doi:10.1016/j.jsmc.2009.07.001

synchronizing cue to maintain proper orientation to the desired nocturnal sleep schedule. Within the context of sleep medicine, "phototherapy" is the term used to denote the intentional use of artificial bright light to shift the intrinsic circadian system to a more appropriate phase relationship with the desired sleep-wake schedule. Although it had been known for some time that changes in the light-dark cycle could shift circadian phase in lower organisms, a pivotal discovery in sleep medicine was the demonstration that artificial bright light could shift phase in the human circadian system.[9] Since that time, it has been demonstrated that there is a dose-response function to the intensity of light used in phototherapy and the degree of resultant phase shifting,[10] such that even average indoor room lighting can accomplish small but significant shifts in phase.[11] Further, building on studies from phase shifting in lower organisms, human studies have provided data on the "phase-response curve" to light.[12–14] The human circadian system is relatively unresponsive to artificial bright light delivered during the middle of the waking day. Phototherapy during the late evening through the middle of the night results in a "phase delay," a shift of the circadian system to a later hour. Phase delaying the circadian system allows for a later bedtime and wake time, such as that desired when traveling from the East Coast to the West Coast of the United States. Phototherapy administered after the trough of core body temperature, near the end of the normal sleep episode or in the early morning hours, results in a "phase advance" or shift of the circadian system to an earlier hour. Finally, full-spectrum lighting was commonly used in phototherapy research, because it was not known what the optimal spectral sensitivity was of the retinal ganglion cells. Recently, research has shown that the circadian system is maximally sensitive to visible light in the blue region of the electromagnetic spectrum.[15,16]

ENDOGENOUS AND EXOGENOUS MELATONIN

The circadian system regulates levels of endogenous melatonin, a pineal hormone. Levels of circulating melatonin seem linked to the timing of the sleep-wake cycle. Melatonin is typically at a very low level during the daytime, and begins to rise near the wake maintenance zone, approximately 2 hours before normal bedtime.[17] Melatonin levels peak near the middle of the nocturnal sleep episode, just before the trough of core body temperature, and decline over the remainder of the sleep episode. Melatonin synthesis seems to be shut off near normal morning wake time by

signaling from the circadian system. Artificial bright light administered during a time of elevated melatonin levels (biologic night), however, can acutely suppress melatonin production.[18] To obtain a robust marker of circadian phase, the Dim Light Melatonin Onset (DLMO) protocol has been established.[17] Blood or saliva samples are obtained at frequent intervals (eg, every half hour) under dim lighting conditions, to prevent light-related suppression of melatonin levels. Sampling is conducted from approximately late afternoon through just after habitual bedtime, to detect the rising limb of the nocturnal release of endogenous melatonin.

Given the coupling of the phase of the melatonin cycle and the sleep-wake cycle, studies have explored the possibility that melatonin may possess a hypnotic or sleep-promoting property. Exogenous melatonin administration has indeed been shown to increase the duration of daytime sleep episodes[19] in normal sleepers, but does not seem to increase the duration of nocturnal sleep in patients with insomnia.[20] In a study where exogenous melatonin was administered in normal sleepers who were scheduled to initiate sleep episodes across a full range of circadian phases, melatonin was ineffective at increasing sleep efficiency when sleep episodes coincided with the circadian night, when endogenous melatonin levels were already elevated. Exogenous melatonin administration did increase the efficiency of sleep episodes scheduled to occur during the circadian day, however, when endogenous melatonin levels were low to nil.[21] Taken together, these results suggest that melatonin administration may act by suppression of the circadian promotion of wakefulness, limiting the efficacy of melatonin as a hypnotic to daytime administration. This holds promise for patients who are attempting to sleep at times when the circadian drive for wakefulness is present, such as shift workers or those with jet lag.

Although less potent than phototherapy, exogenous melatonin has also been shown to possess significant circadian phase shifting properties.[22] The phase-response curve to melatonin is very different, however, than the phase-response curve to light. For melatonin, administration during the late afternoon and early evening hours causes a circadian phase advance. Melatonin given during the latter hours of the night and early morning hours causes a circadian phase delay. In those insensitive to time cues from the environmental light-dark cycle (eg, certain retinally blind individuals), routine administration of exogenous melatonin at the same time every day seems to lead to a stabilization of circadian phase. This is particularly important for free running patients.

CIRCADIAN RHYTHM DISORDERS

Given the preceding review of homeostatic and circadian modulation of sleep and wakefulness, and the review of circadian phase shifting, it is easier to understand the cause and treatment of the circadian rhythm sleep disorders. Jet lag and shift work sleep disorder can be thought of as intentional, albeit mildly to profoundly impactful, misalignment of the desired sleep-wake schedule with the phase of the circadian timekeeping system. The remaining four circadian rhythm sleep disorders are thought to result from dysfunction of the circadian timekeeping system itself. Reference is made frequently to the recent American Academy of Sleep Medicine (AASM) practice parameter for these disorders.[23] An AASM work group reviewed the literature in the area, and graded the study designs used (eg, randomized controlled trials are optimal) and the strength of the findings. Diagnostic procedures and treatments are indicated as "standards" for high-certainty results from good protocol designs; "guidelines" for medium certainty results from less powerful protocols (eg, cohort or case control studies); and "options" for low certainty results or lack of results forcing a consensus opinion from a panel of experts.

SHIFT WORK DISORDER

Although millions of Americans have a shift work schedule, the prevalence of circadian rhythm sleep disorder, shift work type, or shift work disorder (SWD) is unknown. Recent telephone survey data suggest that approximately one third of shift workers report symptoms suggestive of SWD.[24] Patients with SWD often present with complaints of excessive sleepiness during work hours; decreased attention, concentration, and productivity; and difficulties initiating or maintaining daytime sleep. Finally, patients with SWD are likely to present with physical symptoms associated with poor sleep quality including fatigue, headache, and gastrointestinal upset and psychologic symptoms, such as depressed mood.[24] The use of sleep logs is indicated by the AASM practice parameter as a guideline in the assessment of SWD, and when coupled with clinical interview can be used to differentiate SWD from other sleep disorders, such as insomnia.[23] Polysomnography is not indicated as a diagnostic tool for SWD, but can be useful in ruling out other causes of sleep disturbance, such as sleep-disordered breathing and periodic limb movements.[23]

It is presumed that SWD occurs when a patient's internal circadian rhythm is misaligned with their desired sleep-wake schedule, such that patients are attempting to sleep at time of circadian wake-promotion and attempting to work during a time of circadian sleep-promotion. As a result, daytime sleep is often shorter in duration and poorer in quality, as compared with nocturnal sleep, which results in increased homeostatic drive for sleep during work hours, which in turn exacerbates sleepiness. Several studies have suggested that exposure to light during the desired sleep time is a causal factor in maintaining phase misalignment and that appropriately timed exposure to light can shift circadian phase to be consistent with desired sleep-wake pattern and improve adaptation to shift work.[25] A few small studies of shift workers have also suggested, however, that phase misalignment is not necessarily associated with the development of SWD.[26,27] For example, among a study of nurses working the night shift, those who reported poor daytime sleep quality did not differ in circadian phase, as indexed by melatonin onset, from those who reported good daytime sleep quality.[27] These findings, along with findings from simulated shift work studies, have led to the suggestion that individuals vary in their level of tolerance to circadian phase misalignment. A few studies have suggested that increasing age may be associated with decreased tolerance for shift work including increased lapses in attention and concentration.[28,29] In addition, women may experience more difficulty with a shift work schedule given the higher likelihood of daytime responsibilities (eg, childcare) that interfere with quality and quantity of daytime sleep, and hence may experience more health consequences of shift work.[30]

The goals for treating patients with SWD include increasing the duration and quality of daytime sleep, improving alertness while at work, and shifting circadian phase to align better with the desired sleep-wake schedule. Prescribed sleep scheduling is indicated as a treatment standard according to the AASM.[23] Sleep scheduling includes the use of short naps before and during a patient's shift. These naps reduce homeostatic drive for sleep and can be used effectively to decrease sleepiness and accidents related to sleepiness while at work without negatively impacting ability to fall asleep during desired sleep time.[31,32] Medications are also indicated to improve daytime sleep and increase nighttime alertness. Laboratory studies of simulated shift work suggest that melatonin administered at desired morning bedtime can increase duration of daytime sleep.[33] Traditional hypnotics are indicated as a treatment guideline for the promotion of daytime sleep without detrimental effects on alertness and performance during the night shift work.[34,35] In addition, wake-promoting agents, such as modafinil, can be used to decrease sleepiness and improve alertness during work.[36] Caffeine ingestion[31] has also been identified as a treatment option; however, care must be taken to ensure that the use of any stimulant-like medication does not increase difficulty falling asleep at desired time.

Melatonin has also been identified in the treatment of SWD for its circadian phase-shifting properties. Specifically, in a laboratory simulation study of shift work, Sharkey and Eastman[37] found that administration of melatonin before desired bedtime for 4 days produced subsequent advances in the circadian phase markers of DLMO and core body temperature minimum, indicative of circadian adaptation to shift work schedule. Timed exposure to light during work hours and avoidance of exposure to light during sleep periods can also effectively increase adaptation to shift work schedule as measured by advances in DLMO and the trough of the core body temperature rhythm.[38,39] Smith and Eastman[40] reported on a protocol with 7 days of simulated shift night work, which included a "weekend" in the middle when sleep schedule was modified to include nighttime sleep (from 3:00 AM–12:00 PM). Participants also received exposure to pulses of bright light during simulated night work and decreased exposure to light following the night work shifts using darkened sunglasses. The results showed decreased sleepiness and improved work performance at night as compared with controls. These findings suggest that timed light exposure and prevention of light exposure at other times can be effective for shift workers who work nights but prefer a sleep schedule that includes nighttime sleep on their days off.

JET LAG DISORDER

Along with SWD, jet lag disorder is considered to be one of the "extrinsic" circadian rhythm disorders, meaning that the symptoms are caused by a misalignment between a patient's circadian phase and the new sleep-wake schedule desired at the destination. Attempts to sleep during times of circadian wake promotion lead to insomnia and short sleep times, leading to excessive sleepiness. Additional sleep loss may occur in some individuals, who report difficulty sleeping on airplanes, may have poor sleep before travel because of stress, and may incur sleep loss because of early waking for departure or late activities on arrival. Sleep loss and circadian phase misalignment can cause other symptoms, including fatigue, headache, gastrointestinal distress, and difficulties

with concentration and attention, similar to what is observed in SWD.[41] In addition to sleep loss and circadian phase misalignment, symptoms of jet lag may simply be related to voluntary behaviors, such as decreased water intake and the diuretic effect of caffeine and alcohol consumption, and spending time in a low-humidity, low-pressure airliner cabin; jet travelers often experience dehydration, nasal dryness and congestion, and symptoms of hypoxia, such as dizziness, lightheadedness, and headache. These symptoms can disrupt sleep and further exacerbate other symptoms.

Circadian phase misalignment is eventually resolved by exposure to the new light-dark cycle at the destination. For example, westward travel leads to "evening" light exposure at a time that can cause phase delay, whereas eastward travel can lead to "morning" light exposure at time that can cause phase advance.

Although individuals rarely present to a sleep disorders clinic for treatment of jet lag, given the high rates of long-distance jet travel, symptoms of jet lag have a high prevalence. Researchers have identified several methods for preventing jet lag and reducing impact of jet lag on arrival at the destination (see review by Arendt[42]). For example, prescribed sleep scheduling is indicated as an AASM treatment option and can be used in two ways to counteract jet lag. One approach is to maintain the "home" sleep-wake pattern on arrival at the destination (not shifting to a new sleep-wake schedule), especially if time at the destination is short. In a study of 20 flight attendants, maintenance of home schedule was associated with fewer symptoms of jet lag including sleepiness.[43] This approach is often impractical for travelers, however, because it requires diligent maintenance of sleep and wake times, avoidance of light at certain circadian phase when phase shifting in the wrong direction may occur, and possible conflict of sleep schedule with desired activities at the destination. Alternatively, individuals can preemptively adjust their sleep-wake pattern to be aligned with desired pattern at the destination. Among a sample of healthy adults, Eastman and colleagues[44] found that incremental advancement of sleep schedule by 1 hour per day over 3 days could be used to advance circadian phase in preparation for eastward travel. Participants demonstrated a circadian phase advance, as measured by DLMO, of approximately 90 minutes following 3 days of treatment without demonstrating significant side effects, such as difficulty initiating sleep.

Phototherapy is also indicated as an AASM treatment option and is used to align circadian phase with local time zone. Boulos and colleagues[45] found that circadian phase could be successfully delayed and entrained to local time zone following evening exposure to bright light by specially designed goggles. Specifically, DLMO was delayed by an average of 2.5 hours from pre-exposure to postexposure. The changes in circadian alignment were not associated with significant improvements in subjective ratings of sleep or objective cognitive performance, however, and optimal use of the phototherapy requires knowledge of the individual's current circadian phase, such that light is not delivered during inappropriate times of the phase-response curve to light.

Given its hypnotic and phase shifting properties, melatonin has also been used to combat jet lag and is indicated as an AASM treatment standard.[23] In a study of Air Force reservists, melatonin administered before, during, and after an eastbound flight was associated with faster entrainment to local time as measured by cortisol rhythms.[46] Fast-release melatonin administered at bedtime in the days before departure and days after arrival has been found to decrease symptoms of jet lag, decrease sleep-onset latency at destination, and improve ratings of sleep quality.[47]

Finally, hypnotics and stimulants are indicated as treatment options by the AASM to combat the insomnia and excessive daytime sleepiness associated with jet leg.[23] In a randomized controlled trial, the administration of zolpidem at bedtime was associated with increased total sleep time, decreased sleep fragmentation, and increased sleep quality.[48] In a laboratory simulation study of jet lag, administration of triazolam was associated with faster entrainment to local time as measured by cortisol rhythms.[49] Similarly, caffeine has been indicated as a treatment option for combating the daytime sleepiness associated with jet lag.[50] Care must be taken with pharmacologic options, however, because there may be unwanted side effects, such as increased risk for deep vein thrombosis when hypnotics are taken during flight (possibly because of increased time spent immobile), or increased difficulty initiating sleep when caffeine is taken to combat daytime sleepiness.

DELAYED SLEEP PHASE DISORDER

In delayed sleep phase disorder (DSPD), formerly known as "delayed sleep phase syndrome,"[51] the primary complaints are of difficulty falling asleep until several hours later than the desired bedtime and significant difficulty arising at the desired morning wake time. Typically noted during weekdays when school or work obligations dictate a certain sleep-wake schedule, the inability to fall asleep until several hours past the desired bedtime precludes the patient from obtaining sufficient sleep duration, leading to suboptimal daytime alertness, excessive daytime sleepiness, and possibly impaired mood regulation and interpersonal problems. On weekends or vacations, however, the patient adopts a later, "delayed" sleep-wake schedule, demonstrating the absence of sleep onset problems or impaired sleep maintenance. This pattern of impaired sleep alternating with normal-but-delayed sleep must be demonstrated on at least a week of daily sleep diary-keeping or wrist actigraphic monitoring to confirm the diagnosis.[41]

The research of Carskadon[52] has demonstrated a normal propensity for small delays of the sleep-wake schedule and circadian phase across adolescence. Rather than being a purely biologic process, behavioral (eg, remaining awake to complete homework) and social factors (eg, parental approval to keep a progressively later bedtime as the child ages, or increased availability of evening social activities) also contribute to this delaying of the sleep-wake schedule. DSPD may represent an extreme of this commonly observed delay in sleep schedule across adolescence. In contrast to normally sleeping teenagers or young adults, the DSPD patient has a greatly delayed circadian phase relative to the desired sleep-wake schedule. They are unable to fall asleep during the wake maintenance zone but have to awaken at an early hour for school or work obligations. Total sleep time is reduced and a sleep debt builds across the week, leading to very late wake times on weekends to reduce the sleep debt.

There are several treatment options for patients with DSPD. Perhaps the simplest treatment is known as "chronotherapy." To describe this treatment, a prototypical patient might have a circadian phase position optimally set for a sleep schedule with a 2 AM bedtime and a 10 AM wake time, but a desired bedtime of 10 PM and a wake time of 6 AM. Chronotherapy begins by having the patient delay their sleep schedule on the first day by 3 hours, delaying bedtime until 5 AM and the wake time until 1 PM. Each successive sleep episode is delayed an additional 3 hours (8 AM–4 PM, then 11 AM–7 PM, then 2 PM–10 PM, then 5 PM–1 AM, then 8 PM–4 AM). In this example, a smaller delay of the sleep schedule may be required in the final sleep episode to reach the desired 10 PM to 6 AM routine. The patient is then instructed to maintain strict adherence to the desired sleep schedule 7 days a week. Chronotherapy showed good efficacy in the original case series of five patients, with mean bedtime being advanced 4.5 hours from the pretreatment mean of 4:50 AM.

Similarly, mean wake time was advanced by more than 5 hours, with the new sleep-wake schedule having much better alignment with typical daytime activities.[53] Given that chronotherapy does not entail instructions on exposure to bright or environmental light, it is unlikely that the circadian system is able to delay 3 hours per sleep episode. Hence, the precise mechanism by which chronotherapy achieves its effect in DSPD remains unknown. Chronotherapy is recommended in the AASM practice parameter at the level of an indicated option.[23]

Phototherapy has also been studied as a treatment for DSPD (reviewed in[54]). Some studies have shown only minimal or no effect of administration of artificial bright light, but these protocols likely exposed patients to light during the maximal region of phase delays of the phase-response curve to light, instead of late enough to fall in the phase-advance region of the phase-response curve. Studies have shown the ability to predict DLMO in both normal sleepers[55] and DSPD patients[56] merely from knowledge of their habitual sleep schedule. Given that the phase-advance region of the phase-response curve to light begins approximately 7 hours after DLMO[14] and that DLMO can be estimated from the sleep-wake schedule, a simple conservative strategy for timing phototherapy in DSPD requires only knowledge of the habitual, late sleep schedule.[57] At least 1 hour of phototherapy is recommended to begin following the late, habitual rise time (eg, starting at 10 AM in the previous patient example). This should lead to a small phase advance of the circadian system. Each successive sleep cycle is moved 30 minutes earlier each day, with the hour of phototherapy being linked to that progressively earlier, scheduled wake time. Patients can be maintained on a shorter, 30-minute bout of maintenance phototherapy once reaching their desired sleep-wake schedule. Patients are cautioned to avoid bright light in the 2-hour window before bedtime, lest they inadvertently expose themselves to bright light in the phase-delay region of the phase-response curve, which counteracts the morning phototherapy. Phototherapy is recommended in the AASM practice parameter at the level of an indicated guideline.[23]

Exogenous melatonin administration has been studied to treat DSPD. Given 5 hours before habitual sleep onset[58] or 5 hours before DLMO,[59] during the phase advance region of the phase-response curve for melatonin, melatonin administration may be effective in shortening sleep latency. Return of symptoms was very high, however, after discontinuation of presleep melatonin. In a more recent, randomized controlled trial

in DSPD, Kayumov and colleagues[60] had 20 patients ingest 5 mg melatonin or placebo in the 7 PM to 9 PM window for 4 weeks, then undergo a 1-week washout, and crossover to the other treatment condition. Although melatonin administration did not increase total sleep time, it did significantly decrease sleep latency from baseline during sleep recorded on a fixed 12 AM to 8 AM window at the 4 weeks of treatment. It has also been hypothesized that instead of working merely through melatonin administration causing a phase advance of the circadian system, some of the treatment effect may have been achieved by suppression of the circadian drive for wakefulness late in the day, allowing homeostatic drive for sleep to take over and promote sleep onset at an earlier hour. Oral melatonin is recommended in the AASM practice parameter at the level of an indicated guideline.[23] The use of traditional hypnotics, however, is not recommended.

According to the AASM practice parameters,[23] having the patient maintain a daily sleep log or diary is indicated at the level of a guideline. The use of wrist actigraphy is indicated at the guideline level for the diagnosis of DSPD, and in the monitoring of treatment. There is insufficient evidence to recommend assessment of subjective chronotype or to obtain an objective assessment of circadian phase. Polysomnography is not recommended for the diagnosis of DSPD.

ADVANCED SLEEP PHASE DISORDER

In advanced sleep phase disorder (ASPD), formerly known as "advanced sleep phase syndrome," the primary complaint is the inability to remain awake late enough for the desired bedtime, and awakening well in advance of the preferred rising time.[41] As opposed to DSPD, which is observed predominantly in teenagers and young adults, ASPD is most often seen in older adults. There are several reports of familial ASPD,[61] and putative genetic markers of this circadian sleep disorder.[62] In contrast to the significant progress made in the genetic study of ASPD, there is a paucity of published treatment data.

Chronotherapy may be used in the treatment of ASPD. There is a report of prescribing a short, daily advance to the sleep-wake schedule.[63] Given the scarcity of published data, however, the AASM practice parameter recommends the use of sleep scheduling as an indicated option for ASPD.

Phototherapy can also be used as a treatment for ASPD. The circadian system is presumably misaligned with the desired sleep-wake schedule by being set at an earlier, advanced hour. It is necessary to administer artificial bright light in the presleep hours, falling in the phase-delay region of the phase-response curve to light. Similarly, the patient is cautioned to avoid exposure to bright light in the 2-hour window following awakening, to prevent light exposure within the phase-advance region of the phase-response curve to light. The sleep schedule can be progressively delayed by 30 minutes later per day until reaching the desired timing of the sleep schedule. Given the scarcity of data, phototherapy is only indicated at the level of an option in the AASM practice parameter.[23] Given the lack of evidence, the practice parameter states that the use of oral melatonin in the treatment of ASPD is indicated only as an option.

As with DSPD, the AASM practice parameter[23] recommends a daily sleep log or diary, indicated at the level of a guideline. Wrist actigraphy is indicated at the guideline level for making the diagnosis and monitoring treatment in ASPD. Also as with DSPD, there is insufficient evidence to recommend assessment of chronotype or to collect objective assessment of circadian phase in ASPD. Polysomnography is not recommended for the diagnosis of ASPD.

FREE RUNNING DISORDER

In the absence of external time cues, especially exposure to morning light, an individual's circadian phase may become desynchronized from their desired sleep-wake schedule, as in circadian sleep disorder, non–24-hour type, commonly called "free running disorder" (FRD). FRD differs from other intrinsic sleep disorders, such as ASPD and DSPD, in which the circadian system is misaligned but still on a 24-hour cycle, in that patients with FRD do not demonstrate a 24-hour sleep-wake pattern. Studies using the forced desynchrony protocol, in which individuals are kept in an environment free from time cues for nearly a month and are scheduled a sleep-wake cycle significantly different from normal, have found that the human circadian rhythm oscillates with a period slightly longer than 24 hours, approximately 24.2 hours.[64] For sighted individuals, daily exposure to bright morning light "entrains" the circadian system to a 24-hour light-dark cycle by phase advancing each day. For individuals with retinal blindness, the SCN does not receive this external input from the retinal ganglion cells, and without additional entrainment cues, circadian phase may "free run" by progressively delaying a fraction of an hour each day, possibly leading to later sleep and wake times each day.

FRD is very rare. Most patients with FRD have retinal blindness and hence no light-dark cycle information can reach the SCN. In sighted individuals, FRD can also occur posttrauma,[65] because of pituitary adenoma, or may develop following a diagnosis of DSPD. Patients with FRD commonly present with complaints of recurrent insomnia. Specifically, for a period of time when a patient's circadian phase is in sync with their desired sleep-wake schedule, such that the circadian system is promoting sleep during the night and alertness during the day, they do not experience symptoms of insomnia. As the patient's circadian cycle drifts later and later each day or "free runs," however, it eventually drives the patient to be sleepy during the day and be alert at night, causing difficulty falling asleep at night, consistent with insomnia. As circadian phase continues to drift, the insomnia eventually remits as circadian phase eventually realigns with the desired sleep-wake schedule. Other patients simply give in to the drift of circadian phase, and progressively delay their sleep-wake schedule each day by a fraction of an hour. Sleep logs are indicated as an AASM guideline and actigraphy is indicated as an AASM option in the assessment of FRD.[66]

Indicated treatment for FRD is different for sighted and nonsighted individuals. For sighted individuals, presumably with intact retinal ganglion cells, treatment includes entrainment of the sleep-wake cycle through both the circadian and homeostatic systems. Specifically, exposure to light during the daytime and avoidance of light during nighttime (eg, maintaining a dark bedroom, using light blocking shades) helps to strengthen the amplitude of the circadian system. Carefully timed exposure to bright morning light can be used to advance the circadian phase to combat the progressive delay of circadian phase associated with FRD. In addition, strict adherence to a bedtime and wake time schedule with avoidance of napping and engagement in daytime activity can help to preserve homeostatic drive for sleep and prevent difficulty initiating sleep at desired bedtime.

For nonsighted individuals, unable to benefit from the phase entrainment properties of light, administration of melatonin is indicated as a treatment guideline. Initial studies suggested that a 10-mg dose of melatonin administered at desired bedtime could be used to "capture and lock" the sleep-wake cycle at the desired time.[67] Lewy and colleagues (2005)[68] subsequently found that significantly lower doses (0.3–0.5 mg) were sufficient to synchronize sleep-wake cycles in patients with FRD. Some studies have suggested that the timing of melatonin administration in relation to circadian phase is critical in the effectiveness of melatonin. For example, in a sample of 10 patients who were administered melatonin at a clock time of 9:00 PM, seven patients demonstrated an entrained rhythm as measured by urinary cortisol. Of those who responded (four patients entrained to a 24-hour cycle), two continued to free run several weeks before synchronizing and one demonstrated a less than 24-hour rhythm, suggesting that patients received melatonin at different points on their melatonin phase-response curve.[69] Other studies, however, have found the effect of melatonin is independent of circadian phase.[70]

IRREGULAR SLEEP-WAKE DISORDER

The circadian rhythm sleep disorders previously described assume that the individual's internal circadian pacemaker (SCN) is functional and that sleep dysregulation results from misalignment between external cues and internal circadian phase or from failure of the SCN to receive time cues from the external environment. If there is dysfunction of the SCN itself, however, irregular sleep wake disorder (ISWD) may develop. Patients with ISWD do not demonstrate a clear sleep-wake pattern and may present with excessive daytime sleepiness and frequent daytime napping coupled with severely fragmental nocturnal sleep.[41] These patients present with near-normal total sleep times per 24 hours, but seem physiologically unable to maintain consolidated bouts of nocturnal sleep and consolidated bouts of daytime activity. Actigraphy is particularly useful in identifying the irregular rest-activity pattern in ISWD and is indicated as an AASM assessment guideline.[66] Actigraphy may also be especially useful given that patients with ISWD are often unable reliably to complete sleep logs because of severe cognitive decline.

ISWD is most common among older adults, especially those with progressive neurologic diseases, such as Alzheimer's dementia, and those living in nursing homes. For these patients, ISWD likely has several causes. First, general neurologic deterioration may weaken the circadian system and may make patients less sensitive to external time cues (eg, deterioration of the SCN or the retinohypothalamic tract). Second, the institutionalized elderly often receive limited exposure to bright light and limited daytime activity, which normally serve as strong cues for circadian entrainment. Finally, patients are often taking medications with sedating effects which increase daytime napping which decreases homeostatic drive for nocturnal sleep. Furthermore, napping decreases exposure to bright light and daytime

activity. Damage to the hypothalamus following neurologic insult (eg, stroke, tumor resection) can also result in the development of ISWD.

Exposure to bright light may be effective in the treatment of ISWD, and phototherapy is currently indicated as an AASM treatment option. In a study of 77 nursing home residents assessed with actigraphy, exposure to bright morning light was associated with strengthened circadian rhythms. Bright light exposure, however, did not decrease nocturnal sleep fragmentation or increase daytime alertness.[71] Currently, comprehensive behavioral interventions, which include prescribed sleep-wake schedules and timed exposure to light, are indicated as an AASM treatment guideline for elderly patients with dementia.[66] Martin and colleagues (2007)[72] found that rest-activity rhythms, also assessed by actigraphy, were significantly strengthened among patients who received a 5-day intervention of daytime exposure to outdoor light and physical activity and a nighttime reduction in ambient light and noise as compared with patients who received treatment as usual.

Among an older adult population, melatonin has not been found to have significant effects on consolidating sleep-wake periods,[73] but in one study of 189 patients, melatonin in conjunction with light exposure was associated with decreased nocturnal awakenings and increased nocturnal sleep efficiency.[74] Of note, melatonin alone in this sample was associated with increases in negative mood. The authors suggested the use of melatonin only in combination with light, which may have mood-elevating properties. Melatonin is currently indicated as a treatment option for the treatment of ISWD in younger populations, such as those with severe neurodevelopmental disorders. Currently, there are not sufficient data on the use of stimulant medications to combat daytime sleepiness and napping, or on the use of hypnotic medications to combat nocturnal sleep fragmentation in this population, to recommend routine use, because these medications may have serious side effects in elderly patients.

CIRCADIAN FACTORS IN INSOMNIA

Although insomnia is not a circadian rhythm sleep disorder, circadian factors may play a role in the development, maintenance, and treatment of insomnia. In a study of patients with difficulty initiating sleep (ie, sleep-onset insomnia), core body temperature rhythms were significantly delayed relative to their sleep-wake schedule, as compared with "good sleeper" controls. The habitual bedtime for these patients with insomnia often fell within their circadian wake maintenance zone.[75] Similarly, patients with insomnia of the early morning awakening subtype have been reported to have significantly advanced circadian phase, as assessed by core body temperature and melatonin onset.[76] Findings from these and similar studies have led to the suggestion that the phase-shifting properties of light and melatonin may make phototherapy and melatonin administration effective treatments for insomnia.[77] Furthermore, emerging research examining the role of the Per2, Per3, and Clock genes in the development of circadian rhythm disorders and insomnia suggests that there may be substantial overlap in the etiology of these disorders.[78] Although a full description of circadian rhythms in insomnia is beyond the scope of this article, the etiology, diagnosis, and treatment of insomnia is extensively reviewed in other articles.

SUMMARY

The field of sleep disorders has recognized the importance of the six circadian rhythm sleep disorders, with a recent achievement being the publication of a standard of practice paper from the AASM[23] and two comprehensive evidence review papers.[66,79] As noted in the standard of practice paper and again in this article, many of the diagnostic procedures and treatment options have low levels of evidence; most of the diagnostic procedures and treatments fall short of being indicated at the level of a standard, and are only indicated as guidelines or options. This medium- to low-level of certainty may be viewed as a yardstick of the limited progress achieved by sleep disorders researchers in the circadian rhythm sleep disorders. More optimistically, the same levels of evidence may be seen as a call to action for more research into the diagnostic procedures and treatments used by clinicians to treat these interesting disorders.

REFERENCES

1. Borbely AA. A two process model of sleep regulation. Hum Neurobiol 1982;1(3):195–204.
2. Berson DM, Dunn FA, Takao M. Phototransduction by retinal ganglion cells that set the circadian clock. Science 2002;295(5557):1070–3.
3. Moore RY, Eichler VB. Loss of a circadian adrenal corticosterone rhythm following suprachiasmatic lesions in the rat. Brain Res 1972;42:201–6.
4. Stephan FK, Zucker I. Circadian rhythms in drinking behavior and locomotor activity of rats are eliminated by hypothalamic lesions. Proc Natl Acad Sci U S A 1972;69(6):1583–6.
5. Lavie P. Ultrashort sleep-waking schedule. III. Gates and forbidden zones for sleep. Electroencephalogr Clin Neurophysiol 1986;63(5):414–25.
6. Strogatz SH, Kronauer RE, Czeisler CA. Circadian pacemaker interferes with sleep onset at specific times each day: role in insomnia. Am J Physiol 1987;253(1 Pt 2):R172–8.
7. Stepanski EJ, Wyatt JK. Use of sleep hygiene in the treatment of insomnia. Sleep Med Rev 2003;7:215–25.
8. Wyatt JK, Cajochen C, Ritz-De CA, et al. Low-dose repeated caffeine administration for circadian-phase-dependent performance degradation during extended wakefulness. Sleep 2004;27(3):374–81.
9. Czeisler CA, Allan JS, Strogatz SH, et al. Bright light resets the human circadian pacemaker independent of the timing of the sleep-wake cycle. Science 1986;233(4764):667–71.
10. Boivin DB, Duffy JF, Kronauer RE, et al. Dose-response relationships for resetting of human circadian clock by light. Nature 1996;379(6565):540–2.
11. Boivin DB, Duffy JF, Kronauer RE, et al. Sensitivity of the human circadian pacemaker to moderately bright light. J Biol Rhythms 1994;9(3–4):315–31.
12. Honma K, Honma S. A human phase response curve for bright light pulses. Jpn J Psychiatry Neurol 1988;42(1):167–8.
13. Minors DS, Waterhouse JM, Wirz-Justice A. A human phase-response curve to light. Neurosci Lett 1991;133(1):36–40.
14. Khalsa SBS, Jewett ME, Cajochen C, et al. A phase response curve to single bright light pulses in human subjects. Journal of Physiology 2003;549(3):945–52.
15. Brainard GC, Hanifin JP, Greeson JM, et al. Action spectrum for melatonin regulation in humans: evidence for a novel circadian photoreceptor. J Neurosci 2001;21(16):6405–12.
16. Thapan K, Arendt J, Skene DJ. An action spectrum for melatonin suppression: evidence for a novel non-rod, non-cone photoreceptor system in humans. Journal of Physiology 2001;535(Pt 1):261–7.
17. Lewy AJ, Sack RL. The dim light melatonin onset as a marker for circadian phase position. Chronobiol Int 1989;6(1):93–102.
18. Lewy AJ, Wehr TA, Goodwin FK, et al. Light suppresses melatonin secretion in humans. Science 1980;210(4475):1267–9.
19. Hughes RJ, Badia P. Sleep-promoting and hypothermic effects of daytime melatonin administration in humans. Sleep 1997;20(2):124–31.
20. James SP, Sack DA, Rosenthal NE, et al. Melatonin administration in insomnia. Neuropsychopharmacology 1990;3(1):19–23.
21. Wyatt JK, Dijk D-J, Ritz-De Cecco A, et al. Sleep-facilitating effect of exogenous melatonin in healthy

young men and women is circadian-phase dependent. Sleep 2006;29(5):609–18.

22. Lewy AJ, Ahmed S, Jackson JML, et al. Melatonin shifts human circadian rhythms according to a phase-response curve. Chronobiol Int 1992;9(5):380–92.

23. Morganthaler TI, Lee-Chiong T, Alessi C, et al. Practice parameters for the clinical evaluation and treatment of circadian rhythm sleep disorders. Sleep 2007;30(11):1445–59.

24. Drake CL, Roehrs T, Richards G, et al. Shift work sleep disorder: prevalence and consequences beyond that of symptomatic day workers. Sleep 2004;27(8):1453–62.

25. Eastman CI, Stewart KT, Mahoney MP, et al. Dark goggles and bright light improve circadian rhythm adaptation to night-shift work. Sleep 1994;17(6):535–43.

26. Roden M, Koller M, Pirich K, et al. The circadian melatonin and cortisol secretion pattern in permanent night shift workers. Am J Physiol 1993;265:R261–7.

27. Benhaberou-Brun D, Lambert C, Dumont M. Association between melatonin secretion and daytime sleep complaints in night nurses. Sleep 1999;22(7):877–85.

28. Harma MI, Hakola T, Akerstedt T, et al. Age and adjustment to night work. Occup Enviorn Med 1994;51:568–73.

29. Bonnefond A. Interaction of age with shift-related sleep-wakefulness, sleepiness, performance, and social life. Exp Aging Res 2006;32:185–208.

30. Oginska H, Pokorski J, Oginski A. Gender, ageing, and shiftwork intolerance. Ergonomics 1993;36:161–8.

31. Schweitzer PK, Randazzo AC, Stone K, et al. Laboratory and field studies of naps and caffeine as practical countermeasures for sleep-wake problems associated with night work. Sleep 2006;29(1):39–50.

32. Garbarino S, Mascialino B, Penco MA, et al. Professional shift-work drivers who adopt prophylactic naps can reduce the risk of car accidents during night work. Sleep 2004;27(7):1295–302.

33. Sharkey KM, Fogg LF, Eastman CI. Effects of melatonin administration on daytime sleep after simulated night shift work. J Sleep Res 2001;10:181–92.

34. Porcu S, Bellatreccia A, Ferrara M, et al. Performance, ability to stay awake, and tendency to fall asleep during the night after a diurnal sleep with temazepam or placebo. Sleep 1997;20(7):535–41.

35. Walsh JK, Muehlbach MJ, Schweitzer PK. Acute administration of triazolam for the daytime sleep of rotating shift workers. Sleep 1984;7(3):223–9.

36. Czeisler CA, Walsh JK, Roth T, et al. Modafinil for excessive sleepiness associated with shift-work sleep disorder. N Engl J Med 2005;353:476–86.

37. Sharkey KM, Eastman CI. Melatonin phase shifts human circadian rhythms in a placebo-controlled stimulated night-work study. Am J Physiol 2002;282:R454–63.

38. James FO, Walker CD, Bolvin DB. Controlled exposure to light and darkness realigns the salivary cortisol rhythm in night shift workers. Chronobiol Int 2004;21(6):961–72.

39. Eastman CI, Liu L, Fogg LF. Circadian rhythm adaptation to simulated night shift work: effect of nocturnal bright-light duration. Sleep 1995;18(6):399–407.

40. Smith MR, Eastman CI. Night shift performance is improved by a compromise circadian phase position: study 3. Circadian phase after 7 nights with an intervening weekend off. Sleep 2008;31(12):1639–45.

41. American Academy of Sleep Medicine. International classification of sleep disorders, 2nd edition: diagnostic and coding manual. Westchester (IL): American Academy Sleep Medicine; 2005.

42. Arendt J. Managing jet lag: some of the problems and possible new solutions. Sleep Med Rev 2009;13(4):247–8.

43. Lowden A, Akerstedt T. Retaining home-based sleep hours to prevent jet lag in connection with a westward flight across nine time zones. Chronobiol Int 1998;15(4):365–76.

44. Eastman CI, Gazda CJ, Burgess HJ, et al. Advancing circadian rhythms before eastward flight: a strategy to prevent or reduce jet lag. Sleep 2005;28(1):33–44.

45. Boulos Z, Macchi MM, Sturchler MP, et al. Light visor treatment for jet lag after westward travel across six time zones. Aviat Space Environ Med 2002;73(10):953–63.

46. Peirard C, Beaumont M, Enslen M, et al. Resynchronization of hormonal rhythms after an eastbound flight in human: effects of slow-release caffeine and melatonin. Eur J Appl Physiol 2001;85:144–50.

47. Suhner A, Sclagenhauf P, Johnson R, et al. Comparative study to determine the optimal dosage form for the alleviation of jet lag. Chronobiol Int 1998;15(6):655–66.

48. Jamieson AO, Zammit GK, Rosenberg RS, et al. Zolpidem reduces the sleep disturbance of jet lag. Sleep Med 2001;2:423–30.

49. Buxton OM, Copinschi G, Onderbergern AV, et al. A benzodiazepine hypnotic facilitates adaptation of circadian rhythms and sleep-wake homeostatis to an eight hour delay shift simulating westward jet lag. Sleep 2000;23(7):1–13.

50. Beaumont M, Batejat D, Peirar C, et al. Caffeine or melatonin effects on sleep and sleepiness after rapid eastward transmeridian travel. J Appl Physiol 2003;96:50–8.

51. Weitzman ED, Czeisler CA, Coleman RM, et al. Delayed sleep phase syndrome: a chronobiological

disorder with sleep- onset insomnia. Arch Gen Psychiatry 1981;38(7):737–46.

52. Carskadon MA, Wolfson AR, Acebo C, et al. Adolescent sleep patterns, circadian timing, and sleepiness at a transition to early school days. Sleep 1998;21(8):871–81.

53. Czeisler CA, Richardson GS, Coleman RM, et al. Chronotherapy: resetting the circadian clocks of patients with delayed sleep phase insomnia. Sleep 1981;4(1):1–21.

54. Wyatt JK. Delayed sleep phase syndrome: pathophysiology and treatment options. Sleep 2004; 27(6):1195–203.

55. Burgess HJ, Savic N, Sletten T, et al. The relationship between the dim light melatonin onset and sleep on a regular schedule in young healthy adults. Behav Sleep Med 2003;1(2):102–14.

56. Wyatt JK, Stepanski EJ, Kirkby J. Circadian phase in delayed sleep phase syndrome: predictors and temporal stability across multiple assessments. Sleep 2006;29(8):1075–80.

57. Wyatt JK. Circadian rhythm sleep disorders in children and adolescents. Sleep Med Clin 2007;2:387–96.

58. Dahlitz M, Alvarez B, Vignau J, et al. Delayed sleep phase syndrome response to melatonin. Lancet 1991;337(8750):1121–4.

59. Nagtegaal JE, Kerkhof GA, Smits MG, et al. Delayed sleep phase syndrome: a placebo-controlled crossover study on the effects of melatonin administered five hours before the individual dim light melatonin onset. J Sleep Res 1998;7(2):135–43.

60. Kayumov L, Brown G, Jindal R, et al. A randomized, double-blind, placebo-controlled crossover study of the effect of exogenous melatonin on delayed sleep phase syndrome. Psychosom Med 2001;63(1):40–8.

61. Reid KJ, Chang AM, Dubocovich ML, et al. Familial advanced sleep phase syndrome. Arch Neurol 2001;58(7):1089–94.

62. Toh KL, Jones CR, He Y, et al. An hPer2 phosphorylation site mutation in familial advanced sleep phase syndrome. Science 2001;291(5506):1040–3.

63. Moldofsky H, Musisi S, Phillipson EA. Treatment of a case of advanced sleep phase syndrome by phase advance chronotherapy. Sleep 1986;9(1):61–5.

64. Czeisler CA, Duffy JF, Shanahan TL, et al. Stability, precision, and near-24-hours period of the human circadian pacemaker. Science 1999;284:2177–81.

65. Bolvin DB, James FO, Santo JB, et al. Non-24-hour sleep-wake syndrome following a car accident. Neurology 2003;60:1841–3.

66. Sack RL, Auckley D, Auger RR, et al. Circadian rhythm sleep disorders: part II, advanced sleep

phase disorder, delayed sleep phase disorder, free-running disorder, and irregular sleep-wake rhythm. Sleep 2007;30(11):1484–501.

67. Sack RL, Brandes RW, Kendall AR, et al. Entrainment of free-running circadian rhythms by melatonin in blind people. N Engl J Med 2000;343(15):1070–7.

68. Lewy AJ, Emens JS, Lefler BJ, et al. Melatonin entrains free-running blind people according to a physiological dose-response curve. Chronobiol Int 2005;22(6):1093–106.

69. Hack LM, Lockley SW, Arendt J, et al. The effects of low-dose 0.5 mg melatonin on the free-running circadian rhythms of blind subjects. J Biol Rhythms 2003;18(5):420–9.

70. Lewy AJ, Emens JS, Bernnert RA, et al. Eventual entrainment of the human circadian pacemaker by melatonin is independent of the circadian phase of treatment indication: clinical implications. J Biol Rhythms 2004;19(1):68–75.

71. Ancoli-Isreal S, Martin JL, Kripke DF, et al. Effect of light treatment on sleep and circadian rhythms in demented nursing home patients. J Am Geriatr Soc 2002;50:282–9.

72. Martin JL, Marler MR, Harker JO, et al. A multicomponent nonpharmacological intervention improves activity rhythms among nursing home residents with disrupted sleep-wake patterns. J Gerontol A Biol Sci Med Sci 2007;62(1):67–72.

73. Singer C, Tractenberg RE, Kaye J, et al. A multicenter, placebo-controlled trial of melatonin for sleep disturbance in Alzheimer's disease. Sleep 2003; 26(7):893–901.

74. Riemersma-van der Lek RF, Swaab DF, Twisk J, et al. Effect of bright light and melatonin on cognitive and noncognitive function in elderly residents of group care facilities. JAMA 2008;299(22):2642–55.

75. Morris M, Lack L, Dawson D. Sleep-onset insomniacs have delayed temperature rhythms. Sleep 1990;13(1):1–14.

76. Lack LC, Mercer JD, Wright H. Circadian rhythms of early morning awakening insomniacs. J Sleep Res 1996;5(4):211–9.

77. Lack LC, Wright HR. Treating chronobiological components of chronic insomnia. Sleep Med 2007; 8(6):637–44.

78. Hamet P, Tremblay J. Genetics of the sleep-wake cycle and its disorders. Metabolism 2006;55(10 Suppl 2):S7–12.

79. Sack RL, Auckley D, Auger RR, et al. Circadian rhythm sleep disorders: part I, basic principles, shift work and jet lag disorders. Sleep 2007;30(11): 1460–83.

Correlates and Treatments of Nightmares in Adults

Brant P. Hasler, PhD[a], Anne Germain, PhD[b],*

KEYWORDS

- Nightmares • Sleep • Posttraumatic stress disorder
- Pharmacology • Cognitive-behavioral treatments

This article presents the definition of nightmares and diagnostic features, followed by a discussion on the prevalence and frequency of nightmares and related methodological issues. The potential etiologic factors of nightmares, associated features, and available pharmacologic and cognitive-behavioral treatment strategies are reviewed.

Current diagnostic classifications define nightmares as frightening dreams that awaken the sleeper. However, fear is not the only emotion reported in nightmares; and the importance of the awakening criterion for functional and sleep impairments associated with nightmares has been debated in the literature. These points are briefly summarized here. In this article, the term *nightmare* is broadly used to refer to disturbed dreaming that may or may not be accompanied by an awakening, and that is associated with clinically meaningful levels of daytime distress, functional impairments, or sleep disruption.

In reviewing available data on nightmare prevalence and frequency estimates, the need for more unified methodological approaches and longitudinal designs in future studies is highlighted. Although the literature is limited on the etiology of nightmares that occur outside the context of stress or traumatic responses, this article presents hypotheses previously suggested on the correlates and potential underlying mechanisms of nightmares. Selected associated features of nightmares (ie, psychopathology and sleep disturbances) are presented, and available and promising treatment strategies are described. Some pharmacologic and cognitive-behavioral treatments of nightmares have been shown to effectively reduce and eliminate nightmares, but few rigorous, randomized controlled clinical trials have been conducted. Finally, future directions for methodological consideration, research investigations, and clinical practice are offered.

DEFINITION

The Diagnostic and Statistical Manual of Mental Disorders, fourth edition, text revision (DSM-IV-TR)[1] and the International Classification of Sleep Disorders, second edition (ICSD-II)[2] converge on defining nightmares as "intensely disturbing dreams that awaken the dreamer to a fully conscious state and generally occur in the latter half of the sleep period." However, these diagnostic classifications also differ on 2 key points. Firstly, they differ on whether nightmare-associated emotions are limited to fear and anxiety (DSM-IV-TR) or can include all dysphoric emotions, such as anger or despair (ICSD-II). Secondly, only the DSM-IV-TR specifies a criterion that the nightmare or resulting sleep disturbance is associated with significant distress or impairment in waking functioning.

This work was supported by the Department of Defense Congressionally Directed Medical Research Program (PR054093-W81XWH-06-1-0257 and PT073961-W81XWH-07) and the National Institutes of Health (MH083035).
[a] Department of Psychiatry, University of Pittsburgh School of Medicine, 3811 O'Hara Street, Pittsburgh, PA 15213, USA
[b] Department of Psychiatry, University of Pittsburgh School of Medicine, 3811 O'Hara Street, Room E-1124, Pittsburgh, PA 15213, USA
* Corresponding author.
E-mail address: germaina@upmc.edu (A. Germain).

Sleep Med Clin 4 (2009) 507–517
doi:10.1016/j.jsmc.2009.07.012
1556-407X/09/$ – see front matter © 2009 Elsevier Inc. All rights reserved.

The expansion of nightmare-associated emotions beyond fear and anxiety is well recognized in the literature, although fear is the most commonly reported emotion in nightmares.[3] In contrast, the absence of a distress criterion in the ICSD-II has been criticized, because of evidence that distress is more important than frequency in determining whether nightmares are associated with negative outcomes, including sleep disturbance, psychopathology, or health behavior problems.[4]

The awakening criterion has stimulated significant controversy in the field. Historically, distressing dreams that do not lead to an immediate awakening (at least one that is remembered by the dreamer) have been labeled as bad dreams.[5] Theorists have suggested that dreaming serves an extinction function, and that the awakenings associated with nightmares, but not bad dreams, disrupts this extinction process.[4,6] Consequently, many studies dichotomize nightmares and bad dreams as distinct phenomena. However, evidence concerning the importance of awakening to associated distress or psychopathology remains mixed and raises questions about the clinical usefulness of this distinction. Specifically, available treatments to reduce unpleasant dreams usually focus on the extinction of distressing content, rather than on the extinction of these associated awakenings.

Some have argued that all dysphoric dreams fall on a continuum; in this view, nightmares are more intense than bad dreams, both being versions of the same basic phenomenon. Others support the view that the distinction between nightmares and bad dreams relates to underlying differences in the intensity of the emotional content.[7] However, findings from studies that have investigated differences in dream content intensity between nightmares and bad dreams show small differences between the 2 phenomena. For example, Blagrove and Haywood[8] reported that dreams judged to have caused awakenings were rated as more unpleasant (in line with nightmares as more intense versions of bad dreams). However, the statistically significant differences in emotion intensity ratings were less than 0.3 on a 7-point scale. A similarly small difference (approximately 0.7 on a 9-point scale) in ratings of emotional intensity in nightmares compared with bad dreams was also reported by Zadra and colleagues.[9] These small differences in dream intensity between nightmares and bad dreams suggest that dream intensity may not be the primary mechanism that distinguishes nightmares from bad dreams.

The reliability of patients' nocturnal awakening memories is another important, though minimally considered, aspect of the awakening criterion's clinical significance in defining nightmares. It is possible that bad dreams lead to much shorter awakenings, leading to amnesia of the arousal. For instance, awakenings less than 3 minutes in duration are often associated with retrograde and anterograde amnesia.[10] Blagrove and Haywood[8] attempted to address this concern by assessing the dreamers' subjective certainty about whether their disturbing dreams woke them up, and they found that participants were generally confident making this decision and particularly so when dreams were very unpleasant. Nevertheless, the lack of objective measures to accurately evaluate the duration of these awakenings makes it difficult to ascertain that bad dreams associated with an awakening are less subject to memory biases.

As indicated earlier, there is divergence between the diagnostic classifications of nightmare distress. Some have argued that nightmare-related distress is more clinically relevant than nightmare frequency to daytime functioning and psychopathology.[4] From this perspective, nightmares are viewed as a manifestation of the cross-state continuity of distress from waking to sleeping. In support of this assertion, distress is only weakly related to nightmare frequency,[11] but it may be more robustly associated with sleep disturbance[12] and measures of psychopathology[13,14] than with frequency. However, assessments of nightmare distress are vastly underrepresented in the literature,[4] being limited to 1 validated scale, the Nightmare Distress Scale,[11] which may potentially confound nightmare distress with nightmare frequency.[15] Again, longitudinal studies with reliable frequency and distress measures are necessary to fully evaluate the clinical significance of nightmare distress.

Neither classification system includes a criterion for the duration of the nightmare problem, perhaps because the cause of distressing nightmares is often undetermined, or because the clinical meaningfulness of duration of the nightmare problem has not yet been assessed empirically.

Nightmares should not be confused with other distressing nocturnal phenomena. Nightmares are most readily distinguished from other similarly distressing nocturnal events by the extent of mental content, the confusion or disorientation upon awakening, and the presence or absence of memory of the event on the following morning. Sleep recordings show that these distressing nocturnal episodes generally occur in different sleep stages. The particular treatments that are effective for each category of event also vary.

Sleep terrors are associated with intense autonomic arousal. They can begin with a piercing scream, but they are paradoxically associated with difficulty in awakening the sleeper from the episode and in the sleeper returning to deep sleep after the episode.[2] In contrast, there is little confusion or disorientation upon awakening from nightmares, and episodes are vividly recalled the following morning. For sleep terrors, if the sleeper has any recall of the event, recollections the next morning are, at best, vague or fragmented descriptions of frightening images.[16] Although nightmares primarily originate in rapid eye movement (REM) sleep, sleep terrors occur in non-REM sleep, specifically the slow-wave sleep of stages 3 and 4.

In contrast to nightmares and sleep terrors, nocturnal panic attacks often occur in the first few hours of the night during the transition from light (stage 2) sleep to deep (stage 3) sleep. Intense arousal is inherent in nocturnal panic attacks, leading to abrupt and complete awakening from sleep in a state of panic, without an obvious trigger and usually without screaming; the panic attacks are associated with a difficulty in returning to sleep.[17] Complicating differential diagnosis is the co-occurrence that has been documented between these parasomnias, such as an association between monthly nightmares and an increased incidence of night terrors.[19] Although sleep terrors and nocturnal panic attacks share a common predisposing condition—sleep deprivation leads to an increased incidence of both[17,18]—the existing evidence suggests that nightmares lead to sleep disturbance rather than the reverse (see later discussion on association with sleep disturbance).

PREVALENCE AND FREQUENCY

Nightmares are most prevalent during childhood and young adulthood and decline thereafter.[4] However, prevalence estimates in the general population in all age ranges vary and overlap substantially. From childhood through to early adolescence, between 5% and 50% of children have nightmares, with the prevalence of nightmare "problems" generally falling into the 20% to 40% range. In comparison, up to 85% of adults report at least 1 nightmare within the previous year, 8% to 29% report monthly nightmares, and 2% to 6% report weekly nightmares.[19–21] The estimates of weekly prevalence of nightmares have proved consistent across cultures.[12,20–22] Similarly robust are findings of a lower prevalence of nightmares among the elderly, who report at levels 20% to 50% of that of young adults.[23–25]

The variability in estimates is due, in part, to differences in the criteria used, the definition of nightmares, the time frame of assessments, the emphasis on distress or nightmares as a "problem" across studies, and the type of informants (eg, patients, primary care physicians, parents). In studies of children, the information, generally gathered from mothers, may show underestimation in the prevalence of nightmares and may be confounded by the occurrence of other common childhood parasomnias, such as sleep terrors. Nightmare prevalence estimates are derived nearly entirely from cross-sectional data.

Sex differences in nightmare prevalence are one of the most consistent findings in the literature,[26] with a higher percentage of women reporting nightmares; unacknowledged exceptions do exist.[27] Researchers have offered various explanations that are not mutually exclusive for this difference: (1) self-report biases in women, (2) greater vulnerability to risk factors including abuse in women, (3) anxiety and mood disorders in women, (4) sex differences in coping styles, and (5) biologic differences in emotion processing.[4,11,28–30] Together, these findings highlight the need for conducting longitudinal studies using established diagnostic definitions, an important future step to establishing prevalence rates over the life span. Longitudinal studies would also provide new information on the potential modulators (eg, sex, coping styles, biologic factors) that may contribute to enhanced vulnerability or resilience to chronic nightmares. Although the developmental trajectory remains to be clarified, all estimates to date indicate that nightmares are a prevalent problem, underscoring the need for appropriate clinical identification, assessment, and treatment.

Data concerning the frequency of nightmares are also characterized by substantial variability, mostly because of differences in the assessment methods used across studies. Common methods to assess nightmare frequency are prospective nightmare logs or retrospective estimates of the number of nightmares that occurred over a predetermined period of time (usually 1 month to 1 year). Daily dream/nightmare logs that are completed on awakening in the morning can be a simple checklist or a more extensive dream diary used to record nightmare narratives.

Numerous studies have assessed nightmare frequency, using retrospective or prospective measures. The differences between retrospective and prospective methods affect frequency estimates. Specifically, retrospective estimates have yielded frequency estimates ranging from less than once per year to once per month,[27] whereas prospective measures have consistently provided higher nightmare frequency estimates, particularly when compared with 1-year retrospective nightmare frequency measures.[27] Studies that have compared both assessment methods have reported that retrospective questionnaires underestimate nightmare frequency by a factor of 2.5 to 10.[7,13,31] Many of these studies have been conducted with undergraduates who are in their first semester of college, a time of social and emotional upheaval for many. The latter method may provide overestimates of nightmare frequency in noncollege populations. Differences in frequency estimates that are derived from retrospective and prospective measures are generally interpreted as indicating that retrospective measures underestimate nightmare prevalence. Monitoring of nightmares could potentially increase or decrease their frequency. Nevertheless, prospective nightmare measures have been recommended as the gold standard.[4,27]

The most sophisticated study on the topic evaluated the comparability of frequency estimates for nightmares and bad dreams, when assessed by 1-year and 1-month retrospective measures and by narrative and checklist prospective measures.[28] Including both types of prospective measures was intended to address the question of whether intensive monitoring (with narrative logs) results in higher frequencies than a less demanding approach (using checklist logs). In contrast to predictions, narrative logs produced lower nightmare frequency estimates than checklist logs that did not significantly differ from the 1-month retrospective measure and were possibly higher than the 1-year retrospective measure. When examining bad dreams, both prospective measures produced higher estimates than the retrospective measures, but the prospective and retrospective estimates for bad dreams were not significantly different from one another.

Attempts to assess nightmares via polysomnographic (PSG) recordings in the laboratory have been difficult, because nightmares tend to occur less frequently under these conditions.[32] Even posttraumatic nightmares (see the etiology section) have a low incidence (1%–10% vs up to 85% of nights) in the sleep laboratory relative to naturalistic conditions.[33,34] A pilot study, using ambulatory PSG recording, suggested that the presence of the PSG, rather than the setting, is the crucial factor in the lower observed frequency. In a sample of 12 inpatients in a psychiatric clinic, Spoormaker and colleagues (unpublished data, 2004) found a significantly lower nightmare incidence (8% vs 34.5%) using ambulatory PSG over two 24-hour recordings compared with daily logs over 7 days. However, the generalizability of this study outside of inpatient settings is uncertain, and PSG studies of nightmares remain too few to draw firm conclusions.

ETIOLOGY

Nightmares are associated with a range of psychiatric symptoms, full-blown psychiatric disorders such as posttraumatic stress disorder (PTSD), and sleep disturbances. Although some psychiatric, personality, sleep, and biologic correlates of nightmares have been described, most extant studies are cross-sectional, precluding conclusive determination of causality and etiology. Although longitudinal studies are awaited, findings suggest that traumatic events, waking psychological distress, or sleep disturbance may contribute to the onset and maintenance of nightmares. Some theories that have been offered on the etiology of nightmares are briefly summarized in the following sections.

Idiopathic Versus Posttraumatic Nightmares

An important etiologic distinction made to date is the difference between idiopathic and posttraumatic nightmares. Idiopathic nightmares refer to nightmares with unknown cause that are unrelated to a specific traumatic event or PTSD. Posttraumatic nightmares refer to dreaming disturbances that are part of the stress reaction following exposure to a traumatic event, either during the acute stress response or over the course of PTSD. Nightmares are a core feature of PTSD, with up to 90% of individuals with PTSD reporting disturbing dreams with some degree of resemblance to the actual traumatic event. Nightmares may occur as frequently as 6 nights a week in individuals with PTSD,[35] and they may continue for up to 40 to 50 years after the original trauma.[36,37]

The distinction between idiopathic and posttraumatic nightmares has not been firmly established in most of the literature available to date. Given the emerging evidence that persistent nightmares in the wake of a traumatic incident predict later posttraumatic symptoms,[38] making a differential diagnosis may be particularly important for early intervention to ward off PTSD. In addition, these 2 types of nightmares may differ in their associated sleep disturbance (see the following section on associated features) and in the timing of their occurrence during the sleep period. Further research is necessary to characterize fully the etiology, phenomenology, trajectory, and functional consequences of these ostensibly different categories of nightmares.

Nightmares Due to Thin Psychological Boundaries?

Hartmann and colleagues[39,40] proposed the constructs of "thin" and "thick" psychological boundaries to characterize chronic (idiopathic) nightmare sufferers versus those with little or no nightmare experience. Frequent nightmare sufferers tend to be more emotionally sensitive, open, and reactive to elements of their internal and external environments. Individuals with no nightmares, on the other hand, tend to be less reactive to internal and external influences. Several subsequent studies have reported positive findings on the relationship between clinical features of schizophrenia-spectrum disorders and nightmare frequency.[41,42]

Disturbance in a Generally Adaptive Process?

A prevailing assumption is that dreaming is adaptive,[43] and thus nightmares may constitute an anomaly in the adaptive process, also described as "a failed dream."[43] However, the evidence in support of this hypothesis is scant. Flanagan[44] suggested that sleeping, not dreaming per se, is an adaptive process. In contrast, it has also been suggested that nightmares themselves might be the adaptive process. For example, Picchioni and colleagues[45] reported that nightmares are positively associated with waking attempts to cope with stress, suggesting that nightmares may serve a beneficial function. However, the absence of a direct assessment of successful outcomes of coping in this study makes it difficult, at best, to relate nightmares to functional outcomes. The potential specific role of nightmares in adapting to waking stressors and the specific conditions and mechanisms that contribute to successful or unsuccessful adaptation to stress through dreaming disturbances remain to be investigated.

Genetic Predisposition to Nightmares?

A single study has investigated the possible genetic contributions to nightmares. Using data from the Finnish Twin Cohort study, a nationwide questionnaire study that included 1298 monozygotic and 2419 dizygotic twins aged 33 to 60 years, Hublin and colleagues[46] found a genetic influence on nightmares that differed slightly between childhood and adult nightmares. Genetic effects accounted for an estimated 45% of the phenotypic variance in childhood and for an estimated 37% in adulthood. The odds ratios for associated psychiatric disorders also varied by age group; children most frequently experiencing nightmares were 3.67 times more likely to have

a psychiatric disorder than those who never experienced nightmares, whereas adults with frequent nightmares had an odds ratio of 5.87. This suggests that nightmares during adulthood have a strong association with psychopathology. Again, these findings highlight the need for longitudinal studies to rigorously assess the moderators and predictors of the trajectory of nightmares and their clinical outcomes over time.

ASSOCIATED FEATURES

Nightmares are associated with sleep disturbance, but longitudinal studies are required to ascertain the directionality of this association. Sleep disruption as a consequence of nightmares is implicit in their definition, given the criterion of awakening to a fully conscious state. Empirical data bear this out, because frequent nightmares are associated with increased reports of sleep-onset and sleep-maintenance insomnia, more frequent nocturnal awakenings, and worse sleep quality.[21,26,47] Breathing problems (eg, asthma) and snoring are linked to idiopathic nightmares,[48] whereas an association with full-blown sleep apnea has been reported in posttraumatic nightmares.[49] Although longitudinal data are limited, 1 prospective study found that posttraumatic nightmares occurring 3 months after a motor vehicle accident were associated with current sleep-onset and sleep-maintenance problems and predicted sleep maintenance difficulties after 1 year.[50]

Objective indices of sleep disruption, as measured by PSG, suggest that idiopathic and posttraumatic nightmares have been associated with different effects on sleep. Although both nightmare types share an association with elevated numbers of periodic limb movements, posttraumatic nightmares are related to longer and more frequent awakenings[51] this relationship is a possible consequence of a lowered arousal threshold during sleep in PTSD,[52] although the evidence on this is mixed.[53] In addition, posttraumatic nightmares may occur earlier in the night than idiopathic nightmares,[54] but this was not replicated in a recent study.[51] Individuals with idiopathic and posttraumatic nightmares also did not differ on total sleeping time, sleep onset latency, slow-wave sleep, number of microarousals, or any of several REM-related parameters.[51]

Waking Disturbance and Psychopathology

Perhaps most relevant to clinical discussions of nightmares is their relationship to waking disturbance or psychopathology. In general, nightmares appear to be linked to a greater incidence of mental complaints in healthy and clinical populations.

An important part of the nightmare literature has focused on the relationships between personality traits and nightmare frequency. The association between nightmares and anxiety has been most widely investigated. Modest associations between different measures of trait and state anxiety (eg, death anxiety scales, ego strength scales, manifest anxiety scales, and nightmare frequency assessed retrospectively) have been reported.[7,31,55–60] However, the association between nightmare frequency and anxiety is weakened when assessed with daily nightmare logs instead of retrospective questionnaires.[7,31] Nightmare-related distress, rather than nightmare frequency, seems to be more strongly related to anxiety.[13,14,31] In general, studies have consistently reported mild-to-moderate correlations between nightmare frequency and distress and general symptoms of anxiety, mood, somatization, and hostility.[7,13]

As mentioned previously, nightmares are a core feature of PTSD and may be implicated in the pathophysiology of the disorder. In addition, a pretrauma history of nightmares (possibly idiopathic nightmares) predicts the severity of PTSD.[61] PTSD-related nightmares are often resistant to first-line PTSD treatments, but they respond well to pharmacologic and cognitive-behavioral treatments (see the following section).

Nightmares have also been linked to suicidality. Cross-sectional studies have demonstrated an association between nightmares and both suicidal ideation[62,63] and actual suicide attempts[63]; nightmares were the only sleep variable associated with suicidality in a sample of suicide attempters, after controlling for Axis I disorders (including PTSD) and symptom intensity.[64] One prospective study found that nightmare frequency, per 1-month retrospective self-reports, was related to the risk of suicide, with a 57% higher risk among those reporting occasional nightmares and a 105% higher risk among those reporting frequent nightmares.[65] Although all of these studies were statistically controlled for possible confounding factors such as sex, depression, and insomnia, only 1 study was controlled for PTSD.[65] This is an important limitation because PTSD is also linked to suicidality.[66]

TREATMENTS

Most available pharmacologic and psychological literature on the treatments of nightmares is derived from case reports and clinical trials targeting nightmares occurring in the context of PTSD.[67]

Although very few studies have evaluated the effects of these treatments on nightmares of unspecified causes, there is little evidence suggesting that different outcomes would be observed.

Pharmacologic Treatments of Nightmares

By far, the most common treatments of nightmares involve pharmacotherapy. There have been numerous open-label trials, with various agents for the treatment of nightmares. To date, the most effective of available treatments of PTSD-related nightmares is prazosin. Prazosin is an alpha1-noradrenergic antagonist, which is used nightly and associated with clinically meaningful improvements in nightmares, accompanied by reductions in other sleep disturbances and daytime PTSD symptoms. Placebo-controlled studies of prazosin have consistently reported positive effects on nightmares in military and civilian samples.[68–73] However, nightmares recur with prazosin discontinuation.

Several other pharmacologic approaches have also been used with mixed results. Tricyclic antidepressants and monoamine oxidase inhibitors were among the first agents tested for nightmares because of the suppressant effects on REM sleep, but side effects and contraindications limit their clinical use. Selective serotonin reuptake inhibitors (SSRIs), such as paroxetine, sertraline, and fluoxetine, are Food and Drug Administration (FDA)-approved as first-line recommended PTSD treatments, but their efficacy for nightmares is inconsistent across clinical trials. Trazodone and nefazodone, 2 serotonin-potentiating non-SSRI agents, have been associated with moderate-to-large beneficial effects on nightmares in open-label and controlled trials.[74–77]

Cyproheptadine, an antihistamine with serotonin receptor antagonist properties, has not been found effective for reducing PTSD-related nightmares in a randomized controlled study.[78,79] Similarly, guanfacine, an alpha2-adrenergic receptor agonist, was not found to be effective in reducing nightmares in patients with PTSD in 2 randomized controlled trials.[80,81]

Benzodiazepines are often prescribed to patients with PTSD, possibly as agents to manage sleep disturbances,[82–84] despite lack of evidence as to their effectiveness. Two randomized controlled trials found no support for the efficacy of benzodiazepines as treatment for nightmares in PTSD.[85,86] Although benzodiazepines can reduce nightmares associated with REM sleep behavior disorder,[87] their efficacy in alleviating nightmares from other causes is unknown.

Atypical antipsychotic drugs have also been tested in the treatment of PTSD-related nightmares in military veterans with PTSD. Studies conducted with risperidone, olanzapine and quetiapine have yielded mixed results.[88–90] Zolpidem (nonbenzodiazepine imidazopyridine[91]), gabapentin,[92] and mirtazapine[93] show some promise but await more rigorous evaluation.

Cognitive-behavioral Treatments of Nightmares

Cognitive-behavioral treatments of nightmares have focused on 2 general approaches. The first approach is derived from the literature and treatment methods for anxiety disorders. Specifically, desensitization is implemented with the use of repeated exposure to the fearful nightmare content and with habituation to the emotional response triggered by nightmare imagery. Three controlled studies[94–96] have assessed the efficacy of desensitization in reducing nightmare frequency, nightmare intensity, psychological symptoms (eg, anxiety, fear, depression, hostility, and general psychological distress), and sleep complaints. Although desensitization studies did not specify the cause of nightmares in patients enrolled in these trials, all have consistently reported improvements in nightmares and also in sleep disturbances and daytime symptoms of anxiety.[96] Desensitization studies that used nightmare recording or relaxation[94] as control treatment conditions also noted posttreatment improvements in nightmares. Improvements in nightmares were also found over the periods of follow-up assessments for patients randomized to the desensitization groups, which ranged from 1 to 7 months after treatment. Together, these studies suggest that desensitization can be an effective treatment for nightmares. The efficacy of desensitization for PTSD nightmares, however, has not yet been evaluated.

The second behavioral approach for the treatment of nightmares is imagery rehearsal therapy (IRT) and its variants. The goal of IRT is to decrease the frequency or intensity of nightmares by (1) repeatedly rehearsing (practicing) new dream scenarios during wakefulness, and (2) revising compensatory cognitions and behaviors that perpetuate nightmares. In comparison to desensitization, IRT does not involve exposure to distressing material. IRT emphasizes rescripting the original nightmare scenarios into new, nondistressing dream scenarios that are then mentally rehearsed several times per day. Exposure to the original nightmare scenarios is discouraged, and repeated sessions of mental rehearsal of new dream scenarios are implemented daily, 1 to 3 times per day. Generally, the instructions on how to create new dream scenarios are minimal. Patients may choose to alter the ending of the dream, to change specific elements of the original content (eg, characters, nature of interpersonal and social interactions), or to create an entirely new dream scenario.

A series of controlled studies showed that rescripting and mentally rehearsing new dream scenarios alone, with limited to no exposure to the distressing dream content or intense emotional reactions, can significantly alleviate idiopathic nightmares and PTSD-related nightmares, in patients reporting at least 1 nightmare per week[98] and sleep complaints.[47,98] A large controlled trial, involving sexual assault survivors with trauma-related nightmares, replicated these findings when compared with women assigned to a wait-list control group, by showing clinically meaningful improvements in nightmare frequency, reduced severity of daytime PTSD symptoms, and improved sleep quality.[99]

A variant of IRT, called Exposure, Relaxation, and Rescripting Therapy (ERRT[100]), has also been associated with long-term improvements in nightmare frequency, depression-symptom severity, PTSD-symptom severity, and sleep quality for trauma-related nightmares, compared with effects observed in a wait-list control group. ERRT is a combination of (1) education about trauma, PTSD, and sleep; (2) exposure to the nightmare content and distressing themes; (3) diaphragmatic breathing and daily progressive muscle relaxation; and (4) rescripting of the nightmare scenario guided by the therapists and other members of the treatment group. Contrary to IRT, ERRT encourages exposure to the distressing nightmare content. Future research is awaited to determine which patients to treat and how much exposure should be given in the treatment of nightmares.

To date, IRT has shown efficacy with PTSD and non-PTSD related nightmares[97,98,101,102] in civilian and military samples.[99,103] However, to fully evaluate and compare the efficacy of different cognitive-behavioral techniques for the treatment of nightmares, more stringent control treatment conditions and direct comparisons between IRT approaches and desensitization or exposure are required.

Other psychological approaches have also been used in the treatment of nightmares. For instance, positive case reports and case series are available in the literature for lucid dreaming,[104] hypnosis,[105] eye movement desensitization and reprocessing,[106] and psychodynamic therapy.[107,108] These approaches await controlled clinical trials to determine efficacy for nightmares and the related impact of sleep disturbances and daytime functional impairments and distress.

SUMMARY

Nightmares, a common experience for most of the general population, are even more prevalent and frequent among clinical populations. This increased prevalence is consistent with converging evidence of their potential clinical significance across diagnostic categories. Accumulating evidence links nightmares to waking distress and psychopathology; prospective studies suggest that nightmares may be a risk factor for PTSD and increased suicidality, offering new venues for prevention and interventions.

Methodological limitations and differences, across studies to date, preclude a more complete understanding of many aspects of this fascinating phenomenon. Thus, more rigorous methods are needed to address numerous areas. Firstly, the variability in assessment methods may have led to imprecise prevalence estimates, and this limits our ability to compare findings across studies. Studies of nightmares under controlled laboratory conditions may provide novel insights into the psychophysiological correlates of these nocturnal events; however, multi-night designs, with larger samples studied under ecologically valid conditions, are required to accurately evaluate the frequency and prevalence of nightmares in the general population and in clinical samples. Such studies would also permit assessments of the relationships between nightmare distress and frequency. Secondly, many questions remain regarding the cause and outcomes of nightmares. Most findings concerning nightmares and waking function are limited to correlations based on cross-sectional observational data. Experimental and longitudinal designs are required to address questions around the relationships between nightmares, sleep disturbance, and psychopathology. Even in the case of posttraumatic nightmares, where a clear event precedes the onset of nightmares, little is known about the biopsychosocial pathways through which the trauma exposure affects dreaming. More randomized controlled studies are necessary (1) to evaluate and compare available and promising treatment strategies and (2) to establish guidelines and algorithms to guide clinicians in the treatment of nightmares. Effective nightmare treatments can be used as probes to test specific hypotheses regarding the psychophysiological mechanisms underlying nightmares.

A small contingent of highly dedicated scientists is responsible for the laudable advancements in the nightmare literature to date. These researchers have also posited some compelling hypotheses that deserve more rigorous testing. Opportunities for novel contributions to and advancement of this important area of clinical investigation await the efforts of the broader research community.

REFERENCES

1. American Psychiatric Association. Diagnostic and statistical manual of mental disorders text revision (DSM-IV-TR). fourth edition. Washington (DC): American Psychiatric Association; 2000

2. American Academy of Sleep Medicine. The international classification of sleep disorders, second edition (ICSD-2): diagnostic and coding manual: Westchester (IL): American Academy of Sleep Medicine; 2005. p. 99.

3. Zadra A, Donderi DC. Affective content and intensity of nightmares and bad dreams. Sleep 2003; 26:A93–4.

4. Levin R, Nielsen TA. Disturbed dreaming, posttraumatic stress disorder, and affect distress: a review and neurocognitive model. Psychol Bull 2007; 133(3):482–528.

5. Halliday G. Direct alteration of a traumatic nightmare. Percept Mot Skills 1982;54(2):413–4.

6. Rothbaum BO, Mellman TA. Dreams and exposure therapy in PTSD. J Trauma Stress 2001;14(3): 481–90.

7. Zadra A, Donderi DC. Nightmares and bad dreams: their prevalence and relationship to well-being. J Abnorm Psychol 2000;109(2):273–81.

8. Blagrove M, Haywood S. Evaluating the awakening criterion in the definition of nightmares: how certain are people in judging whether a nightmare woke them up? J Sleep Res 2006;15(2):117–24.

9. Zadra A, Pilon M, Donderi DC. Variety and intensity of emotions in nightmares and bad dreams. J Nerv Ment Dis 2006;194(4):249–54.

10. Wyatt JK, Bootzin RR, Anthony J, et al. Sleep onset is associated with retrograde and anterograde amnesia. Sleep 1994;17:502–11.

11. Belicki K. Nightmare frequency versus nightmare distress: relations to psychopathology and cognitive style. J Abnorm Psychol 1992;101(3):592–7.

12. Belicki K, Chambers E, Ogilvie RD. Sleep quality and nightmares. Sleep Res 1997;26:637.

13. Blagrove M, Farmer L, Williams E. The relationship of nightmare frequency and nightmare distress to well-being. J Sleep Res 2004;13(2):129–36.

14. Levin R, Fireman G. Nightmare prevalence, nightmare distress, and self-reported psychological disturbance. Sleep 2002;25(2):205–12.

15. Spoormaker VI, Schredl M, van den Bout J. Nightmares: from anxiety symptom to sleep disorder. Sleep Med Rev 2006;10(1):19–31.

16. Mason TB, Pack AI. Sleep terrors in childhood. J Pediatr 2005;147(3):388–92.

17. Craske MG, Isao JC. Assessment and treatment of nocturnal panic attacks. Sleep Med Rev 2005;9(3): 173–84.

18. Ohayon MM, Guilleminault C, Priest RG. Night terrors, sleepwalking, and confusional arousals in the general population: their frequency and relationship to other sleep and mental disorders. J Clin Psychiatry 1999;60(4):268–76; quiz 277.

19. Belicki D, Belicki K. Nightmares in a university population. Sleep Res 1982;11:116.

20. Bixler EO, Kales A, Soldatos CR, et al. Prevalence of sleep disorders in the Los Angeles metropolitan area. Am J Psychiatry 1979;136(10):1257–62.

21. Ohayon MM, Morselli PL, Guilleminault C. Prevalence of nightmares and their relationship to psychopathology and daytime functioning in insomnia subjects. Sleep 1997;20(5):340–8.

22. Fukuda K, Ogilvie RD, Takeuchi T. Recognition of sleep paralysis among normal adults in Canada and in Japan. Psychiatry Clin Neurosci 2000; 54(3):292–3.

23. Nielsen T, Stenstrom P, Levin R. Nightmare frequency as a function of age, gender, and September 11, 2001: findings from an internet questionnaire. Dreaming 2006;16(3):145–58.

24. Partinen M. Epidemiology of sleep disorders. In: Kryger MH, Roth T, Dement WC, editors. Principles and practice of sleep medicine. 2nd edition. Philadelphia: Saunders; 1994. p. 437–52.

25. Salvio MA, Wood JM, Schwartz J, et al. Nightmare prevalence in the healthy elderly. Psychol Aging 1992;7(2):324–5.

26. Levin R. Sleep and dream characteristics of frequent nightmare subjects in a university population. Dreaming 1994;4:127–37.

27. Robert G, Zadra A. Measuring nightmare and bad dream frequency: impact of retrospective and prospective instruments. J Sleep Res 2008;17(2): 132–9.

28. Bradley MM, Codispoti M, Sabatinelli D, et al. Emotion and motivation II: sex differences in picture processing. Emotion 2001;1(3):300–19.

29. Lyubomirsky S, Nolen-Hoeksema S. Effects of self-focused rumination on negative thinking and interpersonal problem solving. J Pers Soc Psychol 1995;69(1):176–90.

30. Stein MB, Walker JR, Hazen AL, et al. Full and partial posttraumatic stress disorder: findings from a community survey. Am J Psychiatry 1997;154(8):1114–9.

31. Wood JM, Bootzin RR. The prevalence of nightmares and their independence from anxiety. J Abnorm Psychol 1990;99(1):64–8.

32. Fisher C, Byrne J, Edwards A, et al. A psychophysiological study of nightmares. J Am Psychoanal Assoc 1970;18(4):747–82.

33. Krakow B, Melendrez D, Johnston L, et al. Sleep-disordered breathing, psychiatric distress, and quality of life impairment in sexual assault survivors. J Nerv Ment Dis 2002;190(7):442–52.

34. Woodward SH, Arsenault NJ, Murray C, et al. Laboratory sleep correlates of nightmare complaint in PTSD inpatients. Biol Psychiatry 2000;48(11):1081–7.

35. Krakow B, Schrader R, Tandberg D, et al. Nightmare frequency in sexual assault survivors with PTSD. J Anxiety Disord 2002;16(2):175–90.

36. Guerrero J, Crocq MA. Sleep disorders in the elderly: depression and post-traumatic stress disorder. J Psychosom Res 1994;38(Suppl 1): 141–50.

37. Kaup BA, Ruskin PE, Nyman G. Significant life events and PTSD in elderly World War II veterans. Am J Geriatr Psychiatry 1994;2:239–43.

38. Foa EB, Riggs DS, Gershuny BS. Arousal, numbing, and intrusion: symptom structure of PTSD following assault. Am J Psychiatry 1995;152(1): 116–20.

39. Hartmann E, Falke R, Russ D, et al. Who has nightmares? Persons with lifelong nightmares compared with vivid dreamers and non-vivid dreamers. Sleep Res 1981;10:171.

40. Hartmann E. The nightmare: the psychology and biology of terrifying dreams. New York: Basic Books; 1984.

41. Hartmann E. Boundaries of dreams, boundaries of dreamers: thin and thick boundaries as a new personality measure. Psychiatr J Univ Ott 1989; 14(4):557–60.

42. Levin R. Nightmares and schizotypy. Psychiatry 1998;61(3):206–16.

43. Nielsen TA, Zadra A. Nightmares and other common dream disturbances. In: Kryger M, Roth N, Dement WC, editors. Principles and practice of sleep medicine. 4th edition. Philadelphia: Elsevier; 2005. p. 926–35.

44. Flanagan O. Dreaming is not an adaptation. Behav Brain Sci 2001;23(6):936–8.

45. Picchioni D, Goeltzenleucher B, Green DN, et al. Nightmares as a coping mechanism for stress. Dreaming 2002;12:155–69.

46. Hublin C, Kaprio J, Partinen M, et al. Nightmares: familial aggregation and association with psychiatric disorders in a nationwide twin cohort. Am J Med Genet 1999;88(4):329–36.

47. Krakow B, Kellner R, Pathak D, et al. Imagery rehearsal treatment for chronic nightmares. Behav Res Ther 1995;33(7):837–43.

48. Klink M, Quan SF. Prevalence of reported sleep disturbances in a general adult population and their relationship to obstructive airways diseases. Chest 1987;91(4):540–6.

49. Krakow B, Melendrez D, Pedersen B, et al. Complex insomnia: insomnia and sleep-disordered

breathing in a consecutive series of crime victims with nightmares and PTSD. Biol Psychiatry 2001; 49(11):948–53.

50. Kobayashi I, Sledjeski EM, Spoonster E, et al. Effects of early nightmares on the development of sleep disturbances in motor vehicle accident victims. J Trauma Stress 2008;21(6):548–55.

51. Germain A, Nielsen TA. Sleep pathophysiology in posttraumatic stress disorder and idiopathic nightmare sufferers. Biol Psychiatry 2003;54(10):1092–8.

52. Ross RJ, Ball WA, Sullivan KA, et al. Sleep disturbance as the hallmark of posttraumatic stress disorder. Am J Psychiatry 1989;146(6):607–707.

53. Lavie P, Katz N, Pillar G, et al. Elevated awaking thresholds during sleep: characteristics of chronic war-related posttraumatic stress disorder patients. Biol Psychiatry 1998;44(10):1060–5.

54. Hartmann E. Who develops PTSD nightmares and who doesn't? In: Barrett D, editor. Trauma and dreams. Cambridge (MA): Harvard University Press; 1996. p. 101–13.

55. Feldman MJ, Hersen M. Attitudes toward death in nightmare subjects. J Abnorm Psychol 1967; 72(5):421–5.

56. Lester D. The fear of death of those who have nightmares. J Psychol 1968;69(2):245–7.

57. Haynes S, Mooney D. Nightmares: etiological, theoretical, and behavioral treatment considerations. Psychol Rec 1975;25:225–36.

58. Cellucci AJ, Lawrence PS. Individual differences in self-reported sleep variable correlations among nightmare sufferers. J Clin Psychol 1978;34(3):721–5.

59. Dunn KK, Barrett D. Characteristics of nightmare subjects and their nightmares. Psychiatr J Univ Ott 1988;13(2):91–3.

60. Levin R, Masling J. Relations of oral imagery to thought disorder in subjects with frequent nightmares. Percept Mot Skills 1995;80(3 Pt 2):1115–20.

61. Mellman TA, David D, Kulick-Bell R, et al. Sleep disturbance and its relationship to psychiatric morbidity after Hurricane Andrew. Am J Psychiatry 1995;152(11):1659–63.

62. Bernert RA, Joiner TE Jr, Cukrowicz KC, et al. Suicidality and sleep disturbances. Sleep 2005;28(9): 1135–41.

63. Liu X. Sleep and adolescent suicidal behavior. Sleep 2004;27(7):1351–8.

64. Sjöström N, Waern M, Hetta J. Nightmares and sleep disturbances in relation to suicidality in suicide attempters. Sleep 2007;30(1):91–5.

65. Tanskanen A, Tuomilehto J, Viinamaki H, et al. Nightmares as predictors of suicide. Sleep 2001; 24(7):844–7.

66. Kotler M, Iancu I, Efroni R, et al. Anger, impulsivity, social support, and suicide risk in patients with posttraumatic stress disorder. J Nerv Ment Dis 2001;189(3):162–7.

67. Maher MJ, Rego SA, Asnis GM. Sleep disturbances in patients with post-traumatic stress disorder: epidemiology, impact and approaches to management. CNS Drugs 2006;20(7):567–90.

68. Peskind ER, Bonner LT, Hoff DJ, et al. Prazosin reduces trauma-related nightmares in older men with chronic posttraumatic stress disorder. J Geriatr Psychiatry Neurol 2003;16(3):165–71.

69. Raskind MA, Dobie DJ, Kanter ED, et al. The alpha1-adrenergic antagonist prazosin ameliorates combat trauma nightmares in veterans with posttraumatic stress disorder: a report of 4 cases. J Clin Psychiatry 2000;61(2):129–33.

70. Raskind MA, Thompson C, Petrie EC, et al. Prazosin reduces nightmares in combat veterans with posttraumatic stress disorder. J Clin Psychiatry 2002;63(7):565–8.

71. Taylor F, Raskind MA. The alpha1-adrenergic antagonist prazosin improves sleep and nightmares in civilian trauma posttraumatic stress disorder. J Clin Psychopharmacol 2002;22(1): 82–5.

72. Raskind MA, Peskind ER, Hoff DJ, et al. A parallel group placebo controlled study of prazosin for trauma nightmares and sleep disturbance in combat veterans with post-traumatic stress disorder. Biol Psychiatry 2007;61(8):928–34.

73. Raskind MA, Peskind ER, Kanter ED, et al. Reduction of nightmares and other PTSD symptoms in combat veterans by prazosin: a placebo-controlled study. Am J Psychiatry 2003;160(2):371–3.

74. Neylan TC, Lenoci M, Maglione ML, et al. The effect of nefazodone on subjective and objective sleep quality in posttraumatic stress disorder. J Clin Psychiatry 2003;64(4):445–50.

75. Gillin JC, Smith-Vaniz A, Schnierow B, et al. An open-label, 12-week clinical and sleep EEG study of nefazodone in chronic combat-related posttraumatic stress disorder. J Clin Psychiatry 2001; 62(10):789–96.

76. Mellman TA, David D, Barza L. Nefazodone treatment and dream reports in chronic PTSD. Depress Anxiety 1999;9(3):146–8.

77. Davidson JR, Weisler RH, Malik ML, et al. Treatment of posttraumatic stress disorder with nefazodone. Int Clin Psychopharmacol 1998;13(3):111–3.

78. Clark RD, Canive JM, Calais LA, et al. Cyproheptadine treatment of nightmares associated with posttraumatic stress disorder. J Clin Psychopharmacol 1999;19(5):486–7.

79. Jacobs-Rebhun S, Schnurr PP, Friedman MJ, et al. Posttraumatic stress disorder and sleep difficulty. Am J Psychiatry 2000;157(9):1525–6.

80. Neylan TC, Lenoci M, Samuelson KW, et al. No improvement of posttraumatic stress disorder symptoms with guanfacine treatment. Am J Psychiatry 2006;163(12):2186–8.

81. Davis LL, Ward C, Rasmusson A, et al. A placebo-controlled trial of guanfacine for the treatment of posttraumatic stress disorder in veterans. Psychopharmacol Bull 2008;41(1):8–18.

82. Mohamed S, Rosenheck R. Pharmacotherapy for older veterans diagnosed with posttraumatic stress disorder in veterans administration. Am J Geriatr Psychiatry 2008;16(10):804–12.

83. Mohamed S, Rosenheck RA. Pharmacotherapy of PTSD in the U.S. department of veterans affairs: diagnostic- and symptom-guided drug selection. J Clin Psychiatry 2008;69(6):959–65.

84. Mellman TA, Clark RE, Peacock WJ. Prescribing patterns for patients with posttraumatic stress disorder. Psychiatr Serv 2003;54(12):1618–21.

85. Cates ME, Bishop MH, Davis LL, et al. Clonazepam for treatment of sleep disturbances associated with combat-related posttraumatic stress disorder. Ann Pharmacother 2004;38(9):1395–9.

86. Braun P, Greenberg D, Dasberg H, et al. Core symptoms of posttraumatic stress disorder unimproved by alprazolam treatment. J Clin Psychiatry 1990;51(6):236–8.

87. Mahowald MW, Schenck CH. REM Sleep Parasomnias. Chapter 75. In: Kryger MH, Roth T, Dement WC, editors. Principles and practices of sleep medicine. 4th Edition. Philadelphia: Elsevier Sauders; 2005. p. 897–916.

88. Ahearn EP, Krohn A, Connor KM, et al. Pharmacologic treatment of posttraumatic stress disorder: a focus on antipsychotic use. Ann Clin Psychiatry 2003;15(3–4):193–201.

89. David D, De Faria L, Mellman TA. Adjunctive risperidone treatment and sleep symptoms in combat veterans with chronic PTSD. Depress Anxiety 2006;23(8):489–91.

90. Leyba CM, Wampler TP. Risperidone in PTSD. Psychiatr Serv 1998;49(2):245–6.

91. Dieperink ME, Drogemuller L. Zolpidem for insomnia related to PTSD. Psychiatr Serv 1999;50(3):421.

92. Hamner MB, Brodrick PS, Labbate LA. Gabapentin in PTSD: a retrospective, clinical series of adjunctive therapy. Ann Clin Psychiatry 2001; 13(3):141–6.

93. Lewis JD. Mirtazapine for PTSD nightmares. Am J Psychiatry 2002;159(11):1948–9.

94. Miller WR, DiPilato M. Treatment of nightmares via relaxation and desensitization: a controlled evaluation. J Consult Clin Psychol 1983;51(6):870–7.

95. Burgess M, Gill M, Marks I. Postal self-exposure treatment of recurrent nightmares. Randomised controlled trial. Br J Psychiatry 1998;172: 257–62.

96. Cellucci AJ, Lawrence PS. The efficacy of systematic desensitization in reducing nightmares. J Behav Ther Exp Psychiatry 1978;9:109–14.

97. Neidhardt EJ, Krakow B, Kellner R, et al. The beneficial effects of one treatment session and recording of nightmares on chronic nightmare sufferers. Sleep 1992;15(5):470–3.

98. Kellner R, Neidhardt J, Krakow B, et al. Changes in chronic nightmares after one session of desensitization or rehearsal instructions. Am J Psychiatry 1992;149(5):659–63.

99. Krakow B, Hollifield M, Johnston L, et al. Imagery rehearsal therapy for chronic nightmares in sexual assault survivors with posttraumatic stress disorder: a randomized controlled trial. JAMA 2001;286(5):537–45.

100. Davis JL, Wright DC. Randomized clinical trial for treatment of chronic nightmares in trauma-exposed adults. J Trauma Stress 2007;20(2): 123–33.

101. Germain A, Shear MK, Hall M, et al. Effects of a brief behavioral treatment for PTSD-related sleep disturbances: a pilot study. Behav Res Ther 2007; 45(3):627–32.

102. Kellner R, Singh G, Irigoyen-Rascon F. Rehearsal in the treatment of recurring nightmares in posttraumatic stress disorders and panic disorder: case histories. Ann Clin Psychiatry 1991;3(1): 67–71.

103. Forbes D, Phelps AJ, McHugh AF, et al. Imagery rehearsal in the treatment of posttraumatic nightmares in Australian veterans with chronic combat-related PTSD: 12-month follow-up data. J Trauma Stress 2003;16(5):509–13.

104. Zadra AL, Pihl RO. Lucid dreaming as a treatment for recurrent nightmares. Psychother Psychosom 1997;66(1):50–5.

105. Kingsbury SJ. Brief hypnotic treatment of repetitive nightmares. Am J Clin Hypn 1993;35(3):161–9.

106. Raboni MR, Tufik S, Suchecki D. Treatment of PTSD by eye movement desensitization reprocessing (EMDR) improves sleep quality, quality of life, and perception of stress. Ann N Y Acad Sci 2006; 1071:508–13.

107. Gorton GE. Life-long nightmares: an eclectic treatment approach. Am J Psychother 1988;42(4): 610–8.

108. Reeskamp H. Working with dreams in a clinical setting. Am J Psychother 2006;60(1):23–36.

Insomnia in Caregivers of Persons with Dementia: Who is at Risk and What Can be Done About It?

Susan M. McCurry, PhD[a],*, Laura E. Gibbons, PhD[b],
Rebecca G. Logsdon, PhD[a], Michael V. Vitiello, PhD[c],
Linda Teri, PhD[a]

KEYWORDS

- Sleep • Insomnia • Caregivers
- Alzheimer's disease • Dementia • Depression

Sleep disturbances are common among caregivers of persons with dementia. Cross-sectional studies over the past 15 years indicate that approximately two thirds of dementia caregivers report they are having trouble sleeping.[1] What about the other third? How do caregivers with and without sleep complaints differ from one another? How does their sleep quality change over time? What increases or decreases a caregiver's risk for developing sleep problems? How might this information guide the development of evidence-based treatments to improve caregiver sleep?

It is known that sleep disturbances in caregivers can originate from a complex set of precipitating, predisposing, and perpetuating factors, including nonconducive sleep environments, poor sleep habits, cognitive hyperarousal and rumination, care-recipient nocturnal behaviors, age-related primary sleep disorders, and other comorbid medical or psychiatric conditions.[1] It is also known that caregiver sleep, like that of other older adults, has considerable night-to-night variability,[2,3]

and that caregiver reports of their own or their care-recipient's sleep quality are not always congruent with what is expected based on objective measures of nighttime sleep or activity.[4,5] Given the complexity of the phenomenon, caregiver insomnia research is challenging, but the personal and socioeconomic stakes are high: poor caregiver sleep has been linked to lowered immune function, elevated stress hormones, increased risk for cardiovascular disease, and risk for premature mortality.[6–9] Continuing studies into the development, maintenance, and treatment of caregiver sleep disturbances are needed.

This article reviews some of the literature describing the association between caregiver sleep problems, and caregiver and care-recipient demographic, health, and psychosocial variables. Data are presented from a longitudinal study that examined factors associated with self-reported sleep problems in dementia caregivers and care-recipients over a 5-year follow-up period. Also considered is the caregiver sleep treatment outcome literature in light of results from these

[a] Department of Psychosocial and Community Health, University of Washington, 9709 3rd Avenue NE, Suite 507, Seattle, WA 98115–2053, USA
[b] Department of General Internal Medicine, University of Washington, Box 359780, Harborview Medical Center, 325 Ninth Avenue, Seattle, WA 98104, USA
[c] Department of Psychiatry and Behavioral Sciences, University of Washington, Box 356560, Seattle, WA 98195–6560, USA
* Corresponding author.
E-mail address: smccurry@u.washington.edu (S.M. McCurry).

Sleep Med Clin 4 (2009) 519–526
doi:10.1016/j.jsmc.2009.07.005
1556-407X/09/$ – see front matter © 2009 Elsevier Inc. All rights reserved.

cross-sectional and longitudinal studies. Suggestions for future research directions are given.

CROSS-SECTIONAL CORRELATES OF CAREGIVER SLEEP DISTURBANCES

Most caregivers of persons with dementia in the United States are older women.[10] Both increasing age and female gender are associated with a higher prevalence of sleep complaints in community-based samples.[11,12] Older caregivers are also more likely to have a variety of comorbid medical problems, which combined with the medications used to treat these problems increase risk for development of insomnia.[13–15] Finally, primary sleep disorders, such obstructive sleep apnea and restless legs syndrome, are more common in older adults but frequently undiagnosed,[16–18] and so may play an unrecognized role in many caregiver sleep complaints.

In addition to these predisposing and precipitating demographic and medical risk factors for insomnia, a growing body of literature suggests that the unique psychosocial circumstances faced by caregivers, and their emotional and behavioral responses to these circumstances, may perpetuate caregiver sleep complaints. Caregivers are often awakened by their care-recipients at night,[19] and caregivers sleep better when they avail themselves of respite breaks away from the care-recipient.[20] Several studies have shown that care-recipient nocturnal behavioral disturbances are not in themselves, however, necessarily associated with poor caregiver sleep,[2,21] and caregiver sleep problems often continue even after care-recipients are moved out of the home or die.[22] There is also evidence that caregiver objective sleep quality is not significantly different from age-matched noncaregiver samples, although caregivers perceive their sleep to be worse.[23] What may be more important than the actual caregiving role in the development and maintenance of insomnia is caregivers' personal interpretation or appraisal of their situation. In recent years, a number of researchers have begun to consider how modern theories of stress and coping can inform understanding of the relationship between caregiving and caregiver health outcomes, including those important to sleep.[24]

Using structural equation modeling, Brummett and coworkers[25] demonstrated that being a caregiver is related to worse sleep quality, but that this association is mediated by caregiver negative affect, which is also inversely related to perceived social support. Caregivers with good social support and low levels of negative affect may be less likely to develop sleep disturbances. In the Brummett and colleagues[25] study, negative affect was measured based on self-reported depression, anxiety, and stress. Depression and anxiety are both well-known risk factors for insomnia,[26,27] and their prevalence in caregivers is significantly increased compared with noncaregiving adults.[28–31] In caregivers, negative affect also commonly includes nocturnal worry or rumination, grief and bereavement, caregiver vigilance or hyperalertness, and physiologic arousal, all of which have been found to relate to sleep disturbances in older adults.[7,32–34]

The interaction between caregiver sleep disturbances and negative affect potentially flows both ways, creating a negative feedback loop that can be difficult to break. Sleep fragmentation and obstructive sleep apnea in particular cause elevations in stress hormones that further exacerbate risk for development of negative health outcomes, affect, and insomnia.[35] It is possible that intervention strategies that target caregiver cognitions might help interrupt this cycle. Two recent studies show that caregivers with higher self-ratings of personal mastery have lower norepinephrine reactivity and β_2-adrenergic receptor sensitivity in response to stress than caregivers with lower mastery scores.[36,37] Although these studies did not directly measure ratings of caregiver sleep, they do provide further evidence that positive caregiver self-appraisals may reduce the likelihood of developing stress-related physiologic responses that can worsen physical health, negatively impact mood and burden, and both directly and indirectly contribute to poor nightly sleep.

IDENTIFYING DYADS AT GREATEST RISK: LONGITUDINAL STUDIES OF CAREGIVER AND CARE-RECIPIENT SLEEP

The associations presented previously comparing demographic, physical, and other psychosocial correlates of sleep disturbance in caregivers were derived from cross-sectional studies. The factors prospectively associated with the onset of sleep disturbances in caregivers of persons with dementia, however, are largely unknown. The few longitudinal studies that have been conducted have mostly included small sample sizes, nondementia caregivers, relatively short follow-up periods, and a limited range of comparison outcome measures. Carter[38] measured self-reported sleep, depression, and actigraphic sleep quality in 10 caregivers of cancer patients at three sampling points over 10 weeks. She reported that caregiver depression and sleep outcomes varied widely over the 10 weeks, suggesting that accurate assessment of sleep and mood variables requires repeated measurements in this population. Fletcher and coworkers[39] found that baseline levels of sleep disturbance predicted evening fatigue levels, whereas trait anxiety and family support predicted morning fatigue in 60 family caregivers of cancer patients receiving radiation treatment over a 6-month follow-up period. Their analyses, which used hierarchical linear modeling to analyze repeated measures over the study period, further illustrate the interindividual and intraindividual variability in trajectories of caregiver fatigue over time, but did not look at predictors of caregiver or patient nighttime sleep. Matsuda and coworkers[40] evaluated 103 family caregivers of persons with dementia following the care-recipient's placement in a long-term care facility. Significant decreases in the anxiety-insomnia subscale of the General Health Questionnaire were observed for caregivers whose relatives had been in residential care for at least 6 months (N = 41); however, in this study caregivers were only evaluated at two sampling points, no subjective or objective outcomes specific to sleep were included, and there were no analyses examining factors associated with improvement or decline over time.

The largest study to date examining the factors associated with new onset of sleep disturbances in dementia caregivers and care-recipients is an unpublished study by McCurry and coworkers[41] that followed 164 community-dwelling individuals with Alzheimer's disease and their family caregivers over a 5-year interval. Self-report sleep data were collected as part of a longitudinal study examining quality of life in Alzheimer's disease.[42] Subjects were 164 caregivers (mean age 69.3 years, 70% female, 82% spouses of care-recipient) and their family members (mean age 76.7 years, 59% male, average dementia duration 4.5 years) diagnosed with probable or possible Alzheimer's disease.[43]

In the McCurry and colleagues[41] study, caregiver–care-recipient dyads were evaluated at baseline and every 6 months for up to 5 years (mean = 2 years, range = 6–60 months). Assessments included caregiver reports about the care-recipient's sleep, cognitive and functional status, and level of behavioral disturbance. Caregivers also reported on their own nighttime sleep, mood, and burden. A Caregiver Sleep Questionnaire (CSQ) was used to rate the frequency of seven sleep problems occurring during the past month, including being awakened by the dementia patient, being kept awake at night by worry about the caregiving role, and daytime sleepiness or fatigue (**Table 1**). Caregivers also rated their sleep quality and whether they believed they were

getting enough, too much, or too little sleep at night. CSQ scores of 12 points or higher (out of a possible 26), which was equal to the upper twenty-fifth percentile for the sample at baseline, were considered the "sleep disturbed" range.

Care-recipient (Alzheimer's disease patient) sleep disturbance was based on caregiver reports of two or more specific nocturnal behaviors (out of a possible six behaviors, including calling out or yelling, becoming agitated, interrupted breathing spells, "jerky legs" in bed, seeing or hearing things, or snoring). Waking the caregiver in the middle of the night, three or more times a week, as reported on the Revised Memory and Behavior Problems Checklist (RMBPC)[44] was also considered indicative of care-recipient sleep disturbance.

Caregiver mood and burden was evaluated using the Center for Epidemiologic Studies–Depression scale and the Screen for Caregiver Burden (objective and subjective subscales).[45] In addition, caregivers rated their quality of life using the Quality of Life-Alzheimer's Disease scale. Care-recipient cognitive and functional status was evaluated using the Mini-Mental State Examination[46] and the Lawton-Brody Physical and Instrumental Self-Maintenance Scales.[47] Care-recipient mood and behavior were rated using the RMBPC (memory, depression, and disruption subscales).[44] Caregiver and care-recipient demographics included age; gender; and caregiver relationship to the care-recipient (marital partner vs not married).

Cross-sectional associations with baseline caregiver sleep disturbance were evaluated with logistic regression models. Survival analyses were conducted to predict the onset of sleep disturbances in patients and caregivers over the follow-up period. For each outcome, only caregivers or care-recipients reporting no sleep disturbances at baseline (as measured by CSQ, patient sleep disturbance, or RMBPC criteria) were included. Patient cognitive and functional status, depression, behavioral disturbance, and caregiver depression and burden were considered as time-dependent covariates, using the score at the time of the event, the preceding visit (6 months earlier), and the change from the preceding visit to the current one. Caregiver and patient age and gender, and patient marital status, were also evaluated.

Study results showed that baseline caregiver sleep disturbance (CSQ 12 or higher) was associated in logistic regression modeling with higher (worse) scores on the RMBPC-memory scale (odds ratio = 2.69; 95% confidence intervals [CI], 1.43–5.03); objective caregiver burden on the

Table 1
Sleep outcome questionnaires

Caregiver Sleep Questionnaire

Problem frequency (items #1–7)	Sleep quality (Item #8)	Sleep quantity (Item #9)
0 = Never	0 = Very good	0 = Enough
1 = Rarely	1 = Satisfactory	1 = Too much sleep
2 = 2–4x/month or weekly	2 = Troubled	2 = Too little sleep
3 = >once a week or daily (reverse code items #4, 6)	3 = Poor/very bad	

1. Does the care-recipient become more confused or disoriented at night?
2. Is the care-recipient's behavior at night a problem to you or others?
3. Does worrying about your caretaking role ever keep you awake?
4. When you awaken at night, can you fall back to sleep within 10–15 minutes?
5. How often do you usually nap during the day?
6. How often do you fall asleep when you want to stay awake?
7. How often do you use sleeping medication?
8. Overall, how would you rate your sleep at night?
9. Do you feel you get too much sleep, about enough sleep, or too little sleep?

Care-recipient sleep disturbances

At night, does the care-recipient (check if appropriate):

Call out or yell?	Have "jerky legs" in bed?
Become agitated?	See or hear things?
Have interrupted breathing spells?	Snore?

Revised memory and behavior problem checklist, item #10[44]

How often does the care-recipient wake you or other family members up at night?

0 = Never	1 = Not in the past week	2 = 1–2x in the past week
	3 = 3–6x in the past week	4 = Daily or more often

Screen for Caregiver Burden (OR = 2.42; 95% CI, 1.37–4.27 for a five-point change); and male care-recipients (OR = 4.46; 95% CI, 1.56–12.7). Baseline patient sleep disturbance (PSQ two or higher, or waking caregiver three or more times per week) was associated with higher RMBPC-memory scores (odds ratio = 1.53; 95% CI, 1.02–2.28), and lower caregiver quality-of-life ratings (OR = 0.34; 95% CI, 0.15–0.79). Older caregiver age, increased caregiver depression, and female gender were not associated with poor caregiver sleep at baseline.

Over a mean of 24 months of follow-up (range 6–60 months), 18% of caregivers had a new onset of sleep disturbances as measured by a total CSQ score greater than or equal to 12. Current caregiver depression and previous level of objective burden were the strongest predictors of the onset of caregiver sleep problems (**Table 2**). Thirty-eight percent of care-recipients had a new onset of sleep problems as measured by the PSQ (two or more problems) or RMBPC sleep item (waking caregiver three or more times per week). Current care-recipient depression on the RMBPC and higher levels of activities of daily living impairment predicted onset of care-recipient sleep disturbances (see **Table 2**). Caregiver and care-recipient demographics, dementia severity or duration, caregiver subjective burden, and overall level of care-recipient behavioral disturbances were not significant predictors in the survival analysis.

TREATMENT OF SLEEP DISTURBANCES IN CAREGIVERS

A number of reviews over the past decade have examined the impact and quality of evidence-based interventions designed to improve caregiver physical and mental health outcomes.[24,48,49]

Table 2
Survival analyses

Sleep Outcome	Predictor Variables	HR (95% CI)
Caregiver sleep questionnaire: 12+	CES-D[a] (current)	1.42 (1.12–1.80)
	SCB-Objective (previous)	2.33 (1.43–3.78)
Patient sleep disturbances: PSD ≥2 or waking caregiver ≥3x/wk	Lawton-Brody ADL scale (current)	1.55 (1.20–2.00)
	RMBPC-Depression (current)	1.52 (1.09–2.12)

HR = hazard ratio for 5 points, CES-D, and SCB; 1 point ADL and RMBPC.
 Abbreviations: ADL, activities of daily living; CES-D, Center for Epidemiologic Studies–Depression scale; HR, hazard ratio; PSD, patient sleep disturbance; RMBPC, Revised Memory and Behavior Problems Checklist; SCB, Screen for Caregiver Burden.
 [a] Sleep question removed.

T There has been almost no research on the development of treatments to improve caregiver sleep, and almost no studies that have even included caregiver sleep outcomes, let alone targeted them for intervention.

Only two studies published to date have examined the use of cognitive-behavioral insomnia treatment techniques to improve caregiver sleep. McCurry and colleagues[50] randomly assigned 36 caregivers (age 50+ years) of persons with Alzheimer's disease into either wait list control or an active treatment that consisted of standard sleep hygiene, stimulus control, and sleep compression strategies and education about community resources, stress management, and training in the ABCs to reduce patient disruptive behaviors. In deference to caregivers' age and situation (which made it impossible to control the frequency and duration of nighttime awakenings that were caused by the care-recipient), no caregiver was asked to restrict their time in bed to less than 6.5 hours, and daytime naps less than 30 minutes in duration were permitted. Caregivers in active treatment showed significant differences in self-reported sleep on the Pittsburgh Sleep Quality Index (PSQI) total scores at posttreatment and 3-month follow-up, and improvements in weekly diary reports of nightly sleep percent. No significant differences between groups were observed for caregiver mood, burden, or patient behavior problems, suggesting that sleep improvements were not an artifact of improvements in care-recipient nocturnal behaviors or caregiver depression.[50]

Carter[51] subsequently used a repeated-measures experimental design to test the feasibility and effectiveness of a brief behavioral sleep intervention (CAregiver Sleep Intervention [CASI]) that included stimulus control, relaxation, cognitive therapy, and sleep hygiene elements. These standard sleep promotion recommendations were adapted to allow caregivers to set their own sleep and relaxation goals, and to implement behavioral changes at a self-selected pace. Thirty family caregivers of advanced-stage cancer patients were randomized into either CASI or control; both self-report and wrist actigraphy data were collected at baseline, 3 and 5 weeks, and 2-, 3-, and 4-months postbaseline. Caregivers in this study were a wide range of ages (21–85 years), and no data on care-recipients' cognitive or behavioral status were reported. Improvements in both treatment groups were observed, but at 4-month follow-up, CASI subjects had significantly lower PSQI scores and greater actigraph-measured total sleep time than control subjects.

In one other relevant study, King and colleagues[52] randomized 100 older (age 50+ years) women family caregivers of persons with dementia into either a moderate-intensity exercise (brisk walking) program or a nutrition-education attention control condition, and measured stress-induced cardiovascular reactivity; sleep quality (self-rated sleep latency, duration, and sleep quality items from the PSQI); and psychologic distress (stress and depression). Participants were introduced to an exercise training program over the first 6 weeks and then instructed to engage in a minimum of four 30- to 40-minute home-based exercise sessions per week (mostly brisk walking) for 1 year. Exercise produced improvements in systolic blood pressure reactivity and PSQI subjective sleep quality scores in caregiver participants at 1 year. Among exercisers, improvements in sleep quality were related to reductions in perceived stress and subjective caregiver burden. Although caregivers were not recruited into this study based on level of sleep complaints, and sleep was not the specific target of intervention, results add further support to the hypothesized relationship between caregiver sleep disturbances and negative affect or appraisals, mediated by stress-induced cardiovascular reactivity.

The limited treatment literature suggests that intervention strategies that are effective for improving sleep in noncaregiving older adults (eg, sleep restriction, stimulus control, and exercise) can also help caregivers sleep better, despite the unique lifestyle and environmental demands they face. The few treatments that have been developed have largely not included all the components that may be important, however, given what is known about the correlates of sleep problems in caregivers. For example, none of the treatment studies evaluated caregiver self-efficacy; overall health (except for blood pressure in the case of the King and colleagues[52] study); or social support. None included cognitive training to enhance overall caregiver mastery and competence. All three included measures of caregiver depression, stress, and quality of life, but in no case did these measures significantly improve as a result of treatment, perhaps because depressed or distressed caregivers were not specifically recruited for enrollment. Only one study included any measures of physiologic arousal or stress reactivity.

Furthermore, from the standpoint of the broader evidence-based sleep treatment literature, the few studies to date have other significant methodologic problems. None have recruited subjects based on research criteria for insomnia. Study sample sizes to date have been relatively small, and two of the three studies based sleep improvements solely on caregiver self-report. Caregiver samples in the three treatment studies were also quite heterogeneous, representing a wide range of ages, relationships to care-recipients, and care-recipient diagnosis (eg, dementia vs advanced cancer), further limiting the interpretation of findings. Although the existing literature supports the feasibility and potential efficacy of nonpharmacologic treatments for insomnia in caregivers, additional research is needed to understand how caregiver sleep disturbances can best be evaluated, prevented, and reduced.

SUMMARY

This article reviews the literature concerning sleep disturbances in dementia caregivers, including their prevalence, correlates, and treatments. Also provided are new data regarding factors associated with the onset of caregiver sleep disturbances over up to 5 years of caring for a family member with dementia at home. What this review has most clearly revealed, however, is that the study of insomnia and other sleep disturbances in caregivers is still in its infancy.

Although large percentages of caregivers report that they have sleep problems, little is known about their severity, persistence, or symptom profiles. Most research to date that has looked at caregiver health and outcomes has either ignored sleep altogether, or been limited by the diagnostic and assessment strategies used to characterize sleep. Relatively little is known about how or if sleep disturbances in the context of a caregiver-recipient dyad are unique. Persons with dementia and caregivers cohabitating in community settings are often negatively impacted by one another's sleep habits and disruptions. There is growing evidence, however, that being awakened by one's demented or chronically ill spouse or parent does not necessarily lead to insomnia. The cross-sectional and longitudinal data presented in this article provide evidence that caregiver depression, burden, medical morbidity, and appraisal of their situation, and care-recipient depression and functional impairments, may be more important in the development of caregiver sleep problems than care-recipient nocturnal behavioral disturbances.

Sleep has been called the "new vital sign,"[53] because of the growing evidence of its important role to good health. Dementia caregivers, who are "the often forgotten patient"[54] because of their increased risk for medical and psychiatric morbidity, may be particularly at risk to suffer ill consequences from chronic sleep loss superimposed on the stress of their caregiving role. Future research is needed to identify better those caregivers who currently have or who are at risk for developing insomnia. This requires the use of standard research insomnia assessment tools that look at both nighttime sleep and the daytime consequences of sleep loss. Evidence-based interventions need to be developed that target the physical, cognitive, and emotional factors that may be precipitating or perpetuating these sleep problems in an individualized way that is capable of addressing the unique circumstances of each caregiving dyad. Finally, in conjunction with developing individualized treatments, a better understanding is needed of what is considered a clinically meaningful improvement (what truly improves the everyday quality of life) for caregivers with sleep disturbances.

REFERENCES

1. McCurry SM, Logsdon RG, Teri L, et al. Sleep disturbances in caregivers of persons with dementia: contributing factors and treatment implications. Sleep Med Rev 2007;11:143–53.

2. McCurry SM, Pike KC, Vitiello MV, et al. Factors associated with concordance and variability of sleep quality in persons with Alzheimer's disease and their caregivers. Sleep 2008;31(5):741–8.

3. Rowe MA, McCrae CS, Campbell JM, et al. Sleep pattern differences between older adult dementia caregivers and older adult noncaregivers using objective and subjective measures. J Clin Sleep Med 2008;4(4):362–9.

4. Hoekert M, Riemersma-van der Lek R, Swaab DF, et al. Comparison between informant-observed and actigraphic assessments of sleep-wake rhythm disturbances in demented residents of homes for the elderly. Am J Geriatr Psychiatry 2006;14(2):104–11.

5. McCurry SM, Vitiello MV, Gibbons LE, et al. Factors associated with caregiver perceptions of sleep disturbances in persons with dementia. Am J Geriatr Psychiatry 2006;14(2):112–20.

6. Martire LM, Hall M. Dementia caregiving: recent research on negative health effects and the efficacy of caregiver interventions. CNS Spectr 2002;7(11):791–6.

7. Mausbach BT, Ancoli-Israel S, von Kanel R, et al. Sleep disturbance, norepinephrine, and D-dimer are all related in elderly caregivers of people with Alzheimer disease. Sleep Med Rev 2006;29(20):1347–52.

8. Vitaliano PP, Scanlan JM, Zhang J, et al. A path model of chronic stress, the metabolic syndrome, and coronary heart disease. Psychosom Med 2002;64(3):418–35.

9. von Känel R, Dimsdale JE, et al. Poor sleep is associated with higher plasma proinflammatory cytokine interleukin-6 and procoagulant marker fibrin D-dimer in older caregivers of people with Alzheimer's disease. J Am Geriatr Soc 2006;54(3):431–7.

10. National Alliance for Caregiving, American association of retired persons. Caregiving in the U.S.: Executive summary. Bethesda (MD): 2005. Available at: http://www.caregiving.org/data/04execsumm.pdf.

11. Foley DJ, Monjan AA, Brown SL, et al. Sleep complaints among elderly persons: an epidemiologic study of three communities. Sleep 1995;18:425–32.

12. Middlekoop HAM, Smilde-van den Doel DA, Neven AK, et al. Subjective sleep characteristics of 1,485 males and females aged 50–93: effects of sex and age, and factors related to self-evaluated quality of sleep. J Gerontol A Biol Sci Med Sci 1996;51:M108–15.

13. Ancoli-Israel S. Sleep and aging: prevalence of disturbed sleep and treatment considerations in older adults. J Clin Psychiatry 2005;66(Suppl 9):24–30.

14. Taylor DJ, Mallory LJ, Lichstein KL, et al. Comorbidity of chronic insomnia with medical problems. Sleep 2007;30(2):213–8.

15. Vitiello MV, Moe KE, Prinz PN. Sleep complaints cosegregate with illness in older adults: clinical research informed by and informing epidemiological studies of sleep. J Psychosom Res 2002;53(1):555–9.

16. Hornyak M, Feige B, Riemann D, et al. Periodic leg movements in sleep and periodic limb movement disorder: prevalence, clinical significance and treatment. Sleep Med Rev 2006;10(3):169–77.

17. Milligan SA, Chesson AL. Restless legs syndrome in the older adult: diagnosis and management. Drugs Aging 2002;19(10):741–51.

18. Young T, Peppard PE, Gottlieb DJ. Epidemiology of obstructive sleep apnea. Am J Respir Crit Care Med 2002;165:1217–39.

19. McCurry SM, Teri L. Sleep disturbance in elderly caregivers of dementia patients. Clin Gerontol 1995;16(2):51–66.

20. Lee D, Morgan K, Lindesay J. Effect of institutional respite care on the sleep of people with dementia and their primary caregivers. J Am Geriatr Soc 2007;55:252–8.

21. Beaudreau SA, Spira AP, Gray HL, et al. The relationship between objectively measured sleep disturbance and dementia family caregiver distress and burden. J Geriatr Psychiatry Neurol 2008;21(3):159–65.

22. Carter PA. Bereaved caregivers' descriptions of sleep: impact on daily life and the bereavement process. Oncol Nurs Forum 2005;32(4):741.

23. Castro CM, Lee KA, Bliwise DL, et al. Sleep patterns and sleep-related factors between caregiving and non-caregiving women. Behav Sleep Med 2009;7(3):164–79.

24. Schulz R, Martire LM. Family caregiving of persons with dementia: prevalence, health effects, and support strategies. Am J Geriatr Psychiatr 2004;12(3):240–9.

25. Brummett BH, Babyak MA, Siegler IC, et al. Associations among perceptions of social support, negative affect, and quality of sleep in caregivers and noncaregivers. Health Psychol 2006;25(2):220–5.

26. Quan SF, Katz R, Olson J, et al. Factors associated with incidence and persistence of symptoms of disturbed sleep in an elderly cohort: the Cardiovascular Health Study. Am J Med Sci 2005;329(4):163–72.

27. Spira AP, Friedman L, Flint A, et al. Interaction of sleep disturbances and anxiety in later life: perspectives and recommendations for future research. J Geriatr Psychiatry Neuro 2005;18(2):109–15.

28. Cuijpers P. Depressive disorders in caregivers of dementia patients: a systematic review. Aging Ment Health. 2005;9(4):325–30.

29. Flaskerud JH, Carter PA, Lee P. Distressing emotions in female caregivers of people with AIDS, age-related dementias, and advanced-stage cancers. Perspect Psychiatr Care 2000;36(4):121–30.

30. Kochar J, Fedman L, Stone KL, et al. Sleep problems in elderly women caregivers depend on the level of depressive symptoms: results of the Caregiver-Study of Osteoporotic Fractures. J Am Geriatr Soc 2007;55(12):2003–9.

31. Pinquart M, Sorensen S. Differences between caregivers and noncaregivers in psychological health and physical health: a meta-analysis. Psychol Aging 2003;18(2):250–67.

32. Hall M, Buysse DJ, Dew MA, et al. Intrusive thoughts and avoidance behaviors are associated with sleep disturbances in bereavement-related depression. Depress Anxiety 1997;6(3):106–12.

33. Mahoney DF. Vigilance: evolution and definition for caregivers of family members with Alzheimer's disease. J Gerontol Nurs 2003;29(8):24–30.

34. Waldrop DP. Caregiver grief in terminal illness and bereavement: a mixed-methods study. Health Soc Work 2007;32(3):197–206.

35. Shamsuzzaman AS, Gersh BJ, Somers VK. Obstructive sleep apnea: implications for cardiac and vascular disease. JAMA 2003;290:1906–14.

36. Mausbach BT, Aschbacher K, Mills PJ, et al. A 5-year longitudinal study of the relationships between stress, coping, and immune cell beta(2)-adrenergic receptor sensitivity. Psychiatry Res 2008;160(3):247–55.

37. Roepke SK, Mausbach BT, Aschbacher K, et al. Personal mastery is associated with reduced sympathetic arousal in stressed Alzheimer caregivers. Am J Geriatr Psychiatry 2008;16:310–7.

38. Carter PA. Family caregivers' sleep loss and depression over time. Cancer Nurs 2003;26(4):253–9.

39. Fletcher BA, Schumacher KL, Dodd M, et al. Trajectories of fatigue in family caregivers of patients undergoing radiation therapy for prostate cancer. Res Nurs Health 2009;32(2):125–39.

40. Matsuda O, Hasebe N, Ikehara K, et al. Longitudinal study of the mental health of caregivers caring for elderly patients with dementia: effect of institutional placement on mental health. Psychiatry Clin Neurosci 1997;51(5):289–93.

41. McCurry SM, Gibbons LE, Logsdon RG, et al. Longitudinal changes in sleep and psychosocial function in Alzheimer's patients and family caregivers [abstract supplement]. Sleep 2004;27:A121.

42. Logsdon RG, Gibbons LE, Teri L, et al. Quality of life in Alzheimer's disease: longitudinal perspectives [abstract]. Gerontologist 1999;139(Special Issue 1):164.

43. McKhann G, Drachman D, Folstein M, et al. Clinical diagnosis of Alzheimer's disease: report of the NINCDS-ADRDA Work Group under the auspices of Department of Health and Human Services Task Force on Alzheimer's disease. Neurology 1984;34:939–44.

44. Teri L, Truax P, Logsdon RG, et al. Assessment of behavioral problems in dementia: the revised memory and behavior problems checklist. Psychol Aging 1992;7:622–31.

45. Vitaliano PP, Russo J, Young HM, et al. The screen for caregiver burden. Gerontologist 1991;31(1):76–83.

46. Folstein MF, Folstein SE, McHugh PR. Mini-Mental State: a practical method for grading the cognitive state of patients for the clinician. J Psychiatr Res 1975;12:189–98.

47. Lawton MP, Brody EM. Assessment of older people: self-maintaining and instrumental activities of daily living. Gerontologist 1969;9:179–86.

48. Schulz R, O'Brien A, Czaja S, et al. Dementia caregiver intervention research: in search of clinical significance. Gerontologist 2002;42(5):589–602.

49. Zarit SH, Femia EE. A future for family care and dementia intervention research? Challenges and strategies. Aging Ment Health 2008;12(1):5–13.

50. McCurry SM, Logsdon RG, Vitiello MV, et al. Successful behavioral treatment for reported sleep problems in elderly caregivers of dementia patients: a controlled study. J Gerontol B Psychol Sci Soc Sci 1998;53B(2):P122–9.

51. Carter PA. A brief behavioral sleep intervention for family caregivers of persons with cancer. Cancer Nurs 2006;29(2):95–103.

52. King AC, Baumann K, O'Sullivan P, et al. Effects of moderate-intensity exercise on physiological, behavioral, and emotional responses to family caregiving: a randomized controlled trial. J Gerontol A Biol Sci Med Sci 2002;57(1):M26–36.

53. Wilson JF. Is sleep the new vital sign? Ann Intern Med 2005;142(10):877–80.

54. Brodaty H, Green A. Who cares for the carer? The often forgotten patient. Aust Fam Physician 2002;31(9):833–6.

Physicians and Sleep Deprivation

Robert Daniel Vorona, MD[a,b,*], Ian Alps Chen, MD, MPH[a],
J. Catesby Ware, PhD[a,c]

KEYWORDS

- Residents • Sleep loss • Medical errors
- Physician burnout • Physician work hours

Current training programs alert United States medical residents to the consequences of disrupted and restricted sleep. Some of the most notorious examples of disastrous accidents that have been in part attributed to fatigue and sleepiness ct 2 explosion; the Three Mile Island nuclear reactor radiation release; the space shuttle Challenger accident (fatigue of the ground crew); the Exxon Valdez oil spill; and the crash of American Airlines flight 1420. A single physician trainee's or attending physician's error is not likely to lead to death or destruction on the level of these examples. The collective consequences, however, of physicians' sleep deprivation and resultant sleepiness on professional function and the health care of patients are potentially of great moment.

Medical residents are highly trained and carefully selected into their training programs. They are strongly motivated to provide excellent health care to their patients. Presumably, they are equally motivated to maintain their own health. Yet, they regularly endanger their own lives as evidenced by several studies demonstrating increased near-crashes and crashes after extended work shifts.[1–3] Might physicians endanger their own patients? Much of the research concerning sleep deprivation has involved medical residents rather than physicians in active practice. A surprising and glaring paucity of data exist concerning sleep, sleep deprivation, and effects on the activity of practicing physicians.

This article first discusses the history of sleep deprivation and effects on physicians. Then reviewed are data concerning physicians in training and practicing physicians. Finally, the article concludes by stressing the limitations of these data and poses questions for future interested investigators.

HISTORY OF SLEEP LOSS AND FATIGUE IN PHYSICIANS

The Libby Zion case in 1984 continued a debate regarding long work hours for physicians that had simmered since the 1970s.[4] One early study described the difficulty that sleep-deprived interns manifested in the performance of a sustained-attention task. Interns sleeping a mean of 1.8 hours during the preceding 32 hours (as compared with those sleeping 7 hours) were less likely to recognize cardiac arrhythmias on an ECG tape.[5] The interns also described clinical difficulties, and a range of problems that included difficulty thinking, depression, depersonalization, irritability, and memory deficits.[6] Performance deficits also occurred in British house officers on a 3-minute card-sorting task after a sleep deficit of over 3 hours.[7] In 1975, a large survey of 2452 house

[a] Department of Internal Medicine, Eastern Virginia Medical School, 825 Fairfax Avenue, Suite 410, Norfolk, VA 23507, USA
[b] Eastern Virginia Medical School/Sentara Norfolk General Hospital Sleep Disorders Center, 600 Gresham Drive, Norfolk, VA 23507, USA
[c] Department of Psychiatry and Behavioral Medicine, Eastern Virginia Medical School, 825 Fairfax Avenue, Suite 410, Norfolk, VA 23507, USA
* Corresponding author. Department of Internal Medicine, Eastern Virginia Medical School, 825 Fairfax Avenue, Suite 410, Norfolk, VA 23507.
E-mail address: voronard@evms.edu (R.D. Vorona).

Sleep Med Clin 4 (2009) 527–540
doi:10.1016/j.jsmc.2009.07.003

officers from England, Scotland, and Wales established that over one third believed that long duty hours impaired their efficiency.[8] The early 1980s literature for the most part, however, only acknowledged that research on sleep deficiency and physician performance was lacking and required reevaluation.[9]

Libby Zion was an 18-year-old patient whose father was also an ex-prosecutor and *New York Times* reporter. In 1984, she unexpectedly died within 24 hours of admission to New York Hospital. Her father, Sidney Zion, believed that inadequacies in the hospital teaching system were at fault and wrote in a *New York Times* op-ed piece that argued, "You don't need kindergarten to know that a resident working a 36-hour shift is in no condition to make any kind of judgment call – forget about life and death."[10] The subsequent widespread publicity triggered a debate regarding overworked and sleep-deprived housestaff and the state of medical education. Even though a grand jury did not indict the physicians or the hospital, a report critical of the incident helped establish the Bell Commission.[11] This committee's recommendations led to legislative reform of residents' duty hours in New York State, although the committee argued that the more serious and salient problem was actually the lack of resident supervision.[12]

Much debate ensued in the medical community about the consequences of changing work hours and residency training with many arguments promulgated both for and against change.[13] Some arguments against change included the "tradition" of medicine, possible inadequacies in training, problems with patient continuity, and costs.[14–16] Arguments for change included improved patient and physician safety and enhancement of both the work environment and educational training of residents.[17,18] Changes were certainly not widespread, nor always enforced, and progressed at a sluggish pace.[19–22] It was not until approximately 15 years later after Libby Zion's death, in the early 2000s, that many of the issues regarding work hours and residency training gained momentum. Concurrent to all the debate regarding resident work hours, a big push occurred in studying medical errors, patient safety, and health care outcomes. Much of the subsequent knowledge buttressed the arguments for change. For example, in 2000, the Institute of Medicine publicized its' report, "To Err is Human," which focused national attention on patient safety. The Institute of Medicine did not address duty hours specifically, but did discuss medical errors and the prevention of errors.[23] A variety of medical error types occur. They can be classified into different categories: communication failures, diagnostic errors, treatment errors, prophylaxis failure, and follow-up failure.[24] Sleep loss potentially exacerbates many of these error types.

In 2001, several concerned groups petitioned the National Occupational Safety and Health Administration to establish and enforce a federal work hour standard for residents.[25] The accrediting body for residency education, the Accreditation Council for Graduate Medical Education (ACGME), also appointed in 2001 a work group on resident duty hours. Federal legislation, known as the Patient and Physician Safety and Protection Act, proceeded through Congress almost contemporaneously in 2002.[26] In 2002, based on the recommendations of its work group, the ACGME announced that effective July 2003, residency programs are required to meet new duty hour directives. Residents could be scheduled for no more than 80 hours of work per week, averaged over a 4-week period, and were also limited to no more than one overnight call duty every third night on average. They also needed to have 1 day in every 7 free of patient care responsibility, and were to have a 24-hour limit of on-call duty with a follow-up period of 6 hours for transfer of care or educational activities.[27]

The tale of resident work hours did not end, nor was it solved, by the 2003 ACGME requirements. A growing literature investigating the effects of the work hour limitations on residency education developed over the next 5 years. In December of 2008, the Institute of Medicine again revisited the issue of residents' workloads and duty hours. They found that significant changes were still needed to alleviate the effects of fatigue and sleep loss in trainees, and that increased supervision of residents and improved transfer of care processes should occur. The recommendation regarding an 80-hour work week remained unchanged; however, the Institute of Medicine argued for further changes. Specific suggestions included (1) a 5-hour, uninterrupted period of continuous sleep between 10 PM and 8 AM for duty periods running longer than 16 hours; (2) an increase in the minimum time off between scheduled shifts and a suggested maximum frequency of in-hospital night shifts; (3) an increase in the mandatory time off from 4 days per month to 5 days per month; and (4) the recommendation of one full 48-hour period off per month. The committee recognized that substantial costs would ensue and compromises associated with implementing their recommendations. They noted, however, that even today noncompliance with duty hours was "substantial and underreported, and that more intensified monitoring is necessary immediately."[28]

As stakeholders look to the future regarding sleep restriction, consequent sleepiness and fatigue, and work hours for physicians, one might query why changes have been so slow. Limitations in work hours caused by fatigue and sleep have already existed for workers in certain jobs in the United States for many years. For example, commercial drivers are limited in hours based on the Motor Carrier Act of 1935, which noted, "It is obvious that a man cannot work efficiently or be a safe driver if he does not have an opportunity for approximately 8 hours of sleep in 24."[29] Similar limitations in work hours are also in place for airline pilots as established by the Federal Aviation Administration, railroad workers as established by the Federal Railroad Administration, and for maritime workers through the US Coast Guard. In addition, many other countries have already limited the number of hours that medical residents can work. For example, in 2004, work hours for doctors in training in the National Health Service in the United Kingdom were reduced to 58 hours a week. Work hours were to be further reduced by 2009, to 48 hours, similar to other countries in Europe following the European Working Time Directive.[30]

INTERNS AND RESIDENTS

Perhaps because of the Libby Zion case and its associated notoriety,[31] much of the research concerning sleep deprivation and the medical profession involves physicians in training. Little doubt exists that physicians in training are chronically (and acute on chronically) sleep deprived. In 1996 and pre-ACGME mandates, Richardson and colleagues[32] used electroencephalography, electro-oculography, and electromyography to demonstrate that interns obtained just over 3.5 hours of sleep while on call. Attempts to increase sleep time by night float complete coverage from 0200 to 0600 did not achieve success. Multiple sleep latency testing revealed that Stanford anesthesiology residents manifested pathologic sleepiness after call and even at baseline demonstrated increased pressure to sleep.[33]

An expanding body of research suggests that these sleep-restricted interns and residents are more apt to make errors in medical care. Lack of sleep might also jeopardize physicians and patients through changes in health, crashes, impact on professional behavior, and impact on personal life. Literature supports the idea that some benefits may accrue from reducing duty hours of physicians in training. The data are far from unequivocal, however, that reductions in work hours improve the health of patients.

WORK HOURS AND PROFESSIONAL FUNCTION

Barger and colleagues[34] focused their attention on the impact of protracted shifts on interns and "medical errors, adverse events, and attentional failures." In this nationwide study, the authors reported a rough dose-response relationship between number of prolonged shifts within a month's time and interns' report of medical errors. Perhaps more starkly, interns who worked at least five prolonged shifts per month admitted to a tripling of the number of patient deaths associated with "fatigue-related preventable adverse events."

Surgical studies have examined sleep-restricted performance in both simulated surgical tasks and real life tasks with mixed results. Two studies from Europe used a laparoscopic surgery simulator to demonstrate that sleep-deprived residents performed more poorly. Taffinder and colleagues[35] in a small study of six residents established that having a "full night's sleep" led to 20% less errors and 14% greater speed than those trainees "awake all night." The second simulator study revealed that after only 17 hours on call (and median sleep duration of 1.5 hours), 14 surgical trainees worked more slowly and with significantly more mistakes.[36] Eastridge and colleagues[37] from Dallas, Texas, have also found that sleep deprivation impairs simulator performance.

Researchers in the United States hypothesized that surgical residents would learn less effectively on the laparoscopic surgery simulator after sleep deprivation.[38] Their hypothesis was not supported by their findings despite the fact that surgeons were retested after working approximately 34 hours. Only 17 of the 30 surgeons (one participating surgeon was an attending), however, followed through after performing the precall evaluation. Possibly, the trainees more apt to be impaired by sleep loss self-selected out of the postcall portion of the study. A sobering finding of this same study was that even when able to sleep unimpeded, surgical residents admitted to but 6.23 hours of sleep.

Even the most sophisticated simulator study probably cannot mirror stresses, motivations, and results in real life. A study of postoperative complications at Charity Hospital in New Orleans found that postcall status (and attendant sleep restriction to 1.8 hours) was not associated with more complications.[39] Case numbers alone cannot guarantee surgical capability at the end of training. Multiple researchers have explored the possibility, however, that reduced work hours result in less operative experience. A retrospective study from the University of Virginia noted that after institution of the 80-hour duty limitation, among surgical residents only the chief residents demonstrated a decline in operative case load.[40]

Other very recent studies can be found that support or dispute the notion that the ACGME dictates do not reduce surgical case load. For example, a retrospective study of surgical residents at Eastern Virginia Medical School[41] and a study of orthopedic residents[42] found no evidence for a decline in operative cases after July 2003. Another study not only revealed steady operative case experience but also improved American Board of Surgery In-Training Examination scores.[43] On the contrary, a Michigan State study in general surgery[44] and a Tennessee study of orthopedic residents[45] both demonstrated about a 20% decline in resident operative volume.

INJURY IN THE WORKPLACE

Interns are also more likely to harm themselves in the workplace when they work for prolonged ($\geq$32 hours) shifts. Ayas and colleagues[46] revealed that interns were more likely to suffer percutaneous injury after prolonged shifts (OR 1.61). Given the knowledge of circadian rhythms, it is also not surprising that these young doctors were roughly twice as likely to injure themselves during the night as during the day. A Turkish nursing study [47] reinforces these data by revealing that needle stick injuries occurred more frequently in those nurses working longer hours. Interestingly, extended hours in the nursing study referred to those nurses who worked for longer than 8 hours.

HARM OUTSIDE THE HOSPITAL

Long working hours could result in harm beyond the confines of the hospital or office. House officers must often drive home after working extended shifts. Multiple studies establish that being postcall increases the risk for car crashes. Interns have reported more near-miss vehicular accidents (OR 5.9) and car crashes (OR 2.3) after prolonged shifts with a mean of 32 hours.[3] Similar to medical errors, a dose-response relationship was established for number of extended shifts in a month and likelihood of a crash. The authors also made the critical point that these interns were in the hospital for long periods and achieving little sleep (2.6 hours without any night float).

An earlier study of pediatric residents and faculty clearly noted less sleep on call and more accidents for residents than for faculty members. Although a retrospective single institution study, the response rate of both residents and faculty

was high at 87%. On-call residents achieved 4.5 hours less sleep compared with faculty and were almost four times more likely to fall asleep while at a traffic signal (44% vs 12%) and almost twice as likely to report a crash. Accidents arose more frequently driving home than driving to work and were more likely after call than on noncall days. In addition, 23% of residents in this study admitted to falling asleep during driving. The impact of protracted hours was again suggested by the finding that 71% of such episodes occurred after a call night.[48]

Finally, a study of over 1500 emergency physician residents also found that night shift work increased the likelihood of postcall crashes or near misses. The investigators discovered that approximately 75% of crashes and 80% of near crashes occurring in emergency residents transpired after night shift work.[1] These results have import not only for trainee physicians but also for fellow citizens who share the road.

Researchers have also used the driving simulator test to understand the negative consequences of restricted sleep and driving in residents. In a single center and prospective study of driving simulator performance, Ware and colleagues[49] found that male residents seemed to be more impaired than female residents were after call responsibilities. Previous work has also compared sleep restriction with alcohol intake, with 24 hours without sleep equated to a blood alcohol concentration of 0.1.[50] A single center prospective study extended such a construct of comparing sleep restriction and alcohol use to pediatric residents.[51] These residents worked 1 month "heavy call" schedules, defined as 80 to 90 hours per week of work (and every fourth or fifth night call) or 1 month light call schedules, defined as 44 hours per week (without night call save in unusual circumstances). Driving simulator performance in these residents was similar in heavy call and light call with a blood alcohol concentration of 0.04 g% to 0.05 g%. These findings and another nonresident study demonstrating an additive effect of alcohol and sleep loss[52] should also prove cautionary to sleep-deprived residents who might consider driving after consuming alcohol.

PSYCHOLOGIC HARMS

Sleep-deprived residents may also suffer psychologic decrements. A study of United States internal medicine residents probed frequency of "burn out." Before changes in work hours 51% of trainees admitted to depression, 42% to emotional exhaustion, and 61% to depersonalization.[53]

Another study that included 4128 United States physicians in training noted that 61% admitted to more cynicism and 35% manifested "4 or 5 depressive symptoms."[54] Of interest, many of these residents labored under financial stress and 33% admitted to moonlighting. It seems likely that added work burdens reduce the possibility of adequate amounts of replenishing sleep when not on call.

A prospective study of residents from five medical centers used both qualitative and quantitative techniques to assess the consequences of sleep restriction and fatigue. The authors ascertained that insufficient sleep and fatigue were associated with impaired professionalism at work and increased worry about committing errors.[55] These same residents admitted to the toll that sleepiness and fatigue extracted from their personal lives, and the authors pondered the potential long-term effects. As early as 1981, the "House Officer stress syndrome" was reported and consisted of cognitive impairment, chronic anger, family discord, and pervasive cynicism, all potentially exacerbated by sleep loss.[56]

The issue of resident responsibilities and emotional cost has also been investigated outside the United States. A study from Switzerland established an association between stress in residents and hours worked.[57] This study did not tabulate hours of sleep, however, and residents in Switzerland are not supposed to work greater than 50 hours per week (although it was stated that some Swiss physicians in training may work up to 80 hours in a week). A letter from medical students in Pakistan spoke to residents faced with call duties as long as 72 hours and counterproductive coping strategies, such as drug use, denial, and disengagement.[58] Beyond concerns for physicians in training, "burnout" might also have ramifications for patient safety because burnout has been associated with an increased likelihood of subsequent medical errors.[59]

PHYSICIAN TRAINEES POST ACCREDITATION COUNCIL FOR GRADUATE MEDICAL EDUCATION GUIDELINES

Interventional studies and the 2003 ACGME changes in work hour requirements allow investigators to learn if less resident work hours equates to more effective professional and personal lives. Landrigan and colleagues[60] truncated intern work hours in the MICU and critical care unit from 77 to 81 hours, to 63 hours (and removed prolonged shifts of at least 24 hours) and studied error rates. Importantly, the authors addressed the issue of fragmentation of care by using a "sign-out template," although they noted that their efforts did not achieve full success. Nevertheless, the interns working the lesser hours made 36% less "serious medical errors," 57% "nonintercepted serious errors," and 5.6 times less "serious diagnostic errors." In an accompanying article, the same Harvard Work Hours, Health and Safety Group prospectively demonstrated that with a reduction in intern work hours per week from 85 to 65 came 5.8 more hours of sleep per week. Interns in the less onerous schedule slept 7.4 hours per day. The reduced work hours (and increased sleep) were associated with a 50% reduction in attention failures as defined by ambulatory polysomnography.[61]

Horwitz and colleagues[62] used retrospective and nonrandomized methods, but a relatively large database with a control nonteaching service population to explore the effect of ACGME work duration regulations on house staff. These researchers were particularly concerned about the potential of work hour limits to increase "hand offs" and fragment and impair quality of care. Previous data revealed 11% more sign outs after work hour restrictions.[63] After ACGME mandates, the Yale-New Haven teaching service manifested no decrements in care and did show improvements in "ICU stay…, discharge to home or rehabilitation versus elsewhere… and pharmacist interventions to prevent errors." No improvements in mortality were ascertained.[62]

In addition, a University of Michigan single institution study demonstrated that post-ACGME work limitations, residents adhered more closely to quality of care indices for acute coronary syndrome (eg, use of β-blockers). This same study demonstrated reduced 6-month mortality rates but its retrospective nature and the institution of a quality improvement action plan at study outset limit interpretation.[64] By contrast, others in cardiology have provided data that suggest fragmentation of care or perhaps less efficient care with work hour limitations. Congestive heart failure patients admitted to a short-call team spent about 1 day longer in the hospital and obtained significantly less diuretics during the first day in hospital.[65]

Researchers also studied the effects of the institution of ACGME directives on work hours in three pediatric programs.[66] Unfortunately, no improvement in sleep hours, work hours, errors, rates of vehicular crashes, occupational injury, or mood could be demonstrated in this study. A reduction in extended shifts of greater than 30 hours from 81% of residents to 56% did occur. The lack of efficacy in improving function and mood should not be surprising given the stable work and sleep hours.

POST ACCREDITATION COUNCIL FOR GRADUATE MEDICAL EDUCATION MORTALITY DATA

The effects of the ACGME work hours mandate on mortality are ambiguous. A large retrospective study of over 1.5 million patients in the United States found a small but significant reduction in absolute mortality rate (0.25%) in medical patients.[67] No such similar reduction in death rate in surgical patients was noted. The authors posed an intriguing but troubling hypothesis, that shorter work hours for residents might also mean a reduction in transmission of the necessary skills to residents.

Volpp and colleagues[68] have also explored the impact of ACGME work hour regulations on mortality in two large data sets. They found no change in 30-day postadmission mortality in a national study of over 8.5 million Medicare patients admitted to "US nonfederal hospitals" from July 2000 to June 2005. Similar to the data from Shetty and Bhattacharya,[67] this same group found that Veterans Administration acute care hospital medical patients but not surgical patients demonstrated a lower mortality after ACGME work regulations.[69] The authors could not explain the difference between medical and surgical patients' mortality. They suggested such possibilities as more effective transfers or more intensive attending performance in medical services after ACGME changes. Finally, a recent study used National Trauma Data Bank information to demonstrate a very modest decline in trauma patient mortality postinstitution of ACGME guidelines.[70]

POST ACCREDITATION COUNCIL FOR GRADUATE MEDICAL EDUCATION QUALITY OF LIFE

Quality of life has also been explored as a dependent variable of work time reductions with mixed results. In a single institution qualitative study, Lin and colleagues[71] noted that although residents favored limited work times, these same trainees worried about increased fragmentation of care, dilatory follow-up of tests, and less educational opportunities. Another study of internal medicine residents at the University of Washington revealed that after reductions in duty hours came improvements in job gratification and "emotional exhaustion." Some 84% of trainees noted "a positive effect on their well-being." A total of 70% of the same cadre of residents, however, believed that reduced duty hours decreased learning opportunities with their supervising physicians.[72]

OVERSEAS RESTRICTED WORK SCHEDULES

Researchers are looking at more and more restricted duty hours for trainee physicians. A recent study from Great Britain[73] evaluated the impact on errors of limiting work from less than 56 hours to less than 48 hours per week. The same study astutely included measures to urge the use of naps before night work and rotated through evening shifts before night shifts. The numbers of errors did decline by one third on the restricted work week and the evening shift intervention led to greater amounts of sleep (8.7 hours vs 6.9 for day shift sleep). In the intervention group, however, residents again raised concerns about increased transfers of care and less chance for education. Such concerns caused the investigators to alter the intervention schedule after the first 6 weeks of the study.

Interestingly, physician trainees in the previously mentioned study admitted to only 6.75 hours of sleep per night when asked to work the 56 hours scheduled. Ostensibly, a 56-hour work week should allow adequate time for sleep, although Cappuccio and colleagues[73] noted that at times trainees might work as many as 80 hours in a week in this traditional schedule. This still calls into question once again whether residents use shorter work hours to achieve greater amounts of sleep. It also raises the question of whether simply curtailing work hours as opposed to taking a broader look at schedules is more important.

Another study that also looked beyond number of work hours was conducted in New Zealand. Number of nights worked was associated with fatigue-related medical errors, sleepy driving, and elevated Epworth Sleepiness Scale (ESS) score. Increasing hours worked increased risk only for physicians with elevated ESS.[74] The take home message from these last two studies is that factors beyond simple duty hours to include circadian rhythms must be taken into account in a cogent redesign of resident work schedules.

SLEEP LOSS AND PRACTICING PHYSICIANS

Sleep restriction and sleep deprivation affect the performance and the safety of physicians in training. Are attending and practicing physicians affected similarly? This is actually a two-part question: Are practicing physicians subject to the same rigorous work schedules of interns and residents, and are they equally affected by sleep loss when working and driving home after call? It is assumed that their sleep physiology is similar to nonphysicians, although it is not recognized that there may be some self-selection and program selection in some subspecialties of medicine.

AGE EFFECTS

Because physicians in training are younger than physicians who have completed their training (and perhaps in better health), they may better withstand the on-call rigors. Some data indicate, however, that this is not the case. Comparing sleepiness in younger (20–30 years) with older (55–65 years) women after 3 nights of 4 hours of sleep, the younger women were objectively (as measured by the Maintenance of Wakefulness Test) and subjectively more sleepy during the day.[75] This finding in conjunction with the assumption that most practicing physicians have less rigorous schedules than they did as interns and residents suggests that practicing physicians may be less impaired if they are impaired at all.

SUBSPECIALTY

One large retrospective study[76] of cardiac surgeons could not find any impairment related to presumed sleep loss. The study examined a database containing 6751 cases of coronary artery bypass operations. The proxy for sleep deprivation was the start time of the surgery (between 2200 hours and 0500 hours) and the end time of the surgery (between 2300 hours and 0730 hours). Morbidity and mortality rates in sleep-deprived and non–sleep-deprived surgeons did not differ. The authors concluded, "Our opinion is that this study suggests the operative skills of a surgeon are unchanged the day after he has been up the night before operating." The authors argued against the need for physician work restrictions. A letter to the editor in reply was titled, "Sleep Deprivation and Results in Cardiac Surgery: Dangerous Study with Very Dangerous Conclusions."[77] Additionally, another retrospective study of 7323 cases by the same first author failed to find that acute sleep deprivation affected thoracic surgical residents on measures of "operative efficiency, morbidity, or mortality in cardiac surgical operations."[78]

Unlike the report of surgical procedures, an Australian study using a completely different methodology did find evidence of fatigue-related events. This Australian study collected 5600 voluntary, anonymous self-reported incidents and errors by anesthetists. The review of these events found that fatigue was a contributing factor in 2.7% of all reports.[79] Fatigue was reported more often in conjunction with incidents occurring in the late evening or early morning hours. One weakness is that the anesthetists had to recognize that the event was fatigue related. Recognition that fatigue or sleepiness caused an event is not necessarily easily done or correct. Even if fatigue and sleepiness were accurately recognized and even though the reports were anonymous, such a report required an admission of personal failure rather than, for example, equipment failure.

PHYSIOLOGIC ADAPTATION TO SLEEP LOSS

Perhaps practicing surgeons adapt to restricted sleep. Studies do show that a subjective adaptation to restricted sleep may occur (ie, perceived daytime sleepiness quickly plateaus resulting in the perception of acclimization to less sleep). Objective measures of performance continue to deteriorate in chronically restricted sleep conditions.[80,81] Although physicians may believe that they adjust to a restricted sleep schedule, the data indicate that this does not occur, at least in nonmedicine realms. In addition, sleep loss not only affects performance, it can contribute to false memories.[82] The recall of a procedure could be that it went differently than it actually did. Interestingly, caffeine seems to negate this false memory effect.[82]

Possibly, overlearning by repetition during training and further experience in practice reduces sleep deprivation errors. This, however, seems unlikely given the ubiquitous effects of sleep loss. For surgeons, a combination of practiced motor skills and ongoing decision making direct the motor activity and determine the outcome. Sleep loss potentially affects the motor skills and the complex decision making. Studies with even simple tasks, such as the frequently studied Psychomotor Vigilance Test, show that performance decreases as sleep loss increases.[83]

BEHAVIORAL ADAPTATION TO SLEEP LOSS

As an alternative to adjusting physiologically to restricted sleep, practicing physicians might learn that napping, judicious use of caffeine, use of other alerting agents, and practiced teamwork can compensate for impairment from sleep loss. Unfortunately, the data that caffeine and stimulant drugs can negate sleep loss or maintain performance in the face of sleep loss are limited and not straightforward. In nonphysicians, sleep loss seems to reduce risk-taking behavior, and dextroamphetamine restores risky behavior to baseline levels.[84] How this affects physician behavior and judgment is unknown. One overlooked aspect of the most commonly used stimulant, caffeine, is that of the negative effects of withdrawal from caffeine in the face of sleep loss. A study examining executive functioning found that the sleep-loss-caffeine group made 57% more errors during acute withdrawal than the placebo group.[85] In a study looking at chronic use of caffeine (1.75 mg/kg three times a day) and placebo during 4 weeks in normal and sleep-deprived conditions, caffeine did not enhance function or negate the effects of sleep loss.[86] Napping, however, when compared with placebo does improve perceptual learning similarly to the effects of caffeine, although caffeine had a negative effect on motor learning compared with naps.[87] Napping to compensate for lost sleep seems to the most appropriate defense against insufficient sleep at night.

RECENT RESULTS

Overall, little is known about the performance of the practicing physician in the face of sleep loss because so few studies address this important issue. The authors recently conducted a study of 180 attending physicians (mostly 36–55 years old) in academic (N = 58) and private practice settings (N = 122). The sample was composed of seven specialties including mainly family practice and internal medicine physicians (54%); obstetrics and gynecology and surgical specialties (15%); and emergency medicine physicians (9%). An "other" category included 14% of respondents. Twenty-three percent of all responders had abnormally high ESS scores of 11 or greater (mean = 7.8 ± 4). Most (89%) of those with abnormal ESS scores worked under 80 hours per week. Thirteen percent of the total sample reported working more than 80 hours per week. In addition to completing the ESS, the physicians reported the number of hours that they slept and number of hours that they worked. Reduced sleep, but not hours worked, was associated with increased sleepiness.[88] Some reports do suggest, however, that measures of work hours affect job performance and satisfaction.[89,90] The finding of 13% of physicians working more than 80 hours per week is low compared with some studies. A survey of 592 full-time surgeons found that 20% reported working more than 80 hours per week.[91] Even more than surgeons, a survey of 100 Houston, Texas, obstetrician-gynecologists found that 62% worked more than 80 hours per week.[92]

Table 1 provides a comparison of ESS scores with other groups. In the authors' physician survey, private practice based and surgically based subspecialties had higher ESS scores.[88] One problem with using the ESS in sensitive groups is that it is apparent to the test taker how to answer questions to affect the score. Physicians who do not want work mandated restrictions might minimize their scores, whereas overworked and exhausted residents might exaggerate their scores. This ESS transparency could also affect comparisons between surgeons and nonsurgeons and academic and nonacademic specialties.

Most studies of physicians do not measure performance or confirm work hours objectively, although this could be done with actigraph technology. Given the uncertainties of subjective measures, however, those physicians who were sleepier according to the ESS were more likely to associate sleep loss with medical errors and driving impairment.[88] Nearly half (48%) agreed or strongly agreed that they have been "worried about having a car accident driving home post-call." Surprisingly, 24% agreed or strongly agreed that they have "made medical errors because of sleep loss and fatigue" and 77% agreed or strongly agreed with the statement that they have "heard about others making medical error due to sleep loss and fatigue." In a French sample of anesthesiology deaths, 9 (2%) of 419 deaths were thought possibly to be fatigue related.[97] The problem is that the ability accurately to determine fatigue-related deaths is extremely limited.

INSOMNIA AND BURNOUT

Although sleepiness gets much of the attention, physicians are not immune to insomnia and its consequences. Stress and irregular bed times that commonly occur in training and in practice can precipitate and potentiate insomnia. A study using a representative sample of 240 physicians in Madrid, Spain, divided them into low-burnout (N = 55) and high-burnout (N = 58) groups using the Pittsburgh Sleep Quality Index to measure sleep along with the Shirom-Melamed Burnout Questionnaire. Those in the high-burnout group had significantly more disturbed sleep and insomnia. Although determination of a cause-effect relationship is not possible, this study does raise the possibility that disturbed sleep besides affecting performance and patient outcome on a specific day, may negatively globally affect one's career.[98] A qualitative study of nurses experiencing burnout found that before burnout, some nurses purposely reduced sleep to focus better on work.[99]

FATIGUE-RELATED MORBIDITY AND MORTALITY

At least 44,000 people and perhaps as many as 98,000 people die in hospitals each year because of medical errors that could have been prevented.[23] In an automobile, where drivers are presumably highly motivated not to crash, there are 40,000 to 50,000 deaths each year. One indirect way to estimate medical errors that are

Table 1
Epworth Sleepiness Scale scores in different populations

N	Population	X	SD	Reference
188	Normal sleepers	4.5	3.3	93
507	Normal sleepers	4.6	2.8	94
996	Truck drivers	5.7	3.3	95
180	Practicing physicians	7.8	4.0	88
362	Second-year medical students	9.0	3.6	(Ware JC, unpublished data, 2005)
616	Medical students	10.0	3.7	96
135	Residents	14.6	4.5	55
183	Narcoleptics	19.6	3.0	93

caused by fatigue and sleepiness is to look at highway accidents. The National Highway Traffic Safety Administration attributed 1653 fatalities (2.8% of total fatalities) to fatigue, sleepiness, and illness.[100] Can one expect this to be different for medical error deaths?

Because physicians' livelihood and self-esteem depend on the quality of their performance, they have strong motivation to balance work with adequate sleep. Likewise, nonphysicians have strong motivation to obtain adequate sleep for their driving safety. A poll of a representative sample of 750 Ontario drivers found, however, that most (58.6%) admitted that they occasionally drive while under the influence of fatigue or sleepiness. In addition, 14.5% admitted that they had fallen asleep or "nodded off" while driving and nearly 2% were involved in a fatigue or drowsy driving-related crash within the past year.[101] Medical injuries in the United States may be 1 million per year.[102] If one uses 2% as a proxy for the number of medical errors from fatigue, this suggests that 20,000 occurred. If one uses 14.5% as the proxy, 145,000 medical errors resulted from sleepiness and fatigue.

BEHAVIORAL INTERVENTIONS FOR PHYSICIANS

The authors argue that behavioral interventions can be productively applied to the physician work force. The following are preventative behavioral strategies (before work) and operational countermeasures (on the job).

Preventative Behavioral Strategies

Because sleep loss accumulates, it is critical to avoid beginning work duties with a sleep debt. Tracking one's total sleep against the number of needed hours of sleep can give a rough gauge of impairment and the importance of devoting time for a nap. In terms of sleepiness, a 4-hour sleep

loss approximates an alcohol level of 0.095 BrEC%.[103] To help reduce the likelihood of drastic sleep debt and performance impairing sleepiness, 2 nights of unrestricted sleep (weekends) are important. One can even "bank" sleep by spending longer than the usual amount of time in bed before a more challenging rotation.

If possible, one should obtain the same amount of sleep on a working as a nonworking day. This may require using more than one sleep period but probably reduces potentially severe consequences of strenuous schedules. For split schedules, understanding the circadian cycle is helpful (ie, there is a physiologic basis for the afternoon siesta). Taking a nap if possible when sleepy is the most efficient method of napping. Bright light exposure before work, particularly with blue spectrum light, is alerting.[104] Limit napping just before work to 30 minutes to reduce sleep inertia problems. Sleep inertia is likely to be more severe when waking from deep sleep. In theory, a longer nap allows for the completion of an entire 90-minute sleep cycle and is more restorative.

When sleeping at home during the day, educate the household about sleep and the importance of undisturbed sleep. The family should help protect sleep from neighbors, pets, and delivery persons. Techniques that help also include unplugging or turning off the phone, turning off the television or setting it to a channel for white noise, using earplugs, darkening the bedroom, using eyeshades, and sleeping in a cool environment.

Operational Countermeasures

Social interactions (working as a team), chewing snacking, singing, and physical exercise all can help to maintain alertness. The use of short breaks with exercise (eg, stair climbing) of at least 6 minutes and working in brightly lit spaces are recommended.

Finally, it should also be noted that caffeine is alerting. Physicians should avoid caffeine when already alert and consume caffeine approximately 30 minutes before an expected decline in alertness (eg, 0300–0500). Alerting drugs are banned for airline pilots and controversial for physicians. Roughly, 600 mg caffeine equals 20 mg dextroamphetamine equals 400 mg of modafinil for restoring simple psychomotor performance and objective alertness. Physicians should remember that it is unclear if these drugs restore executive functions after sleep deprivation[105] and it remains nebulous for how long one can continue to use alerting agents to compensate for insufficient sleep.

SUMMARY

In the absence of data, it is relatively easy to argue any conclusion. In the case of sleep loss and physician performance, the data (although burgeoning) often are sparse and the data that do exist are often weak with few prospective controlled studies. Even when investigating a specific medical error, there is no objective and exacting way to measure the contribution of sleepiness at the time of the error. The constellation of studies on physicians and nonphysicians, however, do not support a continuation of the traditional model of unfettered duty hours. They do support the following conclusions: (1) sleep loss negatively affects performance; (2) physicians suffer sleep loss in the course of their training and practice; (3) physicians are not immune to sleep loss; (4) sleep loss, in addition to effects on mood and physiology, affects all realms of performance; and (5) impaired performance leads to errors and less than optimal outcomes.

Conservative and circumstantial estimates suggest that 2% to 3% of medical errors are related to fatigue and sleepiness. When trying to correct these errors, however, one need to remember that health care interventions may also result in risk. Implementing work hour restrictions to reduce errors may deprive patients of needed care or deprive residents of needed training. An extreme example occurs in war zones. Wounded soldiers and soldiers under attack may die if a sleep-deprived pilot does not risk flying a rescue or support mission. The risk-benefit ratio varies for sleepy highway drivers, sleepy commercial pilots, sleepy rescue pilots, and sleepy doctors. Making good decisions depends on being able to assess these risks and benefits accurately.

It is important to know from a controlled study if indeed that fatigue and sleep loss do not contribute to increased mortality and increased morbidity by cardiac surgeons. Although Institutional Review Boards presumably would not allow a study comparing sleep deprived and nonsleep deprived surgeons, simulated patient surgery may help to answer some answers just as it has with flight simulator and driving simulator studies. Simulators might increase learning and training efficiency by allowing residents to schedule learning "procedures" when they are alert. Rather than residents dealing with the variety of patients who haphazardly present during clinical rotations or procedures, clinical rotation time might be supplemented with systematic presentations from a core group of computer-simulated patients

Many other questions still exist. A sample of these follows:

- Can practicing physicians better judge their capabilities than airline pilots, truck drivers, and medical residents to implement countermeasures?
- Because surgeons stand and rounding hospital physicians are up and periodically moving, does this impart greater resistance to fatigue and sleepiness? Does this activity explain why reports note that nearly 3% of errors in anesthesia are fatigue related and none in some studies of surgery?
- What are the consequences of intrinsic sleep disorders (eg, obstructive sleep apnea syndrome in sleep deprived physicians)?
- Do work restrictions of pilots and truck drivers reduce errors? Would work restriction in practicing physicians reduce errors? Should greater efforts be expended in duty hour restriction or in sleep hours extension?
- Will a more nuanced approach to duty hour limitation that incorporates greater amounts of sleep with attention to schedule rotation and nights worked be more effective?
- Does it make sense that society is stricter with airline pilots than surgeons?
- Does education regarding the consequences of insufficient sleep have a beneficial effect? What are the effects (if any) of duty hour limits on the ethos of medicine?
- Would judicious use of alerting agents by physicians reduce errors?

The basic questions are, how often do sleep-related or fatigue-related errors occur, and what can be done to mitigate the problem. For now, although computer-based training may improve education and reduce training hours, attending physicians and medical residents care for the patients, something even the highest powered computer cannot. More well-trained and well-rested physicians (along with auxiliary medical personnel) engaged in data-driven duty hours may be the answer particularly as an aging population requires more care in an increasingly complex profession of medicine.

REFERENCES

1. Steele MT, Ma OJ, Watson WA, et al. The occupational risk of motor vehicle collisions for emergency medicine residents. Acad Emerg Med 1999;6(10): 1050–3.

2. Kowalenko T, Kowalenko J, Gryzbowski M, et al. Emergency medicine resident related auto accidents: is sleep deprivation a risk factor? Acad Emerg Med 2000;7(10):1171.

3. Barger LK, Cade BE, Ayas NT, et al. Extended work shifts and the risk of motor vehicle crashes among interns. N Engl J Med 2005;352(2):125–34.

4. Asch DA, Parker RM. The Libby Zion case: one step forward or two steps backward? N Engl J Med 1988;318(12):771–5.

5. Friedman RC, Bigger JT, Kornfeld DS. The intern and sleep loss. N Engl J Med 1971;285(4):201–3.

6. Friedman RC, Kornfeld DS, Bigger TJ. Psychological problems associated with sleep deprivation in interns. J Med Educ 1973;48(5):436–41.

7. Poulton EC, Hunt GM, Carpenter A, et al. The performance of junior hospital doctors following reduced sleep and long hours of work. Ergonomics 1978;21(4):279–95.

8. Wilkinson RT, Tyler PD, Varey CA. Duty hours of young hospital doctors: effects on the quality of their work. J Occup Psychol 1975;48:219–29.

9. Asken MJ, Raham DC. Resident performance and sleep deprivation: a review. J Med Educ 1983; 58(5):382–8.

10. Lerner BH. A case that shook medicine: how one man's rage over his daughter's death sped reform of doctor training. Washington Post. November 28, 2007; HE01.

11. Report of the Fourth Grand Jury for the April/May term of 1986 concerning the care and treatment of a patient and the supervision of interns and junior residents at a hospital in New York County. New York: Supreme Court of the State of New York, County of New York; 1986. p. 50.

12. Bell BM. Prospects for the future. Bull N Y Acad Med 1991;67(4):385–8.

13. Wallack MK, Chao L. Resident work hours: the evolution of a revolution. Arch Surg 2001;136(12): 1426–31.

14. Holzman IR, Barnett SH. The Bell Commission: ethical implications for the training of physicians. Mt Sinai J Med 2000;67(2):136–9.

15. Laine C, Goldman L, Soukup JR, et al. The impact of a regulation restricting medical house staff working hours on the quality of patient care. JAMA 1993;269(3):374–8.

16. Petersen LA, Brennan TA, O'Neil AC, et al. Does housestaff discontinuity of care increase the risk for preventable adverse events? Ann Intern Med 1994;121(11):866–72.

17. Working conditions and supervision for residents in internal medicine programs: recommendations. American College of Physicians. Ann Intern Med 1989;110(8):657–63.

18. Weinger MB, Ancoli-Israel S. Sleep deprivation and clinical performance. JAMA 2002;287(8):955–7.

19. Zion S. Arrogant docs keep violating my Libby's law. New York Daily News. November 18, 1999.

20. Assessment of hospital compliance with resident working hour and supervision requirements. Albany (NY): New York State Department of Health; 1998.

21. Johnson T. Limitations on residents' working hours at New York teaching hospitals: a status report. Acad Med 2003;78(1):3–8.

22. Kennedy R. Residents' hours termed excessive in hospital study. The New York Times. May 19, 1998; Section A1.

23. Institute of Medicine. To err is human: building a safer health system. Washington, DC: National Academies Press; 2000.

24. Leape LL, Lawthers AG, Brennan TA, et al. Preventing medical injury. QRB Qual Rev Bull 1993;19(5): 144–9.

25. Petition to the occupational safety and health administration requesting that limits be placed on hours worked by medical residents (HRG publication #1570). Washington: Public Citizen Health Research Group; 2002. Available at: http://www.citizen.org/publications/release.cfm?ID=6771. Accessed February 13, 2009.

26. 107th Congress, 1st session H.R. 3236: Patient and Physician Safety and Protection Act of 2001, November 6th, 2001. Available at: http://thomas.loc.gov/cgi-bin/query/z?c107:H.R.3236. Accessed February 13, 2009.

27. Accreditation Council for Graduate Medical Education, Report of the Work Group on Resident Duty Hours and the Learning Environment, June 11, 2002. Available at: http://www.acgme.org. Accessed February 13, 2009.

28. Institute of Medicine. Resident duty hours: enhancing sleep, supervision, and safety. Washington, DC: National Academies Press; 2008.

29. Federal Register, vol 65, No 85, May 2, 2000. p. 25540–611.

30. Pickersgill T. The European working time directive for doctors in training. BMJ 2001;323:1266.

31. Spritz N. Oversight of physicians' conduct by state licensing agencies: Lessons from New York's Libby Zion case. Ann Intern Med 1991;115(3):219–22.

32. Richardson GS, Wyatt JK, Sullivan JP, et al. Objective assessment of sleep and alertness in medical house staff and the impact of protected time for sleep. Sleep 1996;19(9):718–26.

33. Howard SK, Gaba DM, Rosekind MR, et al. The risks and implications of excessive daytime sleepiness in resident physicians. Acad Med 2002; 77(10):1019–25.

34. Barger LK, Ayas NT, Cade BE, et al. Impact of extended-duration shifts on medical errors, adverse events, and attentional failures. PLoS Med 2006;3(12):e487.

35. Taffinder NJ, McManus IC, Gul Y, et al. Effect of sleep deprivation on surgeon's dexterity on laparoscopy simulator. Lancet 1998;352:1191.

36. Grantcharov TP, Bardram L, Funch-Jensen P, et al. Laparoscopic performance after one night on call in a surgical department: prospective study. BMJ 2001;323:1222–3.

37. Eastridge BJ, Hamilton EC, O'Keefe GE, et al. Effect of sleep deprivation on the performance of simulated laparoscopic surgical skill. Am J Surg 2003;186(2):169–74.

38. DeMaria EJ, McBride CL, Broderick TJ, et al. Night call does not impair learning of laparoscopic skills. Surg Innov 2005;12(2):145–9.

39. Haynes DF, Schwedler M, Dyslin DC, et al. Are postoperative complications related to resident sleep deprivation? South Med J 1995;88(3):283–9.

40. McElearney ST, Saalwachter AR, Hedrick TL, et al. Effect of the 80-hour work week on cases performed by general surgery residents. Am Surg 2005;71(7):552–5.

41. Shin S, Britt R, Britt LD. Effect of the 80-hour work week on resident case coverage: corrected article. J Am Coll Surg 2008;207(1):148–50.

42. Baskies MA, Ruchelsman DE, Capeci CM, et al. Operative experience in an orthopaedic surgery residency program: the effect of work-hour restrictions. J Bone Joint Surg 2008;90(4): 924–7.

43. Durkin ET, McDonald R, Munoz A, et al. The impact of work hour restrictions on surgical resident education. J Surg Educ 2008;65(1):54–60.

44. Damadi A, Davis AT, Saxe A, et al. ACGME duty-hour restrictions decrease resident operative volume: a 5-year comparison at an ACGME-accredited university general surgery residency. J Surg Educ 2007;64(5):256–9.

45. Weatherby BA, Rudd JN, Ervin TB, et al. The effect of resident work hour regulations on orthopaedic surgical education. J Surg Orthop Adv 2007; 16(1):19–22.

46. Ayas NT, Barger LK, Cade BE, et al. Extended work duration and the risk of self-reported percutaneous injuries in interns. JAMA 2006;296(9): 1055–62.

47. Ilhan MN, Durukan E, Aras E, et al. Long working hours increase the risk of sharp and needlestick injury in nurses: the need for new policy implication. J Adv Nurs 2006;56(5):563–8.

48. Marcus CL, Loughlin GM. Effect of sleep deprivation on driving safety in housestaff. Sleep 1996; 19(10):763–6.

49. Ware JC, Risser MR, Manser T, et al. Medical resident driving simulator performance following a night on call. Behav Sleep Med 2006;4(1):1–12.

50. Dawson D, Reid K. Fatigue, alcohol and performance impairment. Nature 1997;388:235.

51. Arnedt JT, Owens J, Crouch M, et al. Neurobehavioral performance of residents after heavy night call vs after alcohol ingestion. JAMA 2005;294(9): 1025–33.

52. Arnedt JT, Wilde GJ, Munt PW, et al. Simulated driving performance following prolonged wakefulness and alcohol consumption: separate and combined contributions to impairment. J Sleep Res 2000;9(3):233–41.

53. Gopal R, Glasheen JJ, Miyoshi TJ, et al. Burnout and internal medicine resident work-hour restrictions. Arch Intern Med 2005;165(22):2595–600.

54. Collier VU, McCue JD, Markus A, et al. Stress in medical residency: status quo after a decade of reform? Ann Intern Med 2002;136(5):384–90.

55. Papp KK, Stoller EP, Sage P, et al. The effects of sleep loss and fatigue on resident-physicians: a multi-institutional, mixed method study. Acad Med 2004;79(5):394–406.

56. Small GW. House officer stress syndrome. Psychosomatics 1981;22(10):860–9.

57. Buddeberg-Fischer B, Klaghofer R, Stamm M, et al. Work stress and reduced health in young physicians: prospective evidence from Swiss residents. Int Arch Occup Environ Health 2008; 82(1):31–8.

58. Kasi PM, Kassi M, Khawar T. Excessive work hours of physicians in training: maladaptive coping strategies. PLoS Med 2007;4(9):e279.

59. West CP, Huschka MM, Novotny PJ, et al. Association of perceived medical errors with resident distress and empathy: a prospective longitudinal study. JAMA 2006;296(9):1071–8.

60. Landrigan CP, Rothschild JM, Cronin JW, et al. Effect of reducing interns' work hours on serious medical errors in intensive care units. N Engl J Med 2004;351(18):1838–48.

61. Lockley SW, Cronin JW, Evans EE, et al. Effect of reducing interns' weekly work hours on sleep and attentional failures. N Engl J Med 2004;351(18): 1829–37.

62. Horwitz LI, Kosiborod M, Lin Z, et al. Changes in outcomes for internal medicine inpatients after work-hour regulations. Ann Intern Med 2007; 147(2):97–103.

63. Horwitz LI, Krumholz HM, Green ML, et al. Transfers of patient care between house staff on internal medicine wards: a national survey. Arch Intern Med 2006;166(11):1173–7.

64. Bhavasar J, Montgomery D, Li J, et al. Impact of duty hours restrictions on quality of care and clinical outcomes. Am J Med 2007;120(11): 968–74.

65. Schuberth JL, Elasy TA, Butler J, et al. Effect of short call admission on length of stay and quality of care for acute decompensated heart failure. Circulation 2008;117(20):2637–44.

66. Landrigan CP, Fahrenkopf AM, Lewin D, et al. Effects of the Accreditation Council For Graduate Medical Education duty hour limits on sleep, work hours, and safety. Pediatrics 2008;122(2):250–8.

67. Shetty KD, Bhattacharya J. Changes in hospital mortality associated with residency work-hour regulations. Ann Intern Med 2007;147(2):73–80.

68. Volpp KG, Rosen AK, Rosenbaum PR, et al. Mortality among hospitalized Medicare beneficiaries in the first 2 years following ACGME resident duty hour reform. JAMA 2007;298(9):975–83.

69. Volpp KG, Rosen AK, Rosenbaum PR, et al. Mortality among patients in VA hospitals in the first 2 years following ACGME resident duty hour reform. JAMA 2007;298(9):984–92.

70. Morrison CA, Wyatt MM, Carrick MM. Impact of the 80-hour work week on mortality and morbidity in trauma patients: an analysis of the national trauma data bank. J Surg Res 2009;154(1):157–62.

71. Lin GA, Beck DC, Garbutt JM. Residents' perceptions of the effects of work hour limitations at a large teaching hospital. Acad Med 2006; 81(1):63–7.

72. Goitein L, Shanafelt TD, Wipf JE, et al. The effects of work-hour limitations on resident well-being, patient care, and education in an internal medicine residency program. Arch Intern Med 2005;165(22): 2601–6.

73. Cappuccio FP, Bakewell A, Taggart FM, et al. Implementing a 48 h EWTD-compliant rotation for junior doctors in the UK does not compromise patient's safety: assessor-blind pilot comparison. QJM 2009;102(4):271–82.

74. Gander P, Purnell H, Garden A, et al. Work patterns and fatigue-related risk among junior doctors. Occup Environ Med 2007;64(11):733–8.

75. Stenuit P, Kerkhofs M. Age modulates the effects of sleep restriction in women. Sleep 2005;28(10): 1283–8.

76. Ellman PI, Law MG, Tache-Leon C, et al. Sleep deprivation does not affect operative results in cardiac surgery. Ann Thorac Surg 78(3):906–911 [discussion: 906–11].

77. Totaro P. Sleep deprivation and results in cardiac surgery: dangerous study with very dangerous conclusions. Ann Thorac Surg 80(6): 2420 [author reply 2420–1].

78. Ellman PI, Kron IL, Alvis JS, et al. Acute sleep deprivation in the thoracic surgical resident does not affect operative outcomes. Ann Thorac Surg 2005;80(1):60–4 [discussion: 64–5].

79. Morris GP, Morris RW. Anaesthesia and fatigue: an analysis of the first 10 years of the Australian Incident Monitoring Study 1987–1997. Anaesth Intensive Care 2000;28(3):300–4.

80. Balkin TJ, Rupp T, Picchioni D, et al. Sleep loss and sleepiness: current issues. Chest 2008;134(3): 653–60.

81. Van Dongen HP, Maislin G, Mullington JM, et al. The cumulative cost of additional wakefulness: dose-response effects on neurobehavioral functions and sleep physiology from chronic sleep restriction and total sleep deprivation. Sleep 2003;26(2):117–26.

82. Diekelmann S, Landolt HP, Lahl O, et al. Sleep loss produces false memories. PLoS One 2008;3(10): e3512.

83. Dinges DF, Pack F, Williams K, et al. Cumulative sleepiness, mood disturbance, and psychomotor vigilance performance decrements during a week of sleep restricted to 4-5 hours per night. Sleep 1997;20(4):267–77.

84. Killgore WD, Grugle NL, Killgore DB, et al. Restoration of risk-propensity during sleep deprivation: caffeine, dextroamphetamine, and modafinil. Aviat Space Environ Med 2008;79(9):867–74.

85. Killgore WD, Kahn-Greene ET, Killgore DB, et al. Effects of acute caffeine withdrawal on Short Category Test performance in sleep-deprived individuals. Percept Mot Skills 2007;105(3 Pt 2):1265–74.

86. Keane MA, James JE. Effects of dietary caffeine on EEG, performance and mood when rested and sleep restricted. Hum Psychopharmacol 2008; 23(8):669–80.

87. Mednick SC, Cai DJ, Kanady J, et al. Comparing the benefits of caffeine, naps and placebo on verbal, motor and perceptual memory. Behav Brain Res 2008;193(1):79–86.

88. Chen I, Vorona R, Chiu R, et al. A survey of subjective sleepiness and consequences in attending physicians. Behav Sleep Med 2008;6(1):1–15.

89. Attarian H, Schuman C. Excessive daytime sleepiness among practicing physicians. J Clin Sleep Med 2007;3(1):87.

90. Umehara K, Ohya Y, Kawakami N, et al. Association of work-related factors with psychosocial job stressors and psychosomatic symptoms among Japanese pediatricians. J Occup Health 2007; 49(6):467–81.

91. Gadacz TR, Bason JJ. A survey of the work effort of full-time surgeons of the Southeastern Surgical Congress. Am Surg 2005;71(8):674–81.

92. Promecene PA, Schneider KM, Monga M. Work hours for practicing obstetrician-gynecologists: the reality of life after residency. Am J Obstet Gynecol 2003;189(3):631–3.

93. Parkes JD, Chen SY, Clift SJ, et al. The clinical diagnosis of the narcoleptic syndrome. J Sleep Res 1998;7(1):41–52.

94. Johns M, Hocking B. Daytime sleepiness and sleep habits of Australian workers. Sleep 1997;20(10): 844–9.

95. Maycock G. Sleepiness and driving: the experience of heavy goods vehicle drivers in the UK. J Sleep Res 1997;6(4):238–11.

96. Aloe F, Pedroso A, Tavares SM. Epworth sleepiness scale outcome in 616 Brazilian medical students. Arq Neuropsiquiatr 1997;55(2):220–6.

97. Mion G, Ricouard S. Mortality related to anesthesia and sleep deprivation in medical doctors. Anesthesiology 2007;107(3):512 [author reply 512].

98. Vela-Bueno A, Moreno-Jimenez B, Rodriguez-Munoz A, et al. Insomnia and sleep quality among primary care physicians with low and high burnout levels. J Psychosom Res 2008; 64(4):435–42.

99. Ekstedt M, Fagerberg I. Lived experiences of the time preceding burnout. J Adv Nurs 2005;49(1): 59–67.

100. NHTSA (2006). Traffic Safety Facts 2004: a compilation of motor vehicle crash data from the fatality analysis reporting system and the general estimates system.

101. Vanlaar W, Simpson H, Mayhew D, et al. Fatigued and drowsy driving: a survey of attitudes, opinions and behaviors. J Safety Res 2008;39(3):303–9.

102. Weingart SN, Wilson RM, Gibberd RW, et al. Epidemiology of medical error. BMJ 2000;320(7237): 774–7,

103. Roehrs T, Burduvali E, Bonahoom A, et al. Ethanol and sleep loss: a "dose" comparison of impairing effects. Sleep 2003;26(8):981–5.

104. Lockley SW, Brainard GC, Czeisler CA. High sensitivity of the human circadian melatonin rhythm to resetting by short wavelength light. J Clin Endocrinol Metab 2003;88(9):4502–5.

105. Wesensten NJ, Kilgore WD, Balkin TJ. Performance and alertness effects of caffeine, dextroamphetamine, and modafinil during sleep deprivation. J Sleep Res 2005;14(3):255–66.

Cognitive Mechanisms in Chronic Insomnia: Processes and Prospects

Katherine A. Kaplan, MA, Lisa S. Talbot, MA,
Allison G. Harvey, PhD*

KEYWORDS

- Insomnia • Cognition • Worry • Rumination
- Monitoring • Misperception of sleep

AN OVERVIEW OF COGNITIVE PROCESSES

Cognition broadly incorporates all mental processes, including attention, perception, memory, attributions, expectations, and beliefs. In part because of the seminal work of Aaron T. Beck (eg, see Ref[1]), cognitive theories and treatments for psychological disorders have become increasingly well-recognized. Insomnia, too, has received attention from cognitive theorists and therapists for more than 40 years. Each decade of empirical inquiry has introduced and refined our understanding of cognitive processes in chronic insomnia.

Some of the earliest research on cognitive processes focused on the role of attribution and expectation on sleep onset latency and continuity.[2,3] At around the same time, researchers began to notice perceptual processes at play; several different groups reported that individuals who had insomnia tended to overestimate wakefulness and underestimate total sleep time.[4,5] In line with these findings, early research suggested that individuals who had insomnia, relative to good sleepers, were more likely to report having been awake when roused from stage 2 sleep.[6,7] Empirical work in the 1980s began to explore the role of cognitive arousal in insomnia (eg, see Ref[8]) along with intrusive and worrisome pre-sleep thoughts.[9] Seminal work in the 1990s highlighted the importance of unhelpful beliefs about sleep[10] and delineated the content of pre-sleep intrusive thoughts.[11,12] The last decade has ushered in an increase in empirical attention to other cognitive mechanisms in insomnia, including attention to threat and the use of safety behaviors to allay perceived threats.[13–15]

This article summarizes the state of the evidence on cognitive mechanisms in chronic insomnia. It focuses on five established processes: worry and rumination, monitoring for threat, misperception of sleep, unhelpful beliefs, and the safety behaviors that prevent disconfirmation of those unhelpful beliefs. Promising areas of future research on emerging and proposed cognitive processes are discussed. The article concludes with a treatment update on the potential to incorporate current empirical evidence into cognitive behavioral therapy for insomnia (CBT-I).

At the outset, the authors emphasize that every disorder—insomnia included—is likely to have contributions at every level of explanation; cognitive, physiological, genetic, cultural, social, and personality factors likely interact to produce a pattern of chronic insomnia. As such, the focus here is on the cognitive level of explanation, but with the explicit recognition that an exciting and fertile domain for future research will be to delineate the ways in which various levels of representation interact so that integrated models reflecting the true complexity of the disorder can be proposed.

COGNITIVE PROCESSES IN CHRONIC INSOMNIA

The authors have reviewed the empirical status of several cognitive processes in other publications.[14,15] This section focuses on updating the evidence accrued over the previous 5 years.

Department of Psychology, University of California, Berkeley, 3210 Tolman Hall #1650, Berkeley, CA 94720-1650, USA
* Corresponding author.
E-mail address: aharvey@berkeley.edu (A.G. Harvey).

Sleep Med Clin 4 (2009) 541–548
doi:10.1016/j.jsmc.2009.07.007
1556-407X/09/$ – see front matter. Published by Elsevier Inc.

Thought Processes: Worry and Rumination

Summary

It is well established that individuals who have chronic insomnia worry while in bed about a range of topics, including the failure to fall asleep (eg, see Ref[12]). A cognitive model implicating worry[16] posits that worry activates the sympathetic nervous system and corresponding physiological arousal, which hinders sleep onset.[13] Rumination is a related cognitive process that may also disrupt sleep. Rumination and worry may be distinguished temporally: whereas worry has been operationalized as distress regarding future events, rumination concerns thoughts of previous events or current symptoms.[17] Both worry and rumination may heighten physiologic arousal, thereby inhibiting sleep.

State of the evidence

Over several decades we know that experimental manipulations designed to increase worry in good sleepers result in an increase in sleep-onset insomnia,[9,18] and that experimental manipulations designed to decrease worry in patients who have insomnia shorten sleep-onset insomnia.[19,20] A creative set of studies has been published more recently that confirms and extends these findings. Research in this area has continued to move toward causal experimental designs, primarily by way of manipulating pre-sleep worry to observe subsequent effects on sleep.

One recent experimental study sought to manipulate the approach to pre-sleep worries. Individuals who had insomnia were asked to either (1) produce solutions to worries ("constructive worry") in the early evening, or (2) to list their worries and fill out worry questionnaires. The constructive worry group reported less cognitive arousal before bedtime and spent less time awake overall.[21] Such evidence suggests that structured evening problem solving can reduce pre-sleep cognitive arousal.

In a recent study designed to test the relationship between sleeplessness and worry, 96 undergraduates grouped into high or low worriers based on their responses on the Penn State Worry Questionnaire were given either 300 mg caffeine (to induce sleeplessness) or a placebo before sleep. High worriers displayed less total sleep time as measured by actigraphy, suggesting worry may be a risk factor in promoting sleeplessness. High worriers did not report increased worry thoughts compared with low worriers in the face of sleeplessness, suggesting insomnia can occur in both worried and nonworried individuals.[22]

In a cross-sectional study designed to evaluate the relationship between worry and poor sleep in relatively new (poor sleep 3–6 months) and chronic (poor sleep 7–12 months) insomnia sufferers, sleep-related worries were associated with poorer perceived sleep in individuals who had chronic, but not new, insomnia. This finding suggests that worries about sleep become tied to perceived poor sleep over time.[23]

Given that the relationship between pre-sleep intrusive worry and pre-sleep ruminative thoughts is still unclear, researchers have begun to incorporate both of these constructs in a single experimental paradigm. Although not specifically focused on insomnia, Guastella and Molds[24] examined the relationship between rumination and sleep quality following a stressful midterm examination in an undergraduate sample. Individuals who had high-trait and low-trait ruminative response styles[17] were asked to either ruminate about the examination ("think about how you felt when you were taking the test today") or distract ("think about clouds forming in the sky") before sleep. The following morning, participants filled out questionnaires on intrusive pre-sleep worry thoughts and overall sleep quality. A significant interaction was found, such that individuals who had high-trait rumination asked to ruminate before sleep reported reduced sleep quality. Intrusive pre-sleep worry was increased in high-trait ruminators but was not increased by the experimental manipulation (ie, no interaction was found). Such results suggest that high-trait ruminators experience more pre-sleep worry and, if in a ruminative state, suffer from poorer sleep quality.

Providing further support for the role of rumination in insomnia, a correlation study revealed that self-reported poor sleepers were more likely to ruminate.[25] Moreover, the content of this rumination was symptom specific, related to feelings of sadness, impaired concentration, and fatigue.

Attentional Processes: Monitoring for Threat

Summary

Attentional processes have been incorporated into several theoretical models of insomnia.[13,16,26] The experimental evidence suggests that, when anxious, individuals attend to a narrower range of environmental stimuli, so attention becomes preferentially focused on potential threats.[26] Within the context of insomnia, the potential threats are sleep-related. These sleep-related threats can be internal, such as unpleasant bodily sensations, or external, such as environmental noises or conditions. Because physiological arousal heightens the bodily sensations one might detect, monitor for, and attend to, arousal symptoms create further impetus for worry and rumination, resulting in an escalating vicious cycle.[16]

State of the evidence

Generally the research on attentional processes in insomnia has fallen into two categories: computerized information processing tasks (which examine reaction times to make inferences regarding attentional processes) and studies that have used subjective measures (eg, interviews and questionnaires). Taking the former first, in the Emotional Stroop Task participants are presented with a word or list of words, some neutral and some affectively valenced (in this case, sleep-related), printed in various colors.[27] Participants are required to read aloud the color in which the words are printed but to ignore the content of the word. The length of time it takes for the participant to name the color of the ink is examined. An attention bias is inferred if the participant takes longer to name the color of the ink in the sleep-related words. Three studies have used the Stroop task to examine an attentional bias for sleep-related words in insomnia. In two earlier studies (see review in Ref[14]), one study did not find evidence for a sleep-related attentional bias in patients who had primary insomnia,[28] whereas another found that a persistent insomnia group did demonstrate a sleep-related insomnia bias.[29] More recently, an insomnia group was compared with a healthy control group and a sleep expert group (to control for "frequency of concept usage"). The insomnia group demonstrated a sleep-related attentional bias compared with the control group, indicating that the bias likely originates not merely from an enhanced sleep focus but from a more emotional and cognitive involvement with sleep-related stimuli.[30] Moreover, a recent study with sleep-deprived healthy participants did not produce a sleep-related attention bias, suggesting that the attentional bias in patients who have insomnia is unlikely to be primarily explained by the effect of sleepiness.[31]

Another information processing task that has recently been used to examine attention biases in insomnia is the flicker paradigm (eg, see Ref[32]). The flicker paradigm for inducing change blindness (eg, see Ref[33]) involves presenting a visual scene with both bedroom environment and neutral objects. The scene flickers back and forth between the two scenes with one object changing. This process continues until the participant identifies the change. Attentional bias is inferred based on change-detection latency. Two recent insomnia studies have used this methodology. In the first, participants who had primary insomnia exhibited a sleep-related attentional bias (ie, detected the sleep-related object change more quickly than the non-sleep object), whereas good sleepers did not.[34] In the second, individuals who had insomnia exhibited a sleep-related attentional bias relative to both good sleepers and individuals who had delayed sleep phase syndrome (DSPS).[35]

The dot probe[36] is a third information-processing task to assess attentional bias. Two stimuli—one sleep-related word and one neutral—are presented on a screen briefly (eg, 500 milliseconds) following the presentation of a fixation cross. The words then disappear and a dot appears in the location of one of the stimuli. Participants' reaction time to the dot indicates attentional bias (if the participant is faster to respond to the dot when it appears where the sleep-related word previously appeared). Using this paradigm MacMahon and colleagues[37] found a sleep-related attentional bias in the primary insomnia group relative to good sleepers and individuals who had DSPS.

Most studies using information processing tasks thus suggest the existence of an attentional bias in insomnia. An advantage of these studies is that the methodology does not rely on self-report. A disadvantage is that they rely on inference to indicate attentional bias, which has been debated in the literature,[38] and therefore may lack some ecological validity.

A complementary line of research has examined the role of attentional biases using varied methodologies (eg, diary, interview, questionnaire, experimental manipulation), with subjective outcome measures. For example, an experimental manipulation study demonstrated that a form of monitoring—clock monitoring—resulted in more pre-sleep worry and longer sleep onset latency.[39] An interview study provided evidence for an association between monitoring and increased negative thoughts and use of safety behaviors at night and during the day in patients who had insomnia.[40] Together these studies provide initial evidence that individuals who have insomnia are more prone, compared with good sleepers, to selectively attend to or monitor for external and internal sleep-related threats. Moreover, they suggest that monitoring has adverse consequences for sleep[41] and contributes to a vicious cycle of cognitive processes.[40]

More recently, two studies provide support for the role of attentional processes—and in particular, monitoring—as a cognitive mechanism in insomnia. In the first, participants who had insomnia were randomly assigned to either a monitoring group or a no-monitoring group. On waking in the morning, the monitoring group was instructed to monitor body sensations throughout the day, and the other group was instructed to distract from body sensations. Results indicated that the monitoring group reported more negative thoughts, safety behaviors, and daytime sleepiness.[42] A second recent study examined the association between coping disposition (eg, tendency to monitor) and insomnia. Results indicated that individuals who had primary insomnia were more likely to use monitoring as a coping strategy.[43]

In sum, accumulating evidence suggests that attentional biases are present in insomnia. Such attentional biases not only contribute to insomnia but also can exacerbate perceived daytime impairment.

Perceptual Processes: Misperception of Sleep

Summary

Several research studies have documented a tendency toward a discrepancy between objective estimates of sleep parameters and an individual's subjective perception of sleep continuity and duration in insomnia (eg, see Refs[44,45]). Although it may be argued that traditional methods of sleep measurement may not be sufficiently sensitive, it may also be the case that individuals may become more anxious about, and consumed with, their perceived sleep problem. Such vigilance toward the sleep state may lead the individual to overestimate the amount of time spent awake and underestimate the time spent asleep. These two accounts of sleep state misperception (ie, a measurement problem versus a perceptual problem) are not mutually exclusive (see Ref[15] for specific mechanisms and further explanation).

State of the evidence

Notably, an experimental study showed that the misperception of sleep is not attributable to insomnia patients' exhibiting general deficits in time estimation abilities.[46] Another study replicated this finding by demonstrating that there were no differences between good and poor sleepers in estimating time in non-sleep settings.[47] This study also indicated that poor sleepers underestimate their sleep and overestimate their time spent awake, whereas good sleepers do the opposite.[41]

Many of the cognitive processes discussed in this article are interrelated. For example, two experimental studies illustrate the contribution of monitoring to misperception. In the first study, participants were randomly assigned to a clock monitoring group or a digital display monitoring group as they were trying to get to sleep. The clock monitoring group exhibited a greater discrepancy between their subjective estimate of sleep onset latency and the objective estimate; that is, participants overestimated their sleep onset latency

when they monitored the clock.[39] In the second study,[48] three groups of individuals who had insomnia were randomly assigned to a self-focus group, a monitoring group, or a no-instruction group. Participants in the self-focus group were instructed to "pay attention to your image on the TV monitor" and in the monitoring group to "pay attention to your thoughts, body, mood, and ability to perform" while completing a battery of challenging mental tasks. Self-focus was defined as focusing on internal thoughts and feelings—both present and past—whereas monitoring was explained as focusing on cues presenting a current threat. The results indicated that the self-focus group perceived their performance as worse on the test compared with the no-instruction group, although their performance did not in fact differ. Together, these results demonstrate that monitoring is one mechanism contributing to misperception. Moreover, misperception among individuals who have insomnia adversely affects daytime functioning.

Attributional Processes: Unhelpful Beliefs About Sleep

Summary

In seminal research from the 1990s, Morin (eg, see Ref[10]) highlighted the role of unhelpful beliefs about sleep in insomnia. It has been suggested that these unhelpful beliefs may exacerbate intrusive and worrisome thoughts throughout the day and night, contributing to the development and maintenance of sleep disturbance.[16] An unhelpful belief in insomnia might take the form of an individual's believing he or she needs to sleep through the night with no awakenings to feel refreshed. Such a belief is unhelpful in that awakenings are a natural part of nocturnal sleep (eg, see Ref[49]); worry related to this belief might take the form of an individual who, once awakened at night, believes that this fragmented sleep will result in impaired work performance the following day.

State of the evidence

The vast majority of research on unhelpful beliefs in insomnia has used the Dysfunctional Beliefs and Attitudes About Sleep Scale.[50–52] CBT-I treatment trials have reported that that a reduction in DBAS scores predicts better treatment outcome.[53,54] One recent study explored unhelpful sleep beliefs in insomnia of a short duration (3–12 months). Sixty-four individuals participating in group CBT-I reported pre- and posttreatment DBAS scores.[55] Reductions in DBAS scores were weakly related to the outcome variables. Namely, reductions in unhelpful beliefs related to improvement in diary-reported sleep efficiency and subjective ratings of daytime sleepiness, but beliefs had no predictive relationship to the other sleep or daytime variables surveyed. The insomnia treated in this study was short term and, as such, may not have been chronic enough to germinate the unhelpful beliefs seen in many other studies.

In contrast, one recent large-scale correlative study found strong evidence for the role of unhelpful beliefs in maintaining chronic insomnia. In a random sample drawn from the population of Sweden, Jansson and Linton[56] surveyed unhelpful beliefs about sleep, depression, anxiety and arousal at two time points spaced 1 year apart. Researchers found that unhelpful beliefs about sleep—in particular, beliefs about the long-term negative consequences of insomnia—predicted a chronic pattern of poor sleep over and above arousal, depression, anxiety, and beliefs about short-term consequences. Such research provides strong associative evidence for the relationship between sleep beliefs and chronic insomnia.

Safety Behaviors

Summary

Closely related to unhelpful beliefs are so-called "safety behaviors." Safety behaviors are actions taken to avoid feared outcomes that are maladaptive in two ways: (1) they prevent disconfirmation of the unhelpful beliefs, and (2) they increase the likelihood that the feared outcomes will occur. Individuals who have insomnia, in an attempt to cope with anxiety related to unhelpful beliefs about sleep, often use safety behaviors.[57] In the previous section, we described an individual who endorsed the unhelpful belief that only solid, uninterrupted sleep would allow unimpaired work performance the next day. To prevent nocturnal awakenings, this individual might develop a routine of safety behaviors including never going out in the evening, wearing earplugs, and using a sound machine as she slept. Engaging in these behaviors, although understandable in a general way, prevents the individual from clearly learning that she can get adequate sleep even if the routine is broken. Paradoxically, they may make the feared outcome more likely to occur. Not going out in the evening increases the chance that the person will become preoccupied with her sleep, and may contribute to rumination/worry and sad mood. Earplugs can be effective in certain circumstances, but they can also contribute to sleep problems if they are uncomfortable or if they cause the person to strain to try to hear things in the environment. A sound machine can facilitate awakenings in the night.

State of the evidence

One recent study directly examined the relationship between beliefs about sleep and use of safety behaviors.[58] Forty participants completed standard measures of insomnia severity, depression and anxiety, and the DBAS. Following this, individuals kept a sleep diary for 14 consecutive days and recorded the sleep safety behaviors used each day. Holding more unhelpful beliefs about sleep (ie, higher DBAS scores) predicted the use of daily safety behaviors, although depression explained more of the variance in safety behavior use. Such research provides evidence for the hypothesized relationship between sleep beliefs and safety behaviors and suggests depression as a third construct of importance in understanding chronic insomnia.

TREATMENT IMPLICATIONS

The most recent detailed review of treatments for insomnia conducted by the American Academy of Sleep Medicine concluded that cognitive therapy has received insufficient evaluation.[59] Since then an open trial of cognitive therapy for insomnia has been published (n = 19).[60] The therapy was derived from a cognitive model.[16] It aimed to reverse the five cognitive maintaining processes reviewed in this article during both the night and the day. Assessments were completed pretreatment, posttreatment, and at 3-, 6-, and 12-month follow-up. The significant improvement in both nighttime and daytime impairment evident at the posttreatment assessment was retained up to the 12-month follow-up. These preliminary results suggest that cognitive therapy is (1) acceptable to patients who have insomnia, (2) improves sleep, and (3) improves daytime functioning. The results were strongest for measures of daytime functioning and moderate for measures derived from the sleep diary. We await replication of these findings within a sufficiently powered randomized controlled trial, however.

FUTURE PROSPECTS IN COGNITIVE PROCESSES
Savoring and Gratitude

One promising area for future research involves the use of savoring to displace pre-sleep worry and negative associations. Savoring consists of attending to, appreciating, and enhancing positive experiences had during the day.[61,62] Savoring may be helpful in multiple ways. First of all, associating the bed and the pre-sleep period with positive thoughts may work against conditioned arousal. Second, training in recalling pleasant imagery or visualization in the pre-sleep period may also replace pre-sleep worry.[63] Third, this approach is also consistent with Brewin's[64] review of the evidence that conditioned fear reactions in animals can easily be reinstated or renewed by re-exposing the animal to the unconditioned stimulus, placing it in a new context, and then representing the conditioned stimulus. Traditionally, therapies such as CBT aim to modify negative information in memory. Given the animal learning data, Brewin suggested that therapies may be more effective if they work to more explicitly train quick connections to positive material so that the therapy is changing the relative activation of the positive versus negative representations, such that the positive ones are the most easily accessible.

Interestingly, recent research suggests that gratitude may also have beneficial effects on sleep.[65,66] In a series of studies, participants were instructed to write "up to five things in your life that you are grateful or thankful for"[56] weekly or daily. Gratitude was associated with greater positive affect and well-being. In a third study, 65 individuals who had neuromuscular diseases kept daily logs of health behaviors and affect; half were also instructed to list things they were grateful for in the early evening. Of relevance to sleep disturbance, individuals in the gratitude condition reported more hours of sleep and feeling more refreshed on waking than the non-gratitude group.[55] Further, another study showed that higher scores on trait-gratitude predicted better sleep outcomes and, importantly, the relationship between gratitude and better sleep was mediated by more positive and fewer negative pre-sleep cognitions.[56] Taken together, gratitude represents one promising area of for future research.

Expectations

Expectations about sleep episodes may also play a role in the development and maintenance of insomnia. Expectations are operationalized here as specific thoughts, beliefs, and attitudes about the immediate sleep episode. These expectations differ from unhelpful beliefs about sleep in that they are specific to the imminent sleep period. For example, there is evidence that expecting to wake at a certain time may set off physiologic processes, including the release of cortisol, that prepare the body to wake up at the expected rise time.[67] In insomnia, expectations may have deleterious consequences. The insomnia sufferer who strongly endorses being "up like an alarm clock at 4:30 AM" may actually be promoting his or own pattern by stimulating the release of cortisol in accordance with the expected wake-up time. Although intriguing, this proposal has yet to be empirically validated in patients who have insomnia.

Daytime Cognitive Processes

It is clear that processes operating during the daytime are important to the maintenance of insomnia (eg, see Ref[10]). Indeed, daytime processes may be as important as nighttime processes in the maintenance of insomnia.[16] To date, there has been little research investigating daytime cognitive processes in chronic insomnia. Three such studies are reviewed here to highlight the promise of research in this area.

In the first study, the authors tested the prediction that, relative to good sleepers, patients who have insomnia catastrophize more and that this catastrophizing is associated with increased negative affect and heightened perception of threat.[68] Although we theorized at the time that the procedure and result indicated the catastrophizing that might occur in bed, it is equally plausible that this research, conducted during the daytime period, more accurately characterized insomnia patients' thought processes in the day.

Providing further evidence for the importance of daytime processes, we evaluated the role of sleep perception on daytime functioning. Individuals who had insomnia slept with actigraphy and, on waking, were given either positive or negative feedback about their sleep. Those who received negative feedback (ie, that sleep quality was poor) exhibited more negative thoughts, sleepiness, monitoring for sleep-related threat, and safety behaviors throughout the day.[69] In other words, daytime processes related to the experimental manipulation that was delivered rather than to veridical sleep.

Sleep quality and daytime functioning were further evaluated in a recent study using a "speak freely" procedure, interview, and sleep diary. Results suggested that both individuals who had insomnia and normal sleepers use subjective feelings the day after sleep (tiredness on waking and throughout the day, feeling rested and restored on waking, and number of awakenings during the night) as the most important criteria for judging their previous night's sleep quality. Insomnia patients considered a greater number of variables as important for judging their sleep quality, however.[70]

In sum, it will be the exciting task of future research to delineate daytime cognitive processes that contribute to the development and maintenance of chronic insomnia.

REFERENCES

1. Beck AT. Cognitive therapy and the emotional disorders. New York: International Universities Press; 1976.

2. Bootzin RR, Herman CP, Nicassio P. The power of suggestion: another examination of misattribution and insomnia. J Pers Soc Psychol 1976;34:673–9.

3. Steinmark SW, Borkovec TD. Active and placebo treatment effects on moderate insomnia under counterdemand and positive demand instructions. J Abnorm Psychol 1974;83:157–63.

4. Bixler EO, Kales A, Leo LA, et al. A comparison of subjective estimates and objective sleep laboratory findings in insomnia patients [abstract]. J Sleep Res 1973;2:143.

5. Carskadon MA, Dement WC, Mitler MM, et al. Self-reports versus sleep laboratory findings in 122 drug-free subjects with complaints of chronic insomnia. Am J Psychiatry 1976;133(12):1382–8.

6. Rechtschaffen A, Kales A. A manual of standardized terminology, techniques and scoring system for sleep stages of human subjects. Bethesda (MD): U.S. Dept. of Health Education and Welfare; 1968.

7. Borkovec TD, Lane TW, VanOot PH. Phenomenology of sleep among insomniacs and good sleepers: wakefulness experience when cortically asleep. J Abnorm Psychol 1981;90:607–9.

8. Lichstein KL, Rosenthal TL. Insomniacs' perceptions of cognitive versus somatic determinants of sleep disturbance. J Abnorm Psychol 1980;89:105–7.

9. Gross RT, Borkovec TD. Effects of a cognitive intrusion manipulation on the sleep-onset latency of good sleepers. Behav Ther 1982;13:112–6.

10. Morin CM. Insomnia: psychological assessment and management. New York: Guilford Press; 1993.

11. Watts FN, Coyle K, East MP. The contribution of worry to insomnia. Br J Clin Psychol 1994;33:211–20.

12. Wicklow A, Espie CA. Intrusive thoughts and their relationship to actigraphic measurement of sleep: towards a cognitive model of insomnia. Behav Res Ther 2000;38(7):679–93.

13. Espie CA. Insomnia: conceptual issues in the development, persistence, and treatment of sleep disorder in adults. Annu Rev Psychol 2002;53:215–43.

14. Harvey AG, Tang NKY, Browning L. Cognitive approaches to insomnia. Clin Psychol Rev 2005; 25:593–611.

15. Harvey AG. A cognitive theory of and therapy for chronic insomnia. An International Quarterly. J Cognit Psychother 2005;19:41–60.

16. Harvey AG. A cognitive model of insomnia. Behav Res Ther 2002;40:869–94.

17. Nolen-Hoeksema S. Responses to depression and their effects on the duration of depressive episodes. J Abnorm Psychol 1991;100:569–82.

18. Ansfield ME, Wegner DM, Bowser R. Ironic effects of sleep urgency. Behav Res Ther 1996;34:523–31.

19. Levey AB, Aldaz JA, Watts FN, et al. Articulatory suppression and the treatment of insomnia. Behav Res Ther 1991;29:85–9.

20. Haynes SN, Adams A, Franzen M. The effects of presleep stress on sleep-onset insomnia. J Abnorm Psychol 1981;90:601–6.

21. Carney CE, Waters WF. Effects of a structured problem-solving procedure on pre-sleep cognitive arousal in college students with insomnia. Behav Sleep Med 2006;4(1):13–28.

22. Omvik S, Pallesen S, Bjorvatn B, et al. Night-time thoughts in high and low worriers: reaction to caffeine-induced sleeplessness. Behav Res Ther 2007;45(4):715–27.

23. Jansson M, Linton SJ. The development of insomnia within the first year: a focus on worry. Br J Health Psychol 2006;11(Pt 3):501–11.

24. Guastella A, Moulds M. The impact of rumination on sleep quality following a stressful life event. Pers Individ Dif 2007;42:1151–62.

25. Carney CE, Edinger JD, Meyer B, et al. Symptom-focused rumination and sleep disturbance. Behav Sleep Med 2006;4(4):228–41.

26. Dalgleish T, Watts FN. Biases of attention and memory in disorders of anxiety and depression. Clin Psychol Rev 1990;10:589–604.

27. Williams J, Mathews A, MacLoed C. The emotional Stroop task and psychopathology. Psychol Bull 1996;120:3–24.

28. Lundh L-G, Fröding A, Gyllenhammar L, et al. Cognitive bias and memory performance in patients with persistent insomnia. Scand J Behav Ther 1997; 26:27–35.

29. Taylor LM, Espie CA, White CA. Attentional bias in people with acute versus persistent insomnia secondary to cancer. Behav Sleep Med 2003;1(4): 200–12.

30. Spiegelhalder K, Espie C, Nissen C, et al. Sleep-related attentional bias in patients with primary insomnia compared with sleep experts and healthy controls. J Sleep Res 2008;17(2):191–6.

31. Sagaspe P, Sanchez-Ortuno M, Charles A, et al. Effects of sleep deprivation on color-word, emotional, and specific stroop interference and on self-reported anxiety. Brain Cognit 2006;60:76–87.

32. Rensink RA, O'Regan JK, Clark JJ. To see or not to see: the need for attention to perceive changes in scenes. Psychol Sci 1997;8:368–73.

33. Rensink RA. Change detection. Annu Rev Psychol 2002;53:245–77.

34. Jones BT, Macphee LM, Broomfield NM, et al. Sleep-related attentional bias in good, moderate, and poor (primary insomnia) sleepers. J Abnorm Psychol 2005;114(2):249–58.

35. Marchetti LM, Biello SM, Broomfield NM, et al. Who is pre-occupied with sleep? A comparison of attention bias in people with psychophysiological insomnia, delayed sleep phase syndrome and good sleepers using the induced change blindness paradigm. J Sleep Res 2006;15:212–21.

36. MacLeod C, Mathews A, Tata P. Attentional bias in emotional disorders. J Abnorm Psychol 1986;95:15–20.

37. MacMahon KMA, Broomfield NM, Espie CA. Attentional bias for sleep-related stimuli in primary insomnia and delayed sleep phase syndrome using the dot-probe task. Sleep 2006;29:1420–7.

38. Harvey AG, Watkins E, Mansell W, et al. Cognitive behavioural processes across psychological disorders: a transdiagnostic approach to research and treatment. Oxford (UK): Oxford University Press; 2004.

39. Tang NKY, Schmidt DE, Harvey AG. Sleeping with the enemy: clock monitoring in the maintenance of insomnia. J Behav Thor Exp Psychiatry 2007;48:40–55.

40. Semler CN, Harvey AG. An investigation of monitoring for sleep-related threat in primary insomnia. Behav Res Ther 2004;42:1403–20.

41. Tang NK, Harvey AG. Correcting distorted perception of sleep in insomnia: a novel behavioural experiment? Behav Res Ther 2004;42:27–39.

42. Neitzert Semler C, Harvey AG. An experimental investigation of daytime monitoring for sleep-related threat in primary insomnia. Cogn Emot 2007;21(1):146–61.

43. Voss U, Kolling T, Heidenreich T. Role of monitoring and blunting coping styles in primary insomnia. Psychosom Med 2006;68:110–5.

44. Chambers MJ, Keller B. Alert insomniacs: are they really sleep deprived? Clin Psychol Rev 1993;13:649–66.

45. Mercer JD, Bootzin RR, Lack LC. Insomniacs' perception of wake instead of sleep. Sleep 2002; 25(5):564–71.

46. Tang NKY, Harvey AG. Time estimation ability and distorted perception of sleep in insomnia. Behav Sleep Med 2005;3:134–50.

47. Fichten CS, Creti L, Amsel R, et al. Time estimation in good and poor sleepers. J Behav Med 2005;28(6): 1–17.

48. Neitzert Semler C, Harvey AG. Daytime functioning in primary insomnia: does attentional focus contribute to real or perceived impairment? Behav Sleep Med 2006;4(2):85–103.

49. Akerstedt T, Billiard M, Bonnet M, et al. Awakening from sleep. Sleep Med Rev 2002;6:267–86.

50. Morin CM, Stone J, Trinkle D, et al. Dysfunctional beliefs and attitudes about sleep among older adults with and without insomnia complaints. Psychol Aging 1993;8:463–7.

51. Espie CA, Inglis S, Harvey L, et al. Insomniacs' attributions: psychometric properties of the dysfunctional beliefs and attitudes about sleep scale and the sleep disturbance questionnaire. J Psychosom Res 2000;48:141–8.

52. Morin CM, Vallieres A, Ivers H. Dysfunctional beliefs and attitudes about sleep (DBAS): validation of a brief version (DBAS-16). Sleep 2007;30(11):1547–54.

53. Edinger JD, Wohlgemuth WK, Radtke RA, et al. Does cognitive-behavioral insomnia therapy alter dysfunctional beliefs about sleep? Sleep 2001;24:591–9.

54. Morin CM, Blais F, Savard J. Are changes in beliefs and attitudes about sleep related to sleep improvements in the treatment of insomnia? Behav Res Ther 2002;40:741–52.

55. Jansson-Frojmark M, Linton SJ. The role of sleep-related beliefs to improvement in early cognitive behavioral therapy for insomnia. Cogn Behav Ther 2008;37(1):5–13.

56. Jansson M, Linton SJ. Psychological mechanisms in the maintenance of insomnia: arousal, distress, and sleep-related beliefs. Behav Res Ther 2007;45(3): 511–21.

57. Salkovskis PM. The importance of behaviour in the maintenance of anxiety and panic: a cognitive account. Behav Psychother 1991;19:6–19.

58. Woodley J, Smith S. Safety behaviors and dysfunctional beliefs about sleep: testing a cognitive model of the maintenance of insomnia. J Psychosom Res 2006;60(6):551–7.

59. Morin CM, Bootzin RR, Buysse DJ, et al. Psychological and behavioral treatment of insomnia: an update of recent evidence (1998–2004). Sleep 2006;29: 1396–406.

60. Harvey AG, Sharpley A, Ree MJ, et al. An open trial of cognitive therapy for chronic insomnia. Behav Res Ther 2007;45:2491–501.

61. Bryant FB, Veroff J. Savoring: a new model of positive experiences. London (UK): Lawrence Erlbaum; 2007.

62. McMakin DL, Siegle GJ, Shirk SR. Positive emotion regulation coaching for depression. Manuscript submitted for publication.

63. Harvey AG, Payne S. The management of unwanted pre-sleep thoughts in insomnia: distraction with imagery versus general distraction. Behav Res Ther 2002;40:267–77.

64. Brewin CR. Understanding cognitive behaviour therapy: a retrieval competition account. Behav Res Ther 2006;44(6):765–84.

65. Emmons RA, McCullough ME. Counting blessings versus burdens: an experimental investigation of gratitude and subjective well-being in daily life. J Pers Soc Psychol 2003;84(2):377–89.

66. Wood A, Joseph S, Llloyd J, et al. Gratitude influences sleep through the mechanism of pre-sleep cognitions. J Psychosom Res 2009;66(1):43–8.

67. Born J, Hansen K, Marshall L, et al. Timing the end of nocturnal sleep. Nature 1999;397:29–30.

68. Harvey AG, Greennall E. Catastrophic worry in primary insomnia. J Behav Ther Exp Psychiatry 2003;34:11–23.

69. Neitzert Semler C, Harvey AG. Misperception of sleep can adversely affect daytime functioning in insomnia. Behav Res Ther 2005;43:843–56.

70. Harvey AG, Stinson K, Whitaker KL, et al. The subjective meaning of sleep quality: a comparison of individuals with and without insomnia. Sleep 2008;31(3):383–93.

Neurobiologic Mechanisms in Chronic Insomnia

Michael Perlis, PhD[a],*, Phillip Gehrman, PhD[a],
Wilfred R. Pigeon, PhD, CBSM[b], James Findley, PhD[a],
Sean Drummond, PhD[c]

KEYWORDS

- Insomnia • Neurobiology • VLPO • ARAS
- Homeostasis • Inhibition of wakefulness

Insomnia has long been conceptualized in psychologic and physiologic terms[1]; hence, the primary diagnostic classification of "psychophysiologic" insomnia. This diagnostic category[2] was adopted to indicate that this form of sleep disturbance was primary (a disorder vs a symptom) and determined by both psychologic and physiologic factors. Psychologic factors were thought to be related to cognitive phenomena, such as worry and rumination, and behavioral processes, such as instrumental and classical conditioning. Physiologic factors were thought to be related to elevated heart rate, respiration rate, muscle tone, and so forth (ie, elevated end-organ tone or increased metabolic rate). The term "psychophysiologic" insomnia (as opposed to the alternative construction "physiopsychologic" insomnia) also carried with it the implication that this form of insomnia occurs primarily as a physiologic phenomenon. This conceptualization not only calls into question the "primacy of cognition"[3] in insomnia, it leads one to wonder whether somatic hyperarousal (or elevated metabolic rate) is appropriately identified as the primary etiologic factor. The emphasis on physiology seems to be more a matter of historical precedent than the likely possibility that somatic arousal is sufficiently elevated in patients with chronic insomnia to interfere directly with sleep initiation and maintenance.

The alternative perspective is, if "sleep is of the brain, by the brain and for the brain,"[4] that insomnia is better conceptualized in terms of abnormal neurobiology. To support this perspective information is provided (1) regarding the brain structures that are implicated in sleep-wake regulation and how abnormal function within these areas may lead to specific insomnia complaints, and (2) the neurophysiologic control of sleep and wakefulness and how dysregulation at the system level may contribute to the incidence and severity of insomnia. Following this, information is provided on what is known about insomnia in terms of neurobiologic abnormalities as assessed with neurophysiologic, neuroendocrine, and neuroimaging measures. This overview is rounded out with a concluding comment about the dual nature of psychophysiologic insomnia.

STRUCTURES IMPLICATED IN SLEEP-WAKE REGULATION AND DYSREGULATION

Although it is beyond the scope of this article to review every brain structure that is thought to play a role in sleep-wake regulation, a short review serves to illustrate that functional neurobiology may inform how one conceives of the clinical entity of insomnia. Toward this end information is provided on the following brain regions: the

[a] Behavioral Sleep Medicine Program, Department of Psychiatry, University of Pennsylvania, Suite 670, 3535 Market Street, Philadelphia, PA 19104, USA
[b] Department of Psychiatry, Sleep and Neurophysiology Research Laboratory, University of Rochester Medical Center, 300 Crittenden Boulevard, Box PSYCH, Rochester, NY 14642-8409, USA
[c] Laboratory of Sleep and Behavioral Neuroscience, UCSD and VA San Diego Healthcare System, 3350 La Jolla Village Drive, MC 151B, Building 13, 3rd floor, San Diego, CA 92161, USA
* Corresponding author.
E-mail address: mperlis@upenn.edu (M. Perlis).

Sleep Med Clin 4 (2009) 549–558
doi:10.1016/j.jsmc.2009.07.002

pons, the thalamus, the frontal cortex, and the basal ganglia.

Pons

The pons is located in the brainstem and contains nuclei that are related to the coordination of eye and facial movements, facial sensation, hearing, balance, respiration, and the genesis of rapid eye movement (REM) sleep. Given that much of the pons is dedicated to the performance of nonautonomic functions, it follows that the behavioral quiescence of non-REM (NREM) sleep is paralleled by global deactivation within this region. An equally important consideration is the extent to which the aminergic and cholinergic components of the ascending reticular activating system (see later) reside within, or traverse through, the pons. The most straightforward consequence of hyperarousal in the pons on NREM sleep is a direct link to the inability to initiate and maintain sleep. At the level of patient report, this is expected to translate to the complaint of feeling alert while desiring to fall asleep.

Thalamus

The thalamus contains a variety of nuclei that are believed both to process and relay sensory information to various parts of the cerebral cortex. For example, visual information from the eyes travels to the thalamus on the way to the occipital cortex. The thalamus also contains structures (the reticular nuclei) whose function is actively to inhibit sensory flow from the thalamus to the cortex. Increased thalamic activation in nuclei related to sensory processing or decreased activity within the reticular nuclei during sleep could lead to more sensory information reaching the cortex and greater sensory processing perisleep onset or during sleep. Presumably, this is related to the tendency of patients with insomnia to be hyperresponsive to environmental stimuli, which in turn may account for patients' difficulties falling and staying asleep or the perception of shallow sleep. This might be the neurobiologic basis of patients' reports of being "light sleepers."

Frontal Cortex

The frontal lobes contain many subregions involved in cognitive processes related to, among other things, working memory, problem solving, the planning of goal-directed activity, and evaluative judgment.[5] Abnormal activity in the frontal cortex depends on the specific subregion involved and whether the area or "circuit" is inhibitory or excitatory. An example of an excitatory subregion is the dorsolateral prefrontal and left limbic areas.

Activation within these areas is associated with anticipatory anxiety.[6] In insomnia, increased activation within this region likely is associated with the worry and rumination that may interfere with sleep initiation and possibly sleep maintenance. An example of an inhibitory subregion is the orbital frontal cortex (and the cortical-striatal-thalamic-cortical loops).[7] Reduced activation in this region or circuit is associated with behavioral, and likely cognitive, disinhibition of subcortical structures. In this instance, hypoactivation may be associated with the tendency of patients with insomnia to be highly ruminative and their complaint of being unable to "turn their minds off."[8–10]

Basal Ganglia

The primary structures of the basal ganglia (caudate, putamen, globus pallidus, substantia nigra, subthalamic nucleus) and more generally the striatum have major projections from the motor cortex and are known to play a well-defined role in the execution of voluntary movement. In addition, the basal ganglia has been implicated in neurobiologic models of obsessive-compulsive disorder,[11] and found to play a role in the homeostatic regulation of sleep.

With respect to sleep homeostasis, Braun and colleagues[12] have hypothesized that the basal ganglia may be actively involved in slow wave sleep regulation by virtue of their ability to modulate cortical arousal.[13] It is possible that structures within the basal ganglia may, in feed forward fashion, modulate the activity of the reticular nucleus of the thalamus, and in so doing contribute to the homeostatic regulation of sleep.[14] One might speculate that the basal ganglia are not only involved in the homeostatic regulation of sleep, but may actually be the "the sleep homeostat." This may be because the basal ganglia are responsible for both the execution of voluntary movement and potentially the modulation of cortical arousal. Accordingly, they are uniquely situated to modulate cortical arousal based on diurnal activity levels.

At the level of symptom complaint, abnormal metabolism within the basal ganglia during sleep may be associated with a variety of clinical phenomena. To the extent that the circuits are related to inhibition and disinhibition, abnormal activity within these regions may be associated with a patient's tendency to ruminate and worry. Alternatively (or perhaps in addition), abnormal activity in the basal ganglia may be related to the homeostatic dysregulation that seems to occur with insomnia. That is, to the extent that the basal ganglia are related to sleep homeostasis, it may account for the occurrence of sleep initiation and maintenance problems on a given night and for the cyclical pattern of symptoms across time.

NEUROPHYSIOLOGIC CONTROL OF SLEEP AND WAKEFULNESS

Based on the early work of Von Economo[15] and Moruzzi,[16–18] it is well established that cortical arousal is regulated by the ascending reticular activating system (ARAS). This system originates in the brainstem and has two major branches. One branch originates from cholinergic cell groups in the upper pons (including the pedunculopontine and the laterodorsal tegmental nuclei); inputs into the thalamus; and activates the thalamic relays, which densely innervate the cortex. This system, and its source neurons, fire maximally during wakefulness and REM sleep and lowest during NREM sleep.[6,19–21] The other branch originates in the lower pons from a series of neurons including the locus coeruleus (norepinephrine), dorsal and medial raphe (serotonin), and tubero-mammillary cells (histamine) to innervate neurons in the lateral hypothalamic area, the basal fore-brain, and throughout the cortex. This ascending aspect of this system is monoaminergic and the end target neurons are cholinergic or GABAergic. Neurons within this system fire maximally during wakefulness, more slowly during NREM sleep,

and are relatively silent during REM sleep. This description of cortical arousal as it is modulated by the cholinergic and monoaminergic systems was, in 2000, significantly amended with the discovery of orexin (also called hypocretin).[22–25] This neurotransmitter seems to augment activity within the monoaminergic branch of the ARAS (particularly the output from the lateral hypothalamus) and is thought to act in concert with the circadian system to promote the consolidation of wakefulness during the diurnal phase of the 24-hour day. **Fig. 1** provides a schematic representation of the aforementioned arousal systems.

Although the previous description serves to delineate the pathways within the ARAS and their relative degree of activation across the wake, NREM, and REM states, the characterization does not suggest how sleep comes to be initiated, maintained, and terminated in favor of new episodes of wakefulness. To comprehend how this might occur it is necessary to posit that there is either a gating system or a related descending system that exerts influence over the structures that initiate cortical arousal. In the case of the cholinergic branch of the ARAS, there is substantial evidence to suggest that the reticular nucleus of the thalamus serves to block ascending inputs and thereby permit cortical synchronization (ie, sleep). In the case of the monoaminergic branch of the ARAS, investigators during the 1980s and

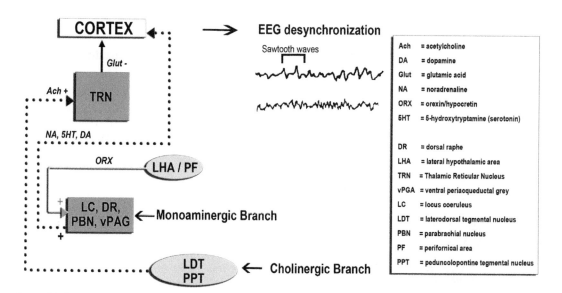

Fig. 1. This figure represents ascending pathways that lead to cortical desynchronization (activation). Although the cholinergic and monoaminergic branches of this system have been well characterized, orexinergic component (and its contribution to the consolidation of wakefulness) is relatively new. One of the many important aspects of this system is that this arousal system is not the same as the ARAS (the fight or flight system) anatomically of functionally. With respect to the latter, the orexin system seems to be under the control of, or intimately related to, the circadian system.

1990s found a candidate mechanism for what might serve as the switch for a "descending de-arousal system," the switch being the ventral lateral preoptic area (VLPO).[6,21] The VLPO is maximally active during sleep; has major outputs to most hypothalamic and brainstem components of the monoaminergic aspect of the ARAS; and contains inhibitory neurotransmitters (ie, galanin and γ-aminobutyric acid [GABA]). The VLPO seems to be uniquely positioned to function as an "off switch" (to inhibit arousal). This putative function was confirmed by Saper and colleagues who have shown that lesions within this region reduce NREM and REM sleep by more than 50%.[6,21]

The Saper group has also demonstrated that the VLPO also has major inputs from the hypothalamic and brainstem components of the monoaminergic aspect of the ARAS and that the VLPO is strongly inhibited by noradrenaline and serotonin. The existence of such inputs and neurotransmitter effects suggests that the VLPO functions not only to inhibit wakefulness but, in turn, is also inhibited by wakefulness. Saper and colleagues[6,21] have likened this reciprocal relationship between the VLPO and the ARAS to the functioning of a "flip-flop circuit." This analogy is taken from electrical engineering and provides a framework for conceptualizing how the wake-promoting and sleep-promoting halves of the circuit are mutually influential. Each half of the circuit strongly inhibits the other, and in so doing creates a bi-stable

feedback loop. When the brain is in a state of wakefulness, sleep is inhibited so that there is a consolidated period of wakefulness. When the switch moves in the sleep direction, wake is inhibited, producing a consolidated period of sleep. This pattern prevents both frequent transitions between sleep and wake and the presence of intermediate states characterized by features of both wakefulness and sleep. **Fig. 2** represents the VLPO's inhibitory influence on the cortex and its bi-stable configuration.

Although elegant, this conceptualization also does not in and of itself explain how sleep is initiated and terminated (ie, it only serves to explain how sleep and wakefulness tend to occur in a consolidated fashion). To accomplish this, there must also be a system that impinges on the circuit and allows for homeostasis and allostasis.

In the case of sleep-wake homeostasis, there must be a process that represents the accumulation of wakefulness or sleep that can act to "trip the switch." The concept of sleep-wake homeostasis (and its interaction with the circadian system) has been described theoretically and tested empirically by Borbely and colleagues.[26–29] In this model, the accumulation of wakefulness is represented by "process S" and is measured in terms of the relationship between the duration of wakefulness and the discharge of slow wave activity during NREM Sleep. To date, the neurobiologic structures that comprise the "sleep homeostat" are unknown. One candidate for a process that may represent

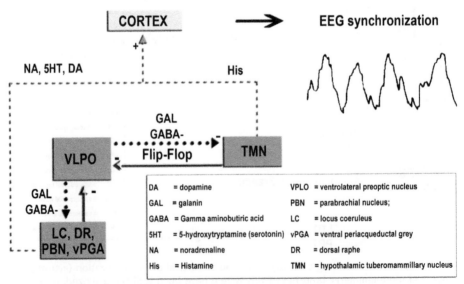

Fig. 2. This figure provides a simplified representation of the "sleep switch", the circuit and ascending pathways that lead to cortical synchronization (deactivation). One of the many important aspects of this system is the mutually inhibitory functioning between the VLPO and the TMN. For a thorough review of this system the reader is referred to Saper and colleagues.[21]

the duration of wakefulness is the accumulation of adenosine within the basal forebrain. Experimental work with this hypothesis has shown that adenosine levels rise in proportion to the duration of wakefulness and when injected into the basal forebrain, adenosine induces sleep and promotes activity within the VLPO.

In the case of sleep-wake allostasis, it has been proposed that orexin neurons within the posterior half of lateral hypothalamus serve to reinforce wakefulness (promote sustained wakefulness) and thereby act as a "finger" on the flip-flop switch that prevents unwanted transitions into sleep (a second possible, albeit highly speculative, candidate mechanism for sleep-wake homeostasis is noted in the discussion regarding the basal ganglia.).

NEUROBIOLOGIC IMPLICATIONS FOR INSOMNIA

The previous description of the normal regulation of sleep and wakefulness suggests that insomnia may occur in association with one of several neurobiologic abnormalities. First, the switch itself may be malfunctioning. Saper and colleagues[6] describe this as follows:

> ...mathematical models show that when either side of a flip-flop neural circuit is weakened, homeostatic forces cause the switch to ride closer to its transition point during both states. As a result, there is an increase in transitions, both during the wake and the sleep periods, regardless of which side is weakened. This is certainly seen in animals with VLPO lesions, which fall asleep about twice as often as normal animals, wake up much more often during their sleep cycle and, on the whole, only sleep for about one-quarter as long per bout - in other words, they wake up and are unable to fall back asleep during the sleep cycle, but also are chronically tired, falling asleep briefly and fitfully during the wake cycle....

This description seems to characterize not so much psychophysiologic insomnia but rather sleep as it occurs in neonates and infants and insomnia as it occurs in the elderly (ie, polyphasic sleep with middle or late insomnia) or in patients with narcolepsy. A malfunctioning switch could also produce an intermediate state characterized by aspects of both sleep and wakefulness. This can be seen in several studies of individuals with insomnia who, compared with good sleepers, show evidence of wakefulness in terms of increased beta EEG activity while otherwise seeming to be asleep (see later).

Second, chronic activation of the monoaminergic branch of the ARAS might lead to some form of desensitization or a compensatory down-regulation which results in insufficient force to trip the switch and a switch that tends to favor the "wake on" position (ie, there is a failure to inhibit wakefulness or substantially more wakefulness is required to flip the switch to the sleep position). In this instance, one might expect decreased activation within the nuclei than input to the VLPO (eg, locus coeruleus, the dorsal or medial raphe, or the tuberomammillary cells). From a neuroendocrine point of view, however, one might expect to see continued evidence of hyperarousal in parallel with the neurobiologic down-regulation (ie, patients with chronic insomnia exhibit hypercortisolemia), or excessive secretion of the monoamines or even hypocretin-orexin, despite diminished central nervous system activity. Evidence for some of these possibilities, which are presaged by the psychobiologic inhibition model,[30] is reviewed next.

Finally, it is possible that the neurobiologic abnormalities that occur with insomnia occur within the cholinergic branch of the ARAS and appear as altered functioning within the thalamus, basal forebrain, and cortex. For example, one might expect (1) reduced activity during wakefulness within the adenosinergic regions of the basal forebrain; (2) overall decreased cortical arousal during wakefulness; (3) increased activity during the sleep period within the thalamic nuclei related to sensory processing and reduced activity within the sensory gating nuclei (ie, the reticular nucleus); and (4) overall increased cortical arousal during sleep.

Alterations within this system may be relevant to sleep, not only for continuity disturbance but also the phenomenon of sleep state misperception as it is known to occur in psychophysiologic insomnia and paradoxic insomnia, and perhaps in all forms of primary insomnia. The evidence for these possibilities, which are presaged by the neurocognitive model,[31] is also reviewed next.

EVIDENCE FOR NEUROBIOLOGIC ABNORMALITIES IN INSOMNIA
Neurophysiologic Measures of Insomnia

To date, there are several studies that have shown that patients with primary insomnia exhibit more cortical arousal than either good sleepers or patients with insomnia comorbid with major depression.[32–38] Specifically, these studies show that patients with primary insomnia exhibit more high-frequency EEG activity (beta and gamma frequencies) at sleep onset and during NREM sleep. These EEG frequencies are associated with active mental information processing during wakefulness, suggesting that patients with insomnia have a failure to terminate mental processing while otherwise asleep. There is also evidence that patients with sleep state misperception (ie, paradoxic insomnia) exhibit more beta EEG activity than good sleepers or patients with primary insomnia,[38] and beta activity is negatively associated with the perception of sleep quality,[39,40] and positively associated with the degree of subjective-objective discrepancy.[37] Taken together, these data suggest that cortical arousal may occur uniquely in association with primary insomnia (ie, one or more of the types of primary insomnia including psychophysiologic insomnia, paradoxic insomnia, idiopathic insomnia, and so forth) and that this form of arousal may be associated with the tendency toward sleep-state misperception.

Comment

Although the data acquired from this measurement strategy seem strongly to support the idea that cortical arousal may be a biomarker for insomnia (and this is theoretically appealing to the extent that the increased occurrence of beta and gamma activity is thought to be permissive of increased sensory and information processing), the lack of replication across larger-scale contemporary investigations[41] and unpublished studies (eg, D. Buysse, personal communication, 2005; and M. Perlis, unpublished data, 2005) suggests that this approach has some limitations. In the authors' hands, the occurrence of beta and gamma activity varies not only with trait considerations (diagnostic category) but also seems to be mediated and moderated by a variety of factors including first night effects[42] prior sleep debt, degree of circadian dysrhythmia, type of insomnia, technical considerations, and the extent to which there is environmental noise. There is also recent evidence that beta and gamma activity varies by gender.[43]

Neuroendocrine Measures of Insomnia

Several studies have begun to examine activation of the stress response system in patients with insomnia, focusing on the hypothalamic-pituitary-adrenal (HPA) axis. These studies provide evidence that insomnia involves, or results from, chronic activation of the stress response system. Other neuroendocrine measures, including norepinephrine, melatonin, and most recently GABA, have also been examined as potential correlates of insomnia.

Urinary measures

An early study of urinary free 11-hydroxycorticosteriods, which are metabolites of HPA axis activity, in young adult good and poor sleepers found that the mean 24-hour rate of 11-hydroxycorticosteriods excretion over 3 days was significantly higher in the poor sleepers.[44] A subsequent study of urinary cortisol and epinephrine in middle-aged good and poor sleepers found no significant differences, although poor sleepers showed a trend toward higher urinary cortisol and epinephrine secretion. More recently, Vgontzas and colleagues[45,46] collected 24-hour urine specimens for urinary free cortisol, catecholamine metabolites (DHPG and DOPAC), and growth hormone and correlated these measures with polysomnography measures of sleep continuity and sleep architecture in subjects with primary insomnia. Urinary free cortisol levels were positively correlated with total wake time, and DHPG and DOPAC measures were positively correlated with percent stage 1 sleep and wake after sleep-onset time. Although not statistically significant, norepinephrine levels tended to correlate positively with stage 1 and wake after sleep onset, and negatively with percentage of slow wave sleep. These data suggest that HPA axis and sympathetic nervous system activity are associated with objective sleep disturbance.

Plasma measures

Plasma measures of ACTH and cortisol have also been compared among patients with primary insomnia and matched good sleepers. In one study, patients with insomnia had significantly higher mean levels of ACTH and cortisol over the course of the 24-hour day, with the largest group differences observed in the evening and first half of the night.[45,46] Patients with a high degree of sleep disturbance (sleep efficiency <70%) secreted higher amounts of cortisol than patients with less sleep disturbance. In contrast to these findings, a recent study of patients with primary insomnia and age- and gender-matched good sleepers found no differences in the mean amplitude or area under the curve for cortisol secretion over a 16-hour period (19:00–09:00 hours).[47]

Comment

Some of the variability of neuroendocrine findings in insomnia may be explained by intrusion of wakefulness into the measured sleep period. This is a particular concern for studies using urinary measures, which integrate biologic activity over a long period of time. This possibility is important when considering causality (ie, whether increased HPA activity leads to insomnia, or whether insomnia leads to increased HPA activity). There is a certain degree of face validity in the association between insomnia and HPA axis activity, given the presumed relationship between stress and insomnia. A recent study investigating a possible animal model of acute insomnia demonstrated that activity in the amygdala, a key brain region for activation of the stress response, is critically necessary for stress-induced insomnia to occur.[48,49] Further, there is evidence that the VLPO contains receptors for the stress hormone corticotrophin-releasing factor, suggesting that stress may have direct effects on the sleep switch.[6] Finally, although the findings from various studies are not entirely consistent, the elevations in ACTH and cortisol before and during sleep in insomnia patients may help to shed light on the intimate association between insomnia and major depression, which is also associated with HPA axis activation. Specifically, insomnia is a risk factor for[11,50–57] a prodromal symptom of[58] and a ubiquitous[59,60] and persistent symptom of major depression.[60] The common link may be that acute stress leads to both an activation of the HPA axis and insomnia, and that chronic insomnia in turn leads to a persistent activation of the HPA axis.

Neuroimaging Measures of Insomnia

To date two brain activity studies that evaluate sleep in patients with insomnia have been undertaken: one using TC-99HMPAO single-photon emission CT (SPECT) and one using fluorodeoxyglucose positron emission tomography (PET). In the SPECT study, imaging was conducted around the sleep-onset interval in patients with primary insomnia and good sleeper subjects. Contrary to expectation, patients with insomnia exhibited a consistent pattern of reduced activity across eight preselected regions of interest, with the most prominent effect observed in the basal ganglia.[61] The frontal medial, occipital, and parietal cortices also showed significant decreases in blood flow compared with good sleepers. In the PET study, imaging data were acquired from patients with chronic insomnia and control subjects for an interval during wakefulness and during consolidated NREM. Patients with insomnia exhibited increased global cerebral glucose metabolism during wakefulness and NREM sleep.[62] In addition, it was found that patients with insomnia exhibited smaller declines in relative glucose metabolism from wakefulness to sleep in wake-promoting regions including the ascending reticular activating system, hypothalamus, and thalamus. A smaller decrease was also observed in areas associated with cognition

and emotion including the amygdala, hippocampus, insular cortex, and in the anterior cingulate and medial prefrontal cortices.

In addition to the brain activity studies, there is one study by Winkelman and colleagues,[63] using proton MR spectroscopy, which assess brain GABA levels in 16 patients with primary insomnia as compared with 16 good sleeper subjects. GABA was measured in terms of global activity within the basal ganglia; thalamus; and the temporal, parietal, and occipital cortical areas. Average brain GABA levels were found to be nearly 30% lower in patients with primary insomnia. Given that GABA is the primary inhibitor neurotransmitter in the brain, this suggests that there was less inhibition (ie, more activation) in the insomnia group. Further, GABA levels were negatively correlated with wake after sleep-onset measures. These data suggest that GABA deficiency may be a neurobiologic characteristic of insomnia and the efficacy of benzodiazepine hypnotics may reside in their potential to increase GABA secretion and activity within the brain.

Comment

Although results from the two brain activity studies seem to be inconsistent, numerous methodologic differences may help to explain differences in the findings. For instance, the SPECT study with its short time resolution may have captured a more transient phenomenon, which occurs when subjects with chronic and severe insomnia first achieve persistent sleep. The PET study with its longer time resolution may have captured a more stable phenomenon that occurs throughout NREM sleep in subjects with moderately chronic and severe insomnia. In addition to the temporal resolution issues, the PET study used a sample of insomnia patients who did not show objective sleep continuity disturbances in the laboratory, whereas the SPECT study included patients with objective sleep continuity disturbances. The samples may have differed with respect to the type of insomnia, the degree of partial sleep deprivation, and the degree of sleep state misperception. Although further studies are needed, these preliminary investigations clearly demonstrate the feasibility of using functional neuroimaging methods in the study of insomnia, and suggest that insomnia complaints may indeed have a basis in altered brain activity. For additional information on how imaging may be informative regarding the neurobiology of insomnia, the reader is referred to an article by Drummond and colleagues, published in 2004.[64]

SUMMARY

Although it is provocative and intellectually challenging to claim that insomnia is "of the brain and by the brain,"[4] the causes and consequences of insomnia are not likely to be so narrowly circumscribed.

First, if one allows that chronic insomnia occurs as the result of abnormal functioning of specific brain regions or the sleep-wake systems, it is still likely that the changes in brain function are permissive of cognitive processes that independently contribute to problems with initiating and maintaining sleep (or perceiving sleep as "sleep"). For example, if the insomnia occurs in relation to altered thalamic activation, the consequent increase in sensory processing (by either increased sensory flow or reduced sensory inhibition) likely independently contributes to insomnia because the individual experiences an increased sensitivity to external stimuli.

Second, if it is demonstrated that insomnia is a neurobiologic condition, it is still likely to be true that insomnia frequency, severity, or chronicity are mediated or moderated by cognitive and behavioral factors. For example, one may not be awake during the preferred sleep phase because of worry or attention bias, but these factors are nevertheless likely to exacerbate the condition in ways that make it more severe, more frequent, and more chronic.

Third, irrespective of the mechanisms that give rise to insomnia, it is likely that the condition interferes with many of the putative functions of sleep. In the end, the causes of chronic insomnia may be primarily related to the brain but the effects of insomnia may span many domains including both the psychologic (eg, mood; daytime fatigue or sleepiness; cognitive capacity, from executive function to long-term memory) and the physiologic domains (eg, immunity, the capacity to recover from traumatic injury, and even longevity in the absence of illness).

In the final analysis, insomnia may be precisely as it has been classically defined: a psychophysiologic thing. Perhaps the only difference between the original concept and the current one is a matter of scope. Originally, it may have been the case that psychologic factors were construed only in terms of mental phenomena like worry and rumination and behavioral phenomena like sleep extension and poor stimulus control, and physiologic factors were construed only in terms of metabolic rate. Today psychologic factors include sensory and information processing abnormalities and attentional bias and physiologic factors include not only end-organ function and tone but the brain abnormalities that may directly give rise to the insomnia condition. Expanding existing frames of reference in this manner may allow clinicians to abandon the mind-brain dichotomies and long-standing discipline-specific research agendas (eg, psychology vs neuroscience) that have long plagued mind-brain research in general and insomnia research in specific. Further, expanding existing frames of reference in this manner may lead to a new approach to the problem of insomnia, one that is more integrative and synthetic.

REFERENCES

1. Perlis ML, Smith MT, Pigeon WR. Etiology and pathophysiology of insomnia. In: Kryger M, Roth T, Dement WC, editors. Principle and practice of sleep medicine. Philadelphia: Elsevier Saunders; 2005. p. 714–25.
2. American Academy of Sleep Medicine. International classification of sleep disorders. Diagnostic and coding manual. 2nd edition. Westchester (IL): American Academy of Sleep Medicine; 2005.
3. Lazarus RS. On the primacy of cognition. Am Psychol 1984;39:124–9.
4. Hobson JA. Sleep is of the brain, by the brain and for the brain. Nature 2005;437:1254–6.
5. Kandel ER, Schwartz JH, Jessel TM. Principles of neural science. 4th edition. New York: McGraw-Hill; 2000.
6. Saper CB, Scammell TE, Lu J. Hypothalamic regulation of sleep and circadian rhythms. Nature 2005; 437:1257–63.
7. Tekin S, Cummings JL. Frontal-subcortical neuronal circuits and clinical neuropsychiatry: an update. J Psychosom Res 2002;53:647–54.
8. Lichstein KL, Rosenthal TL. Insomniacs' perceptions of cognitive versus somatic determinants of sleep disturbance. J Abnorm Psychol 1980;89:105–7.
9. Freedman RR, Sattler HL. Physiological and psychological factors in sleep-onset insomnia. J Abnorm Psychol 1982;91:380–9.
10. Nicassio PM, Mendlowitz DR, Fussell JJ, et al. The phenomenology of the pre-sleep state: the development of the pre-sleep arousal scale. Behav Res Ther 1985;23:263–71.
11. Chang PP, Ford DE, Mead LA, et al. Insomnia in young men and subsequent depression. The Johns Hopkins Precursors Study. Am J Epidemiol 1997; 146:105–14.
12. Braun AR, Balkin TJ, Wesenten NJ, et al. Regional cerebral blood flow throughout the sleep-wake cycle: an $H_2(15)O$ PET study. Brain 1997;120(Pt 7): 1173–97.
13. Lavin A, Grace AA. Modulation of dorsal thalamic cell activity by the ventral pallidum: its role in the

regulation of thalamocortical activity by the basal ganglia. Synapse 1994;18:104–27.

14. Steriade M, Timofeev I, Durmuller N, et al. Dynamic properties of corticothalamic neurons and local cortical interneurons generating fast rhythmic (30–40 Hz) spike bursts. J Neurophysiol 1998;79:483–90.

15. Von Economo C. Sleep as a problem of localization. J Nerv Mental Dis 1949;71:249–59.

16. Moruzzi G. Sleep mechanisms: summary statement. Prog Brain Res 1965;18:241–3.

17. Moruzzi G. Reticular influences on the EEG. Electroencephalogr Clin Neurophysiol 1964;16:2–17.

18. Moruzzi G, Magoun HW. Brain stem reticular formation and activation of the EEG. 1949. J Neuropsychiatr Clin Neurosci 1995;7:251–67.

19. Jones BE. The organization of central cholinergic systems and their functional importance in sleep-waking states. Prog Brain Res 1993;98:61–71.

20. Jones BE. Toward an understanding of the basic mechanisms of the sleep-waking cycle. Behavior Brain Sci 1978;1:495.

21. Saper CB, Chou TC, Scammell TE. The sleep switch: hypothalamic control of sleep and wakefulness. Trends Neurosci 2001;24:726–31.

22. George CF, Singh SM. Hypocretin (orexin) pathway to sleep. Lancet 2000;355:6.

23. Kilduff TS, Peyron C. The hypocretin/orexin ligand-receptor system: implications for sleep and sleep disorders. Trends Neurosci 2000;23:359–65.

24. Siegel JM. Narcolepsy: a key role for hypocretins (orexins). Cell 1999;98:409–12.

25. Takahashi JS. Narcolepsy genes wake up the sleep field. Science 1999;285:2076–7.

26. Borbely AA, Achermann P. Sleep homeostasis and models of sleep regulation. J Biol Rhythm 1999;14:557–68.

27. Borbely AA. Processes underlying sleep regulation. Horm Res 1998;49:114–7.

28. Borbely AA, Achermann P. Sleep homeostasis and models of sleep regulation. In: Kryger M, Roth T, Dement WC, editors. Principals and practice of sleep medicine. 3rd edition. Philadelphia: W.B. Saunders; 2000. p. 377–90.

29. Borbely AA. A two process model of sleep regulation. Hum Neurobiol 1982;1:195–204.

30. Espie CA, Broomfield NM, MacMahon KMA, et al. The attention-intention-effort pathway in the development of psychophysiologic insomnia: an invited theoretical review. Sleep Med Rev 2006;10:215–45.

31. Perlis ML, Giles DE, Mendelson WB, et al. Psychophysiological insomnia: the behavioural model and a neurocognitive perspective. J Sleep Res 1997;6:179–88.

32. Freedman R. EEG power in sleep onset insomnia. Electroencephal Clin Neurophysiol 1986;63:408–13.

33. Merica H, Gaillard JM. The EEG of the sleep onset period in insomnia: a discriminant analysis. Physiol Behav 1992;52:199–204.

34. Merica H, Blois R, Gaillard JM. Spectral characteristics of sleep EEG in chronic insomnia. Eur J Neurosci 1998;10:1826–34.

35. Lamarche CH, Ogilvie RD. Electrophysiological changes during the sleep onset period of psychophysiological insomniacs, psychiatric insomniacs, and normal sleepers. Sleep 1997;20:724–33.

36. Jacobs GD, Benson H, Friedman R. Home-based central nervous system assessment of a multifactor behavioral intervention for chronic sleep-onset insomnia. Behavior Ther 1993;24:159–74.

37. Perlis ML, Smith MT, Orff HJ, et al. Beta/gamma EEG activity in patients with primary and secondary insomnia and good sleeper controls. Sleep 2001;24:110–7.

38. Krystal AD, Edinger JD, Wohlgemuth WK, et al. NREM sleep EEG frequency spectral correlates of sleep complaints in primary insomnia subtypes. Sleep 2002;25:630–40.

39. Hall M, Buysse DJ, Nowell PD, et al. Symptoms of stress and depression as correlates of sleep in primary insomnia. Psychosom Med 2000;62:227–30.

40. Nofzinger EA, Price JC, Meltzer CC, et al. Towards a neurobiology of dysfunctional arousal in depression: the relationship between beta EEG power and regional cerebral glucose metabolism during NREM sleep. Psychiatr Res 2000;98:71–91.

41. Bastien CH, LeBlanc M, Carrier J, et al. Sleep EEG power spectra, insomnia, and chronic use of benzodiazepines. Sleep 2003;26:313–7.

42. Curcio G, Ferrara M, Piergianni A, et al. Paradoxes of the first-night effect: a quantitative analysis of antero-posterior EEG topography. Clin Neurophysiol 2004;115:1178–88.

43. Buysse DJ, Germain A, Hall ML, et al. EEG spectral analysis in primary insomnia: NREM period effects and sex differences. Sleep 2008;31:1673–82.

44. Johns MW. Relationship between sleep habits, adrenocortical activity and personality. Psychosom Med 1971;33:499–508.

45. Vgontzas AN, Tsigos C, Bixler EO, et al. Chronic insomnia and activity of the stress system: a preliminary study. J Psychosom Res 1998;45:21–31.

46. Vgontzas AN, Bixler EO, Lin HM, et al. Chronic insomnia is associated with nyctohemeral activation of the hypothalamic-pituitary-adrenal axis: clinical implications. J Clin Endocrinol Metab 2001;86:3787–94.

47. Riemann D, Klein T, Rodenbeck A, et al. Nocturnal cortisol and melatonin secretion in primary insomnia. Psychiatr Res 2002;113:17–27.

48. Cano G, Saper CB. Mechanisms underlying stress-induced insomnia [abstract]. 35th Annual Meeting

of the Society for Neuroscience. Washington DC, November 12–16, 2005.

49. Cano G, Mochizuki T, Saper CB. Neural circuitry of stress-induced insomnia in rats. J Neurosci 2008; 28:10167–84.

50. Ford DE, Kamerow DB. Epidemiologic study of sleep disturbances and psychiatric disorders: an opportunity for prevention? JAMA 1989;262: 1479–84 [see comments].

51. Dryman A, Eaton WW. Affective symptoms associated with the onset of major depression in the community: findings from the US National Institute of Mental Health Epidemiologic Catchment Area Program. Acta Psychiatr Scand 1991;84:1–5.

52. Breslau N, Roth T, Rosenthal L, et al. Sleep disturbance and psychiatric disorders: a longitudinal epidemiological study of young adults. Biol Psychiatr 1996;39:411–8.

53. Livingston G, Blizard B, Mann A. Does sleep disturbance predict depression in elderly people? A study in inner London. Br J Gen Pract 1993;43:445–8 [see comments].

54. Mallon L, Broman JE, Hetta J. Relationship between insomnia, depression, and mortality: a 12-year follow-up of older adults in the community. Int Psychogeriatr 2000;12:295–306.

55. Roberts RE, Shema SJ, Kaplan GA, et al. Sleep complaints and depression in an aging cohort: a prospective perspective [In Process Citation]. Am J Psychiatr 2000;157:81–8.

56. Vollrath M, Wicki W, Angst J. The Zurich study. VIII. Insomnia: association with depression, anxiety, somatic syndromes, and course of insomnia. Eur Arch Psychiatry Neurol Sci 1989;239:113–24.

57. Weissman MM, Greenwald S, Nino-Murcia G, et al. The morbidity of insomnia uncomplicated by psychiatric disorders. Gen Hosp Psychiatr 1997;19: 245–50.

58. Perlis ML, Giles DE, Buysse DJ, et al. Self-reported sleep disturbance as a prodromal symptom in recurrent depression. J Affect Disord 1997;42:209–12.

59. Perlis ML, Giles DE, Buysse DJ, et al. Which depressive symptoms are related to which sleep electroencephalographic variables? Biol Psychiatr 1997;42: 904–13.

60. Thase ME. Antidepressant treatment of the depressed patient with insomnia. J Clin Psychiatr 1999;60(Suppl 17):28–31.

61. Smith MT, Perlis ML, Chengazi VU, et al. Neuroimaging of NREM sleep in primary insomnia: a Tc-99-HMPAO single photon emission computed tomography study. Sleep 2002;25:325–35.

62. Nofzinger EA, Buysee DJ, Germain A, et al. Insomnia: functional imaging evidence for hyperarousal. Am J Psychiatr 2004;161:2126–8.

63. Winkelman JW, Buxton OM, Jensen JE, et al. Reduced brain GABA in primary insomnia: preliminary data from 4T proton magnetic resonance spectroscopy (1H-MRS). Sleep 2008;31: 1499–506.

64. Drummond SP, Smith MT, Orff HJ, et al. Functional imaging of the sleeping brain: review of findings and implications for the study of insomnia. Sleep Med Rev 2004;8:227–42.

Primary Insomnia: An Overview of Practical Management Using Cognitive Behavioral Techniques

Colin A. Espie, MAppSci, PhD, CPsychol, FBPsS, FCS, FRSM*,
Simon D. Kyle, MA

KEYWORDS

- Primary insomnia • Cognitive behavioral therapy
- Treatment • Assessment • Management

Most people's experiences of poor sleep are memorable, because sleeplessness and its daytime consequences are unpleasant. There are those, however, for whom insomnia is the norm. Persistent and severe sleep disturbance affects at least 1 in 10 adults and 1 in 5 older adults, thus representing a considerable public health concern. Although sleep disruption is central to several medical and psychiatric disorders, it can also be the primary presenting problem, and in practice, most insomnia patients are treated by general practitioners. Differential diagnosis is important, and specialist physicians, psychiatrists, and clinical psychologists might need to be involved. The purpose of this article is to summarize current understanding of primary insomnia, and how it can be evaluated and treated. Particular emphasis is placed on evidence-based practical management.

WHAT IS PRIMARY INSOMNIA?

At the subjective level, the sleep of someone with primary insomnia is regarded as unsatisfactory, both in pattern and quality, and their daytime functioning is impaired. Such individuals typically are overwhelmingly concerned about sleep onset, or about returning to sleep, and about the unpredictability of their sleep. Furthermore, they commonly report daytime consequences attributable to sleep disturbance, such as fatigue, mood, and cognitive impairment, which can result in occupational and interpersonal dysfunction. **Table 1** illustrates the 24-hour nature of insomnia, representing both night and daytime sleep-related distress.[1]

The *Diagnostic and Statistical Manual of Mental Disorders* (Fourth Edition, Text Revision) (DSM-IV-TR)[2] and the *International Classification of Sleep Disorders* (Second Edition) (ICSD-2)[3] provide clinical definitions of the insomnias, and **Table 2** summarizes common criteria that can be applied. One of the differences between the 2 nosologies is that DSM-IV-TR does not differentiate between primary insomnia subtypes, focusing more on the presentation of persistent sleep disturbance in the absence of other mental or physical disorders that might account for it. ICSD-2, however, outlines several primary insomnia phenotypes (**Table 3**). The most common of these is psychophysiological insomnia (for a comprehensive summary on models of insomnia pathogenesis, see, eg, Perlis and colleagues[4]).

HOW COMMON IS INSOMNIA?

Community psychiatric morbidity data show that sleep disturbance is the most common symptom

University of Glasgow Sleep Centre, Sackler Institute of Psychobiological Research, Faculty of Medicine, Southern General Hospital, Glasgow, Scotland, G51 4TF, UK
* Corresponding author.
E-mail address: c.espie@clinmed.gla.ac.uk (C.A. Espie).

Sleep Med Clin 4 (2009) 559–569
doi:10.1016/j.jsmc.2009.07.009

Table 1
Night and daytime experiences of individuals with primary insomnia (focus group and audio-diary qualitative extracts from Kyle et al[1])

Nighttime	Daytime
… its mentally, you know, you're physically shattered, but mentally you just can't switch off	I don't work full time now as a result…I work part time and I don't think I'll ever work full time again…if you have the sort of cumulative effect of night after night of not sleeping, em, you're not functioning well at work, and a job that I could have done without any trouble at all before I had this problem, I find is giving me difficulty
… you're like tossing or turning…and a lot of the time I do check the clock, which is probably not a good thing to do, but I can't help it…and you get frustrated cos you're not going to sleep, and then you try harder and it makes it worse…	Even simple tasks take 3 times as long as they normally would…and reading is another, I need to read quite a lot at work, you find you've read a page and you have no clue what it said, you have to go back and re-read it
I find that once I open my eyes, I'm awake, that's it, whether I've had an hour and half sleep or 4 hours sleep, I'm up and awake and the minds active	I find my mood only kinda starts to be affected after a couple of nights of not having a great sleep…I start to get really snappy, and that's not like my temperament or anything like that, that's not me at all
I always find that I'm quite hyperalert to any noises going on at all when I'm trying to get to sleep	I had planned to go to Edinburgh today but that I had to cancel, my friend came over later on, and I decided against going out because I just felt too tired, I find this all very frustrating, I'm a pretty sociable person…so it doesn't suit me at all

of mental disease, regardless of age, sex, or ethnic group. Indeed insomnia is more common than worry, and twice as common as anxiety or depressive symptoms.[5] Insomnia affects one-third of adults occasionally, and 9% to 12% on a chronic basis.[6–8] Insomnia is more commonly reported in women, shift workers, and patients with medical and psychiatric disorders. Among older adults, prevalence has been estimated at 25%, although comorbid conditions and hypnotic drugs are factors in this increased prevalence. Primary insomnia alone has an estimated prevalence of approximately 3%.[8,9]

THE ASSESSMENT OF PRIMARY INSOMNIA

A thorough history and intake interview is central to assessment (see eg, Chapter 3 in Morin and Espie[10]). This assessment would incorporate sections on the presentation of the complaint, its development and lifetime history (cf idiopathic vs psychophysiological insomnia), its relationship to lifestyle (cf inadequate sleep hygiene), treatment history (including general physical and mental health), and screening questions for the purposes of preliminary differential diagnosis (eg, relating to mood, limb movements, breathing).

Polysomnography (PSG) is normally undertaken only when another sleep disorder is suspected.[11]

Thereafter, if a primary insomnia is the provisional diagnosis, "sleep diary" monitoring of sleep pattern and sleep quality, over 10 to 14 nights, is a recommended staple form of assessment.[12] This assessment is often supplemented by self-report index scales (particularly the Insomnia Severity Index[13] or the Pittsburgh Sleep Quality Index).[14] There is a wide range of self-rating instruments that provide helpful data in support of psychological formulation of insomnia and treatment outcome evaluation. These indices include the Dysfunctional Beliefs and Attitudes about Sleep Scale,[15] the Glasgow Sleep Effort Scale,[16] and the Pre-Sleep Arousal Scale[17] (see Refs.[18,19] for reviews). In addition, wrist actigraphy, which estimates sleep-wakefulness based on body movement, can supplement interview questions in identifying paradoxical insomnia and in recognizing any potential circadian anomalies.[20]

THE TREATMENT OF INSOMNIA: AN EVIDENCE-BASED PERSPECTIVE

There has been relatively little research on the natural course of insomnia. However, emerging

Table 2
Criteria for defining insomnia

A subjective complaint of difficulties initiating or maintaining sleep, nonrestorative sleep
Duration of insomnia is longer than 1 month
The sleep disturbance (or associated daytime fatigue) causes marked distress or impairment in social occupational or other important areas of functioning
The sleep disturbance does not occur exclusively in the context of another mental or sleep disorder, and is not the direct physiologic effect of a substance or a general medical condition
Severity of sleep disturbances: Sleep latency or time awake after sleep onset greater than 30 min; or, List awakening occurring mare than 30 min before desired time and before total sleep time reaches 6.5 h; sleep efficiency is lower than 85%. May not be corroborated by PSG findings
Frequency: Sleep difficulties present 3 or more nights per week
Duration: Insomnia present for more than 1 (DSM-IV) or 6 months (ICSD)
Daytime impairments/marked distress: Score of 2 or 3 on Insomnia Severity Index scale (items 5 and 7).

Abbreviations: DSM-IV, *Diagnostic and Statistical Manual of Mental Disorders* (Fourth Edition); ICSD, *International Classification of Sleep Disorders: Diagnostic and Coding Manual* (Second Edition); PSG, polysomnography.
From Morin CM, Espie CA. Insomnia: A clinical guide to assessment and treatment. New York: Kluwer Academic/Plenum publishers; 2003; with permission.

data suggest that insomnia syndrome persists and is maintained in severity over time.[21] Few studies have characterized those suffering from idiopathic insomnia, but there is some evidence to suggest that this particular subtype may be resistant to intervention.[22] On the other hand, inadequate sleep hygiene associated with lifestyle factors (caffeine, bedroom environment, and so forth) may ameliorate as these are resolved without need for clinical attention. It is important to make the distinction between inadequate sleep hygiene and psychophysiological or paradoxical insomnia subtypes because there is no sound evidence that the latter 2 will respond to sleep hygiene as a single therapy.[23] On the other hand, prognosis with effective treatment can be very good.

Pharmacotherapy

Insomnia traditionally has been treated pharmacologically. Barbiturates were superseded by benzodiazepine (BZ) compounds during the 1960s and 1970s. These drugs were safer in overdose, and were thought to have fewer side effects and to be less addictive. Controlled studies have demonstrated that a considerable number of BZs, of short to intermediate half-life, are effective hypnotic agents. However, from the mid-1970s potential problems became apparent, both during administration and withdrawal. Longer-acting hypnotics were prone to carryover effects of morning lethargy, and shorter-acting drugs could lead to "rebound insomnia."[24] Furthermore, tolerance develops, leading either to increased dosing or switching to alternative medication. Although

Table 3
Classification of primary insomnia subtypes within ICSD-2

Classification	Sleep Disorder	Complaint of Insomnia, Plus...
Insomnias	Psychophysiological insomnia	Learned sleep preventing associations, conditioned arousal, "racing mind" phenomenon
	Paradoxical insomnia	Complaint of poor sleep disproportionate to sleep pattern and sleep duration
	Idiopathic insomnia	Insomnia typically begins in childhood or from birth
	Inadequate sleep hygiene	Daily living activities inconsistent with maintaining good-quality sleep

BZs used for short periods or intermittently can maintain effectiveness, these are not the treatment of choice in chronic insomnia,[25] and are contraindicated in older adults and in cases where insomnia may involve sleep-related breathing disorder because of their potentially depressant effects on respiration. Several BZ compounds have been removed from the market in the United Kingdom, United States, and elsewhere. Contemporary hypnotic therapy has extended to include BZ receptor antagonists (BzRAs; often referred to as "z" drugs), and more recently melatonin receptor agonists (MeRAs) have been introduced. Whereas the place in therapeutics of MeRAs has yet to become established, the BzRAs are often thought to offer more sustained benefit for insomnia and to have fewer adverse effects. Nevertheless, there remains uncertainty about the effectiveness of BzRAs in chronic insomnia, with few data to suggest stability of gains beyond active administration.[26]

Psychological Therapy

Psychological treatment for chronic insomnia, primarily in the form of cognitive behavioral therapy (CBT), has been extensively investigated in over 100 controlled studies during the past 20 years. Indeed, 9 systematic reviews or meta-analyses of CBT have been published in the past 15 years.[26–34] To take 2 examples, the American Academy of Sleep Medicine (AASM [formerly the American Sleep Disorders Association of Sleep]) taskforce reports (1999 and 2006) comprised 85 clinical trials (4194 participants), and indicated that CBT was associated with improvement in 70% of patients, which was sustained for at least 6 months post treatment.[30,33] Of note, there is growing evidence not only that sleep parameters improve but that daytime functioning and health-related quality of life impairments can also be alleviated.[35] These clinical and generalized benefits reflect moderate to large standardized effect sizes (ES), with large ES reported for primary symptom measures of sleep latency and wake time after sleep onset. Moreover, the 2006 review[33] included 12 trials on insomnia associated with medical or psychiatric disorders, suggesting that CBT may be effective also in more complex populations. It is thought that CBT achieves these outcomes because it tackles directly the dysfunctional thoughts and maladaptive behaviors that otherwise maintain insomnia.

In routine practice, the overwhelming majority of insomnia patients are treated with pharmacotherapy rather than CBT. In contrast to CBT, this is not evidence-based for chronic insomnia. There are no data to support the long-term resolution of sleep problems following either short-term or medium-term (up to 6 months) pharmacotherapy, whereas the beneficial effects of CBT are known to persist for months or years after the treatment course is completed. For example, Morin and colleagues[36] compared CBT, medication (temazepam), combined therapy, and a placebo control condition. All 3 active treatments produced short-term improvements in sleep, but the temazepam-only condition regressed to baseline during follow-up. By comparison, both groups treated with CBT exhibited good 12-month outcome, suggesting the durable efficacy of CBT relative to pharmacotherapy. Sivertsen and colleagues[37] reported recently that CBT was associated with greater benefit than zopiclone. Indeed, CBT was associated with a 10% increase in polysomnographic sleep efficiency at posttreatment and 6-month follow-up, relative to no reliable change with zopiclone.

To this end, based on the published evidence, the National Institutes of Health Consensus and State of the Science Statement (2005) concluded that CBT is "as effective as prescription medications are for short-term treatment of chronic insomnia. Moreover, there are indications that the beneficial effects of CBT, in contrast to those produced by medications, may last well beyond the termination of active treatment" (page 14).[25]

Recent data also point to the "real-world" effectiveness of CBT for insomnia, demonstrating successful treatment outcomes in patients across a range of presenting populations. For example, a comparative meta-analysis,[34] comparing CBT outcomes in middle-aged and older adults (55 years plus), reported moderate to large ES, regardless of age, in sleep-onset latency and wake time after sleep onset. Consistent with this, the AASM also recommend CBT as a standard treatment for insomnia in older adults.[38] Likewise, a recent randomized controlled trial has found that CBT is clinically helpful in depressed patients with comorbid insomnia.[39]

In a similar vein, the authors have recently reported on the effectiveness of CBT in post-cancer care,[40] reinforcing the earlier findings of Savard and colleagues[41] that CBT is effective in insomnia associated with cancer. Indeed, much of the authors' work in Glasgow has been in the clinical effectiveness tradition, enrolling relatively unselected patients into the trials program. The authors have randomized 490 patients across 3 clinical trials of CBT versus treatment as usual, and have not found any consistent pattern of demographic or clinical predictors of poor response to CBT.[40,42,43] The findings thus support the effectiveness of CBT for insomnia, obtaining an approximate 70% treatment response regardless of severity or chronicity of presenting characteristics. This result is consistent with other United Kingdom data showing that insomnia in chronic hypnotic users also responds well to CBT.[44] However, despite the recommended preference for CBT relative to medication for chronic insomnia,[25] and these recent demonstrations of CBT working in real-world settings, practical problems remain in making CBT widely available.[45,46]

Based on outcome data, the AASM has published practice parameters statements that endorse stimulus control therapy, progressive muscular relaxation, biofeedback, paradoxical intention therapy, sleep restriction, and 2 (alternative) multicomponent CBT approaches.[38,47] Thus two facts are of particular note. (a) CBT is a treatment modality, just as is sleep pharmacotherapy. The latter comprises a range of licensed medications, and CBT a range of (7) proven psychotherapeutic methods. (b) Sleep hygiene is *not* an endorsed psychological treatment.

Light Therapy and Exercise

The timing of production of the pineal hormone melatonin may be influenced by oral ingestion of melatonin or MeRA agents, and endogenously by exposure to bright light, which is a potent marker for human circadian rhythms. Light exposure enables the resetting of rhythms in circadian rhythm sleep disorders such as advanced sleep phase syndrome and delayed sleep phase syndrome.[48] However, the results of studies investigating the efficacy of bright light relative to psychological treatments for insomnia, or as an additive component to CBT, are awaited.

Athletic people sleep well, although this may be more to do with behavioral patterning than aerobic fitness. Nevertheless, there is evidence that exercise can have positive effects on sleep quality, particularly if taken late afternoon or early evening, and in otherwise relatively fit individuals.[49] Morning exercise can also be an effective modality to encourage the same waking time and early morning light exposure; which help to reset sleep patterns on a daily basis. Again, there is little evidence, and no formal recommendation, that exercise is a specifically supported intervention for insomnia in clinical practice.

THE PSYCHOLOGICAL TREATMENT OF INSOMNIA IN CLINICAL PRACTICE: KEY COMPONENTS

Brief descriptions of effective CBT elements are presented in **Box 1**, and the following text provides some explanation of the techniques themselves along with information on implementation (for further detailed reading of each component see Refs.[10,50]).

Sleep Education and Sleep Hygiene

The simple provision of information may ameliorate the sense of being out of control, but without therapeutic attempts at cognitive restructuring (see later discussion), inaccurate attributions and misunderstandings are likely to remain. In a generic sense sleep hygiene arguably provides patients with a starting point for self-management, but as stated earlier is not a powerful treatment for persistent insomnia.[23]

Stimulus Control Treatment

The principle underlying stimulus control treatment is that it increases the bedroom's cueing potential for successful sleep. For good sleepers, the pre-bedtime period and the stimulus environment trigger positive associations of sleepiness and sleep. For the poor sleeper, however, the bedroom triggers associations with restlessness and lengthy nighttime wakening via a stimulus-response relationship, thereby continuing to promote wakefulness and arousal. The concept is similar to phobic conditions whereby a conditioned stimulus precipitates an anxiety response. Treatment involves removing from the bedroom all stimuli that are potentially sleep-incompatible. Reading and watching television, for example, are confined to living rooms. Sleeping is excluded from living areas and from daytime, and wakefulness is excluded from the bedroom. The individual is instructed to get up if not asleep within 15 to 20 minutes or if wakeful during the night. Conceptually, stimulus control is a reconditioning treatment that enforces discrimination between daytime (waking) and nighttime (sleeping) environments.

Sleep Restriction Therapy

Sleep restriction restricts sleep to the length of time that the person is likely to sleep. This method may be equivalent to promoting "core sleep" at the expense of "optional sleep." Sleep restriction primarily aims to improve sleep efficiency. Because sleep efficiency is the ratio of time asleep to time in bed, it can be improved either by increasing the numerator (time spent asleep) or by reducing the denominator (time spent in bed). People with insomnia generally seek the former, but this may not be necessary, either biologically or psychologically. Sleep restriction first involves recording in a sleep diary and calculating average nightly sleep duration. The aim, then, is to obtain this average

---

Box 1
"Ingredients" of CBT for insomnia

Components of stimulus control and sleep restriction treatment

Define individual sleep requirements

Establish parameters for bedtime period
  ("threshold" time and "rising" time)

Eliminate daytime napping

Differentiate rest from sleep

Schedule sleep periods with respect to needs

Establish 7 days per week compliance

Remove incompatible activity from bedroom environment

Rise from bed if wakeful (>20 min)

Avoid recovery sleep as "compensation"

Establish stability from night to night

Adjust the sleep period as sleep efficiency improves

Components of cognitive intervention

Identify thought patterns and content that intrudes

Address (mis)attributions connecting sleep and waking life

Establish rehearsal/planning time in early evening

Relaxation and imagery training

Distraction and thought blocking

Develop accurate beliefs/attributions about sleep and sleep loss

Challenge negative and invalid thoughts

Eliminate effort to control sleep

Motivate to maintain behavior and cognitive change

Use relapse-prevention techniques

---

each night. This goal is achieved by setting rising time as an "anchor" each day and delaying going to bed until a "threshold time," which permits this designated amount of sleep. Thus, the sleep period is reduced and sleep efficiency is likely to increase. The permitted "sleep window" can then be titrated week by week in 15-minute increments in response to sleep efficiency improvements.

Cognitive Control

This technique aims to deal with thought material in advance of bedtime and to reduce intrusive bedtime thinking. The person with insomnia is asked to set aside 15 to 20 minutes in the early evening to rehearse the day and to plan ahead for tomorrow, thus "putting the day to rest." Cognitive control is a technique for dealing with what might otherwise be "unfinished business" from the day past or from forward thinking for the days to come. Thus it may be most effective for rehearsal, planning, and self-evaluative thoughts that are important to the individual and which, if not dealt with, may intrude during the sleep-onset period.

Thought Suppression

Thought-stopping and articulatory suppression techniques attempt to interrupt the flow of thoughts. No attempt is made actively to deal with thought material per se but rather the goal is to attenuate thinking. With articulatory suppression the patient is instructed to repeat, subvocally, the word "the" every 3 seconds. This procedure is derived from the experimental psychology literature. Articulatory suppression is thought to occupy the short-term memory store used in the processing of information. The type of material most likely to respond is repetitive but nonaffect-laden thinking that is not "powerful" enough (cognitively or emotionally) to demand attention. In addition, this technique may be useful during the night to enable rapid return to sleep.

Imagery and Relaxation

There is a wide range of relaxation methods including progressive relaxation, imagery training, biofeedback, meditation, hypnosis, and autogenic training, but little evidence to indicate the superiority of any one approach. Evidence relating to whether individuals with insomnia are hyperaroused in physiologic terms remains equivocal, and there are no adequate data that relaxation has its effect through autonomic change. Consequently, and at the cognitive level, these techniques may act through distraction or the promotion of mastery and self-efficacy. During relaxation, the mind focuses on alternative themes such as visualized images or physiologic responses. In meditation, the focus is on a "mantra" and in self-hypnosis, on positive self-statements. Relaxation may be effective for thought processes that are anxiety-based or which flit from topic to topic.

Cognitive Restructuring

Cognitive restructuring challenges misattributions about insomnia and its consequences, and the other faulty beliefs that maintain wakefulness and the sense of helplessness that many people with insomnia report. Cognitive restructuring seems to work through appraisal by testing the validity of assumptions against evidence and real-life experience. As an evaluative technique, it may be effective with beliefs that are irrational but compelling. If such thoughts as, for example "I am going to be incapable at work tomorrow" are not challenged, they will create high levels of preoccupation and anxiety, and sleep is unlikely to occur. With cognitive restructuring, the person with insomnia learns alternative responses to replace inaccurate thinking.

Paradoxical Intention

The technique of paradoxical intention is useful in situations in which performance anxiety has developed, that is, when the effort to produce a response inhibits that response itself. The paradoxical instruction is to allow sleep to occur naturally through passively attempting to remain quietly wakeful rather than attempting to fall asleep. Paradox may be regarded as a decatastrophizing technique because it seems to act on the ultimate anxious thought (of remaining awake indefinitely) initially by focusing on and enhancing this thought (a habituation model), and then subjecting it to appraisal through rationalization and experience. By intending to remain awake, and failing to do so, the strength of the sleep drive is reestablished and performance effort is reduced.

Cognitive Behavioral Therapy as an Integrated Psychological Therapy

There is thought to be considerable synergy between the elements of the CBT approach. This synergy is part of the reason that CBT is a psychotherapy method, and not merely a collection of strategies. Some examples may help to illustrate this approach.

In stimulus control therapy, patients are encouraged not to read in bed; but to protect the bedroom environment exclusively for sleep (and sexual activity). Patients often say that they know many people who read in bed who are good sleepers, and so may not understand the instruction, and may not be motivated to apply it. Certainly a rationale can be given, in terms of operant and classic conditioning theory, that serves to explain how these are differing conditioned relationships. However, by considering the synergy across the CBT approach it can also be clarified that there may be differences in personal intention in each case, associated with the habit of reading. Whereas the intention of the good sleeper is normally to remain awake in order to read (and is unable to do so), the intention of the person with insomnia is normally to use reading as a hypnotic aid in order to fall asleep. The good sleeper ultimately is frustrated in this goal, being overtaken by the homeostatic pressure for sleep, and has to put the book down, whereas poor sleepers are ultimately frustrated in their goal, not yet being asleep, and are overtaken by a vicious circle of mental and somatic arousal (which is a pressure for wakefulness). This example, therefore, reveals not only the cognitive behavioral interactions in CBT but also demonstrates how CBT is best applied as a psychobiological therapy.

Another example could be drawn from sleep restriction therapy, which is typically seen as a behavioral strategy. Yet it too may be psychobiological; having cognitive and biologic effects. Reducing the sleep window involves staying up late and getting up early, according to a preplanned, personally tailored protocol. Not only does that preplanning take decision processing out of the equation, it also, inevitably, leads to a series of what strict cognitive therapists would call "behavioral experiments"—tests that might disprove a dysfunctional mental hypothesis. If people follow the instructions, what happens is that they fall asleep quickly (without trying to), that they find it problematic to remain awake leading up to bedtime (when they have to), and that they remain sleepy at rising time (when they don't expect to). However, it is the biologic imperative that permits sleep restriction to work, and homeostatic drive and personal sleep requirement guides the titration process in subsequent weeks.

A final example can be drawn from the emerging therapy area being applied to primary insomnia, which is mindfulness-based therapy (cf Refs.[51,52]). This "third wave" psychological therapy is seen as going beyond a cognitive approach that emphasizes (re-)evaluative strategies to a more acceptance-based model that does not attempt to correct belief and attitude systems. In part, acceptance is seen as a therapeutic goal and outcome that enables the person to move on. However, in the context of existing behavioral strategies for insomnia, this may not be particularly novel. The quarter of an hour rule within stimulus control, for example, involves accepting that you are not asleep, not trying to fix that in any way but rather "giving up" trying to sleep and getting out of bed. This focus could be seen as a similar philosophical position to take in relation to wakeful experiences in bed. Explicitly paradoxical approaches also involve acceptance at some level, or at least adopting an entirely new relationship to a personal problem.

FUTURE DIRECTIONS IN THE PSYCHOLOGICAL MANAGEMENT OF PRIMARY INSOMNIA

There are several current research strands that will further improve the understanding and delivery of psychological treatment for insomnia. The first one relates to "dosage." Any given patient logically requires the necessary amount of intervention (not less and not more) to respond. "Dose" might be determined, for example, by the number of elements in the treatment, the number of sessions, the amount of personal tailoring of treatment, and the qualifications and experience of the therapist. A dose response traditionally is the relationship between the amount of exposure (dose) to a substance, and the resulting changes in body function or health (response). It has been suggested that the therapeutic session is a natural quantitative unit of psychotherapy, that is, the number of sessions is stochastically related to exposure to the active ingredients in any psychotherapy[53] Following this rationale, Edinger and colleagues[54] have shown that a brief CBT intervention (4 sessions) is clinically effective in primary insomnia, but less so in comorbid insomnia, implying that dosing may need to reflect complexity of presentation. More work in this area is needed to further determine the required "dose" (beyond simply number of sessions/ components) to achieve a response that is clinically meaningful. Such work has important implications for cost-effectiveness and utility models (and therefore service provision) of insomnia treatment.

A related issue deals with the "absorbed" dose; in psychological therapies, particularly CBT for insomnia, this would reflect implementation/ adherence with behavioral instructions. It is known, for example, that patients who achieve more consistent bedtimes and rising times have improved sleep efficiency,[55] suggesting that application of therapeutic advice is an important carrier of outcome. Likewise, Vincent and Hameed[56] reported that only adherence explained variance in patients' posttreatment outcome. These findings, coupled with data indicating that sleep restriction is a potent, but least liked, component of the CBT "package,"[57] suggest future research should attempt to understand and identify predictors of adherence, and pilot interventions aimed at improving adherence.[58]

Finally, although much of the literature has focused on the behavioral elements of CBT in accounting for treatment gains, there is an emerging literature on cognitive processes in the development and maintenance of insomnia.[59–61] Indeed, an uncontrolled pilot study[62] of a "pure" cognitive intervention revealed, at 12-month follow-up, large improvements in both sleep and daytime functioning parameters. It will be important to further document such improvements in randomized clinical trials, and to determine how specialized cognitive interventions may be integrated into existing CBT "packages" or as stand-alone treatments for particular primary insomnia phenotypes. This latter point is important; most treatment studies to date have recruited patients using generic (DSM-IV-TR) primary insomnia criteria. There is a dearth of data on treatment response within primary insomnia subtypes.

SUMMARY

Insomnia is a common problem with real individual, societal, and economic consequences.[63] Primary insomnia, a psychological-based disorder of initiating or maintaining sleep, is particularly common, yet undertreated. There is an extensive body of literature demonstrating the effectiveness of both CBT and pharmacologic approaches in improving sleep parameters in the acute treatment phase; CBT, however, has shown durable improvements long after treatment "administration." Despite this evidence base, CBT service provision is poor. Ongoing work continues to address this paradox. Subtypes of primary insomnia are rarely identified or detailed. Future basic work on the pathophysiology of insomnia subtypes will help in the tailoring of treatment. Finally, investigation of the "dose-response" relationship and adherence factors will ultimately aid in further refining the psychological management of insomnia.

REFERENCES

1. Kyle SD, Espie CA, Morgan K. A qualitative analysis of daytime functioning and quality of life in persistent insomnia using focus groups and audio-diaries. Presented at the 22nd Annual meeting of the Associated Professional Sleep Societies. Baltimore, June 7–12, 2008.

2. American Psychiatric Association. Diagnostic and statistical manual of mental disorders. Text revision. 4th edition. Washington, DC: American Psychiatric Press Inc; 2000.

3. American Academy of Sleep Medicine. International classification of sleep disorders: diagnostic and coding manual. 2nd edition. Westchester (IL): American Academy of Sleep Medicine; 2005.

4. Perlis ML, Pigeon WR, Smith MS. Etiology and pathophysiology of Insomnia. In: Kryger MH, Roth T, Dement WC, editors. Principles and practice of sleep medicine. Philadelphia: WB Saunders; 2005. p. 714–25.

5. Singleton N, Bumpstead R, O'Brien M, et al. Psychiatric morbidity among adults living in private households, 2000. UK: Office of National Statistics; 2001.

6. Morin CM, LeBlanc M, Daley M, et al. Epidemiology of insomnia: prevalence, self-help treatments, consultations, and determinants of help-seeking behaviors. Sleep Med 2006;7(2):123–30.

7. Ford DE, Kamerow DB. Epidemiologic-study of sleep disturbances and psychiatric-disorders—an opportunity for prevention. JAMA 1989;262(11):1479–84.

8. Ohayon MM. Epidemiology of insomnia: what we know and what we still need to learn. Sleep Med Rev 2002;6(2):97–111.

9. Ohayon M. Epidemiological study on insomnia in the general population. Sleep 1996;19(3):S7–15.

10. Morin CM, Espie CA. Insomnia: a clinical guide to assessment and treatment. New York: Kluwer Academic/Plenum publishers; 2003.

11. Reite M, Buysse D, Reynolds C, et al. The use of polysomnography in the evaluation of insomnia. Sleep 1995;18(1):58–70.

12. Buysse DJ, Ancoli-Israel S, Edinger JD, et al. Recommendations for a standard research assessment of insomnia. Sleep 2006;29(9):1155–73.

13. Morin CM. Insomnia: psychological assessment and management. New York: The Guildford Press; 1993.

14. Buysse DJ, Reynolds CF, Monk TH, et al. The Pittsburgh sleep quality index—a new instrument for psychiatric practice and research. Psychiatry Res 1989;28(2):193–213.

15. Morin CM, Stone J, Trinkle D, et al. Dysfunctional beliefs and attitudes about sleep among older adults with and without insomnia complaints. Psychol Aging 1993;8(3):463–7.

16. Broomfield NM, Espie CA. Towards a valid, reliable measure of sleep effort. J Sleep Res 2005;14(4):401–7.

17. Nicassio PM, Mendlowitz DR, Fussell JJ, et al. The phenomenology of the pre-sleep state—the development of the pre-sleep arousal scale. Behav Res Ther 1985;23(3):263–71.

18. Morin CM. Measuring outcomes in randomized clinical trials of insomnia treatments. Sleep Med Rev 2003;7(3):263–79.

19. Moul DE, Hall M, Pilkonis PA, et al. Self-report measures of insomnia in adults: rationales, choices, and needs. Sleep Med Rev 2004;8(3):177–98.

20. Morgenthaler TI, Lee-Chiong T, Alessi C, et al. Practice parameters for the clinical evaluation and treatment of circadian rhythm sleep disorders. Sleep 2007;30:1445–59.

21. Morin CM, Belanger L, LeBlanc M, et al. The natural history of insomnia: a population-based 3-year longitudinal study. Arch Intern Med 2009; 169(5):447–53.

22. Edinger JD, Stout AL, Hoelscher TJ. Cluster-analysis of insomniacs MMPI profiles—relation of subtypes to sleep history and treatment outcome. Psychosom Med 1988;50(1):77–87.

23. Stepanski EJ, Wyatt JK. Use of sleep hygiene in the treatment of insomnia. Sleep Med Rev 2003;7(3):215–25.

24. Kripke DF. Chronic hypnotic use: deadly risks, doubtful benefit. Sleep Med Rev 2000;4(1):5–20.

25. State-of-the-Science Panel. National Institutes of Health state-of-the-science conference statement on manifestations and management of chronic insomnia in adults, June 13–15, 2005. Sleep 2005;(28):1049–57.

26. Riemann D, Perlis ML. The treatments of chronic insomnia: a review of benzodiazepine receptor agonists and psychological and behavioral therapies. Sleep Med Rev 2009;13(3):205–14.

27. Morin CM, Culbert JP, Schwartz SM. Nonpharmacological interventions for insomnia—a metaanalysis of treatment efficacy. Am J Psychiatry 1994;151(8):1172–80.

28. Murtagh DRR, Greenwood KM. Identifying effective psychological treatments for insomnia—a metaanalysis. J Consult Clin Psychol 1995;63(1):79–89.

29. Pallesen S, Nordhus IH, Kvale G. Nonpharmacological interventions for insomnia in older adults: a meta-analysis of treatment efficacy. Psychotherapy 1998;35(4):472–82.

30. Morin CM, Hauri PJ, Espie CA, et al. Nonpharmacologic treatment of chronic insomnia. Sleep 1999; 22(8):1134–56.

31. Smith MT, Perlis ML, Park A, et al. Comparative meta-analysis of pharmacotherapy and behavior

therapy for persistent insomnia. Am J Psychiatry 2002;159(1):5–11.

32. Montgomery P, Dennis J. Cognitive behavioural interventions for sleep problems in adults aged 60+. Cochrane Database Syst Rev 2003;1:CD003161.

33. Morin CM, Bootzin RR, Buysse DJ, et al. Psychological and behavioral treatment of insomnia: update of the recent evidence (1998–2004). Sleep 2006;29:1398–414.

34. Irwin MR, Cole JC, Nicassio PM. Comparative meta-analysis of behavioral interventions for insomnia and their efficacy in middle-aged adults and in older adults 55+years of age. Health Psychol 2006;25(1):3–14.

35. Krystal AD. Treating the health, quality of life, and functional impairments in insomnia. J Clin Sleep Med 2007;3(1):63–72.

36. Morin CM, Colecchi C, Stone J, et al. Behavioral and pharmacological therapies for late-life insomnia—a randomized controlled trial. JAMA 1999;281(11):991–9.

37. Sivertsen B, Omvik S, Pallesen S, et al. Cognitive behavioral therapy vs zopiclone for treatment of chronic primary insomnia in older adults—a randomized controlled trial. JAMA 2006;295(24):2851–8.

38. Morgenthaler T, Kramer M, Alessi C, et al. Practice parameters for the psychological and behavioral treatment of insomnia: an update. An American Academy of Sleep Medicine report. Sleep 2006;29:1415–9.

39. Manber R, Edinger JD, Gress JL, et al. Cognitive behavioral therapy for insomnia enhances depression outcome in patients with comorbid major depressive disorder and insomnia. Sleep 2008;31(4):489–95.

40. Espie CA, Fleming L, Cassidy J, et al. Randomized controlled clinical effectiveness trial of cognitive behavior therapy compared with treatment as usual for persistent insomnia in patients with cancer. J Clin Oncol 2008;26(28):4651–8.

41. Savard J, Simard S, Ivers H, et al. Randomized study on the efficacy of cognitive-behavioural therapy for insomnia secondary to breast cancer, part I: sleep and psychological effects. J Clin Oncol 2005;23(25):6083–96.

42. Espie CA, MacMahon KMA, Kelly HL, et al. Randomized clinical effectiveness trial of nurse-administered small-group cognitive behavior therapy for persistent insomnia in general practice. Sleep 2007;30(5):574–84.

43. Espie CA, Inglis SJ, Tessier S, et al. The clinical effectiveness of cognitive behaviour therapy for chronic insomnia: implementation and evaluation of a sleep clinic in general medical practice. Behav Res Ther 2001;39(1):45–60.

44. Morgan K, Dixon S, Mathers N, et al. Psychological treatment for insomnia in the management of long-term hypnotic drug use: a pragmatic randomised controlled trial. Br J Gen Pract 2003;53(497):923–8.

45. Espie CA. 'Stepped care': a health technology solution for delivering cognitive behavioral therapy as a first line insomnia treatment. Sleep, in press.

46. Perlis ML, Smith MS. How can we make CBT-I and other BSM services widely available? J Clin Sleep Med 2008;4(1):11–3.

47. Chesson AL, Anderson WM, Littner M, et al. Practice parameters for the nonpharmacologic treatment of chronic insomnia. Sleep 1999;22(8):1128–33.

48. Bjorvatn B, Pallesen S. A practical approach to circadian rhythm sleep disorders. Sleep Med Rev 2009;13(1):47–60.

49. Singh NA, Clements KM, Fiatarone MA. Sleep, sleep deprivation, and daytime activities—a randomized controlled trial of the effect of exercise on sleep. Sleep 1997;20(2):95–101.

50. Perlis ML, Lichstein KL. Treating sleep disorders: principles and practice of behavioural sleep medicine. New York: Wiley; 2003.

51. Kabat-Zinn J. Full catastrophe living: using the wisdom of your body and mind to face stress, pain, and illness. New York: Delacorte Press; 1990.

52. Ong JC, Shapiro SL, Manber R. Combining mindfulness meditation with cognitive-behavior therapy for insomnia: a treatment-development study. Behav Ther 2008;39(2):171–82.

53. Howard KI, Kopta SM, Krause MS, et al. The dose-effect relationship in psychotherapy. Am Psychol 1986;41(2):159–64.

54. Edinger JD, Wohlgemuth WK, Radtke RA, et al. Dose-response effects of cognitive-behavioral insomnia therapy: a randomized clinical trial. Sleep 2007;30(2):203–12.

55. Riedel BW, Lichstein KL. Strategies for evaluating adherence to sleep restriction treatment for insomnia. Behav Res Ther 2001;39(2):201–12.

56. Vincent NK, Hameed H. Relation between adherence and outcome in the group treatment of insomnia. Behav Sleep Med 2003;1(3):125–39.

57. Vincent N, Lionberg C. Treatment preference and patient satisfaction in chronic insomnia. Sleep 2001;24(4):411–7.

58. Vincent N, Lewycky S, Finnegan H. Barriers to engagement in sleep restriction and stimulus control in chronic insomnia. J Consult Clin Psychol 2008;76(5):820–8.

59. Espie CA, Broomfield NM, MacMahon KMA, et al. The attention-intention-effort pathway in the development of psychophysiologic insomnia: a theoretical review. Sleep Med Rev 2006;10(4):215–45.

60. Espie CA. Understanding insomnia through cognitive modelling. Sleep Med 2007;8(Suppl 4):S3–8.

61. Harvey AG. A cognitive model of insomnia. Behav Res Ther 2002;40(8):869–93.

62. Harvey AG, Sharpley AL, Ree MJ, et al. An open trial of cognitive therapy for chronic insomnia. Behav Res Ther 2007;45(10):2491–501.

63. Daley M, Morin CM, LeBlanc M, et al. The economic burden of insomnia: direct and indirect costs for individuals with insomnia syndrome, insomnia symptoms, and good sleepers. Sleep 2009;32(1):55–64.

Comorbid Insomnia

Bruce Rybarczyk, PhD[a],*, Hannah G. Lund, BA[a],
Laurin Mack, MS[a], Edward Stepanski, PhD[b,c]

KEYWORDS

- Comorbid insomnia • Insomnia • Behavioral treatment
- Secondary insomnia • Self-help

Until recently the prevailing view in sleep medicine was that chronic insomnia most often presented as a secondary effect of another disorder. The goal in evaluating insomnia was to identify the primary disorder causing the insomnia so that treatment could target the parent disorder. If insomnia occurred in the context of a previously diagnosed disorder, it was automatically assumed to be a symptom of that disorder (eg, depression), a secondary effect from another symptom (eg, nocturnal pain), or a side effect from a medication used to treat the disorder (eg, diuretics causing nocturia). It followed that if the primary disorder could be effectively treated, then the insomnia would remit.[1] On the other hand, if the primary disorder was chronic then the insomnia was likely to be viewed as inevitable and possibly treated symptomatically with hypnotic medication. The diagnostic term *secondary insomnia* was applied to these insomnias, separating them from *primary insomnia*, which was assumed to be a stand-alone disorder.

Beginning around the year 2000, a new paradigm gradually emerged for understanding the nature of insomnia occurring in the context of psychiatric and medical illness. Research on understanding the etiology and treatment of these insomnias has led to a reconceptualization of these chronic sleep disturbances as functionally equivalent to primary insomnia in terms of psychological and behavioral factors that maintain the disorder. As a result, the term *comorbid insomnia* (CI) began to replace what was formerly referred to as *secondary insomnia*. This reconceptualization was given official sanction in 2005 with the consensus report of the National Institutes of Health,[2] and has been further reinforced by several reviews[3–5] and a wide range of studies occurring since that time.[6–10]

Behavioral treatments for insomnia have been refined over 3 decades, and have been shown to be highly efficacious in ameliorating primary insomnia.[11,12] However, until recently they were rarely used for the treatment of CI[13,14] because of the expectation that treatment had to target the primary disorder. This expectation limited the utility of CBT, because CI is known to present much more frequently than primary insomnia in sleep clinics and other health settings.[15,16] This situation led to a profound underutilization of a potent behavioral intervention for one of the most common sleep disorders afflicting millions of Americans.[2]

The recent reconceptualization of CI has been largely driven by a wave of research on three fronts. First, there have been a wide range of randomized clinical trials (RCTs) and case series studies documenting the efficacy of behavioral treatments for CI. The limited numbers of studies suggesting some efficacy of behavioral treatments for CI before 2000 were primarily smaller, non-randomized investigations. Second, the basic cause-and-effect relationship between the presumed parent disorder and insomnia has been challenged by the clinical evidence that insomnia often precedes the appearance of other disorders, and that it often continues after the presumed primary disorder has remitted. Finally, some critical etiologic research has been done in specific CI areas, including three conditions with

Preparation of this article was supported in part by National Institute of Aging grant AG017491 awarded to the first author.

[a] Department of Psychology, Virginia Commonwealth University, PO Box 842018, Richmond, VA, 23284-2018, USA
[b] Department of Internal Medicine, University of Tennessee Health Science Center, TN, USA
[c] Accelerated Community Oncology Research Network, Inc (ACORN), Kirby Parkway, Suite 400, Memphis, TN 38138, USA
* Corresponding author.
E-mail address: bdrybarczyk@vcu.edu (B. Rybarczyk).

a high prevalence of CI, namely cancer, depression, and chronic pain.

In this article the authors review the theoretical foundation for the new understanding of CI as an equivalent to primary insomnia, the body of evidence supporting behavioral interventions for CI, research on methods to increase public access to behavioral treatment of CI, and the specific advances in the domain of cancer, depression, and pain disorders.

THEORETICAL RATIONALE FOR THE RECONCEPTUALIZATION OF COMORBID INSOMNIA

The theoretical rationale for viewing CI as a diagnostic and treatment equivalent to primary insomnia can be found in the Spielman's 3-P model of chronic insomnia.[17] This model posits that all insomnias have predisposing, precipitating, and perpetuating factors that vary in importance over time. As such, the factors related to the precipitation of an initial episode of insomnia, such as stressful events, schedule changes, and so forth, are different from those factors that perpetuate and intensify the insomnia. Over time, the initial triggers for insomnia are replaced or eclipsed by cognitive and behavioral factors that maintain or perpetuate the insomnia. These factors include dysfunctional beliefs and cognitions regarding sleep, adoption of sleep-incompatible behaviors, circadian desynchronization, conditioned arousal to the bedroom, and other inhibitory factors (eg, excessive time in bed, increased caffeine consumption). The factors have been carefully delineated for primary insomnia, and interventions have been successfully designed to combat each of them.

Possible precipitators of initial episodes of insomnia in medical populations are varied and numerous. These precipitators include various sleep-disruptive symptoms such as pain, gastrointestinal distress, coughing, and other respiratory difficulties. Medication side effects such as frequent urination or central nervous system stimulation are also cited as catalysts in the onset of insomnia among medical patients who are prone to insomnia. Stress and negative affect related to a new medical diagnosis, and uncertainty about the future can also be triggers for new-onset insomnia in these groups. Medical and psychiatric disorders that are comorbid with insomnia may have played a role in precipitating insomnia, but then become less important as perpetuating factors take root and exacerbate insomnia. Despite the myriad of complex and interacting precipitators, the factors in any given individual need not

be isolated, because behavioral treatment packages are aimed at the perpetuating factors that are common to almost all individuals with insomnia.

Hospitalization has been cited as one possible precipitating factor for CI and, given the frequency of this event for medical patients, merits consideration as a place where new-onset insomnias might potentially be prevented. Excessive noise and light, as well as forced awakenings for taking vital signs or administering medications during sleep hours, are known factors in poor sleep during hospitalization. Hospital personnel typically view these sleep-disrupting problems as necessary evils of the requirements of efficient patient care, and as issues that will resolve for the patient after discharge.[18] However, the presumption that hospitalization-triggered sleep difficulties are transient has been challenged by two recent studies. One study by Smith and colleagues[19] found that among 333 patients hospitalized for burn injuries, 40.5% had sleep-onset insomnia at discharge, and this insomnia doubled the chances of insomnia at 2-year follow-up. A second study of 86 cardiac and orthopedic patients who were assessed before hospitalization for elective surgery and 3 months post hospitalization[18] found that the rate of chronic insomnia nearly doubled during that period, increasing from 10% to 19%. Of note, the latter study found that poor sleep during hospitalization did not predict insomnia at 3 months' follow-up. One possible explanation for the latter finding is that sleep problems began after discharge, when patients are often encouraged to sleep more than usual and to spend time in bed resting to promote recovery, thus promoting the perpetuating factors noted here.

Lastly, in terms of predisposing factors for insomnia, Spielman and colleagues have cited the role of personality factors (anxious, depressive, and emotionally reactive) and physiologic vulnerabilities such as decreased sleep drive and circadian rhythm deficiencies.[17] An additional factor that has received the attention of investigators since the 1960s is physiologic hyperarousal.[20] Bonnet and Arand theorize that an "arousal system" that is independent of the sleep system may be set to a high basal level that predisposes these individuals to chronic insomnia.[21] Others have described hyperarousal as an overactivation of the stress response system, particularly in the hypothalamic-pituitary-adrenal axis.[22,23] Specific evidence has accumulated linking insomnia to higher levels of daytime alertness (despite decreased total sleep time[24]), increased heart rate,[25] increased metabolic rates,[21] increased β activity in the sleep electroencephalogram,[26] and increased heart rate variability.[27] In addition to these studies showing higher levels of arousal, insomniacs have greater physiologic reactivity when completing a stressful task.[28] Unfortunately, due to the assumption that CI is a more complex disorder, most studies investigating hyperarousal thus far have focused exclusively on primary insomnia.

Chronic hyperarousal may also be associated with depression, pain, fatigue, and other medical and psychiatric disorders, and thus may serve as a common factor in the development of these comorbid conditions.[5] In this model, CI is seen as part of a hyperarousal/stress syndrome rather than as a discrete condition secondary to other conditions. For example, insomnia would be related to depression because the risk for both is increased as a result of a cascade of physiologic and psychological events that occur in response to a stressful event. Such a view explains the high co-occurrence of these two conditions, but without the need to see one as the direct cause or consequence of the other. Similar pathologic consequences of hyperarousal stress syndrome could include some pain syndromes, anxiety disorders, posttraumatic stress disorder (PTSD), and various cardiovascular events such as coronary artery disease.[5,29]

RESEARCH ON BEHAVIORAL INTERVENTIONS FOR COMORBID INSOMNIA

Table 1 provides a summary of the 25 published experimental studies testing and substantiating the efficacy for behavioral treatments for CI. These studies were found through a search of PsycINFO and MEDLINE using the key word "insomnia" in combination with "behavior," "behavioral," and a variety of medical and psychiatric diagnostic terms for the years 1965 through February 2009. The authors also examined the citations from studies that were obtained with this search to determine if any investigations were overlooked by this method. A study demonstrating the efficacy of a caffeine reduction strategy among human immunodeficiency virus (HIV) patients[30] was not included in the count because it employed a single sleep hygiene treatment strategy. Overall, these treatments indicate a high level of efficacy, with most of them demonstrating moderate to large effect sizes[3–5] comparable to those found for behavioral treatments of primary insomnia.

Among the 25 studies, 14 were classified as RCTs, with the remainder being quasi-experimental designs, multiple case studies, or multiple baseline case studies. Apart from the first RCT testing cognitive behavioral treatment for insomnia (CBT-I) for insomnia that was comorbid with periodic limb movement disorder,[31] and two that

tested relaxation treatment for CIs,[32,33] all of the other RCTs have been published since the year 2000, with half occurring since 2005. In contrast, by the year 2000 a large body of RCTs established high levels of efficacy for cognitive behavioral treatments for *primary insomnia*, with effect sizes in the moderate to high range.[11,12]

Most of the studies completed since 2000 have used multicomponent CBT-I, which has been established as the gold standard for insomnia intervention. This approach has the advantage of addressing a wide range of potential causative factors, and therefore does not require an accurate assessment of the primary causes of insomnia in each individual.[20] The specific components within the omnibus approach are fairly uniform, including a combination of stimulus control, sleep restriction, sleep hygiene, procedures for discontinuing or reducing hypnotics, and cognitive methods. The one exception is relaxation training, which is not included in some of the multicomponent intervention studies (eg, Refs.[10,34,35]). A recent study with patients who have Alzheimer's disease[36] also employed a necessarily different treatment model, which included caregiver administered modifications in activities, defined intervals for sleep, and light exposure (using a light box).

A variety of common comorbid conditions have been targeted in the recent wave of RCTs. In the domain of medical comorbidity, these studies have included mixed chronic illnesses,[37–39] chronic pain,[34] cancer,[10,35,40] coronary artery disease,[41] osteoarthritis,[41] fibromyalgia,[42] Alzheimer's disease,[36] primary care patients,[43] and pulmonary disease.[41] In the domain of psychiatric comorbidity there have been 3 nonrandomized studies addressing PTSD,[7,44,45] one for mild depression,[6] and one for patients with chronic mental illness.[46] In terms of RCTs, there have been only two with individuals with alcoholism[33,47] and one targeting participants with depression.[8] There is accordingly a critical need for additional RCT research that addresses the efficacy of CBT-I for psychiatric conditions that frequently occur with CI, including but not limited to PTSD, anxiety disorders, bipolar disorder, and nonalcohol substance abuse disorders.

Many investigators have underscored the fact that insomnia exacerbates the symptoms and effects on daytime functioning of coexisting medical and psychiatric conditions.[5] Thus, most intervention studies have hypothesized that secondary daytime medical, mental health, and quality of life benefits should follow from improved sleep. Virtually all of the non-RCT studies presented in **Table 1** found some improvements in daytime functioning in conjunction with

Table 1
Experimental studies of behavioral treatment for comorbid insomnia

Study	Comorbid Diagnosis	Treatment	Outcomes Compared with Controls	Daytime Functioning Outcomes
Multiple baseline or multiple case				
Morin et al (1989)[91]	Chronic pain	CBT	+Log, +PSG	Y
Davidson et al (2001)[74]	Cancer	CBT	+Log, +Quest	Y
Krakow et al (2001)[44]	PTSD	CBT	+Quest	Y
Quesnel et al (2003)[48]	Metastatic breast cancer	CBT	+Log, +PSG	Y
Dopke et al (2004)[46]	Serious mental illness	CBT	+Log, +Quest	Y
DeViva et al (2005)[45]	PTSD	CBT	+Log, +Quest	Y
Taylor et al (2007)[6]	Mild depression	CBT	+Log	Y
Germaine et al (2007)[7]	PTSD	Single session CBT	+Log	Y
Hudson et al (2008)[63]	HIV	Single session stimulus control	+Quest, −Act	Y
Goodie et al (2009)[43]	Primary care patients, >58% with medical diagnoses	Behavioral therapy/bibliotherapy	+Log, +Quest	N/A
Quasi-experimental				
Simiet et al (2004)[40]	Cancer	CBT (without sleep restriction)	+Log	Y
Randomized clinical trials (single treatment group)				
Cannici et al (1983)[32]	Cancer	Relaxation	+Log	N
Edinger et al (1996)[31]	PLMD	CBT	−Log, −Quest, −PSG	N
Greef and Conradie (1998)[33]	Alcoholism	Relaxation	+Quest	N/A
Currie et al (2000)[34]	Chronic pain	CBT	+Log, +Quest, +Act	Y

	Psychiatric and medical diagnoses	CBT (without sleep restriction)		
Lichstein et al (2000)[37]			+Log, −Quest	N
McCurry et al (2005)[36]	Alzheimer disease	Modified behavioral	+Quest, +Act	Y
Rybarczyk et al (2005)[39,41]	Osteoarthritis, coronary artery disease, COPD	CBT	+Log, +Quest	Y
Savard et al (2005)[35]	Breast cancer	CBT	+Log, +Quest, −PSG	Y
Manber et al (2008)[8]	Depression	CBT	+Log, +Quest, +Act	Y
Espie et al (2008)[9]	Cancer	CBT	+Log, +Act	Y
Randomized clinical trials (multiple treatment groups)				
Rybarczyk et al (2002)[49]	Chronic medical illness	CBT HART	CBT: +Log, +Quest, −Act HART: +Log, +Quest, −Act	N
Currie et al (2004)[47]	Alcoholism	CBT SHMT	CBT: +Log, +Quest, −Act SHMT: +Log, +Quest, −Act	N
Edinger et al (2005)[42]	Fibromyalgia	CBT SH	CBT: +Log, +Act SH: +Log, +Act	N
Randomized clinical trial (treatment comparison with single component)				
Epstein and Dirksen (2007)[10]	Breast cancer	CBT SH	+Log, +Act within group −Log, −Act between group	N/A

+, Significant findings; −, Nonsignificant findings.

Abbreviations: Act, actigraphy; CBT, cognitive behavioral therapy; COPD, chronic obstructive pulmonary disease; HART, home audiotape relaxation therapy; Log, sleep log; N, no; N/A, not available; PLMD, periodic limb movement disorder; PSG, polysomnography; PTSD, posttraumatic stress disorder; Quest, sleep habit questionnaire; SH, sleep hygiene; SHMT, self-help multicomponent treatment; Y, yes.

improvements in sleep. In contrast, only half of the 12 RCTs that included measurement of daytime functioning benefits found significant outcomes, with main findings being in two cancer studies,[35,48] and the Alzheimer's disease[36] and depression[8] studies. Rybarczyk and colleagues[41,49] assessed an array of secondary outcome measures that were relevant to chronic illness across two different studies. Only a single global rating of daytime effects of insomnia produced significant effects in one of the two studies.[41] Currie and colleagues[34] found no secondary benefits among chronic pain patients, and Edinger and colleagues[42] found no pain benefits in a fibromyalgia sample when comparing CBT-I to a control condition, although benefits were found for the sleep hygiene only group. A conservative assumption, based on the RCT findings, is that when regression to the mean and other threats to internal validity are controlled for, these daytime benefits are not as significant and widespread as would be assumed based on non-randomized studies and cross-sectional studies that examine the relationship between insomnia and other variables.

The evidence regarding objective changes in sleep following CBT-I is much less decisive than the self-report evidence. Among the three non-randomized and 10 RCT studies that employed objective outcome measures (ie, either actigraphy or polysomnography), 5 found no effects, including 4 that were RCTs.[31,35,47,49] This percentage of null findings is smaller by percentage than those obtained in the CBT-I for primary insomnia literature,[11,12] although effect sizes are consistently smaller in both studies when significant findings are obtained. The lack of ecological validity of laboratory-based polysomnography has been implicated as part of the reason for lower effect sizes for insomnia in CBT-I outcome studies. Also, the failure of several RCT studies to obtain actigraphy outcomes may be partly due to the limitations of the scoring algorithms for specialized populations that may spend more time lying motionless in bed while not asleep, resulting in overestimates of sleep time.[50]

It is worth noting that not only have pharmacologic agents been shown to have lower long-term efficacy relative to behavioral methods for treatment of chronic insomnia,[51,52] but nonpharmacologic interventions are also likely to be more attractive than hypnotics for individuals with CI and their health providers. In addition to usual concerns about dependency and tolerance associated with long-term use of hypnotics, individuals with medical and psychiatric conditions who are potentially taking several medications have an increased risk for drug interactions and adverse events.[53,54] Furthermore, with hypnotic use there is additional concern about and risk of addiction among individuals with psychiatric histories that include drugs or alcohol. With cancer patients, the common symptom of daytime fatigue may be amplified by hypnotic medications, especially longer-acting compounds.[55]

INCREASING ACCESSIBILITY OF COGNITIVE BEHAVIORAL THERAPY FOR COMORBID INSOMNIA

Even though the literature holds much promise for millions of adults with primary insomnia and CI, much work needs to be done to increase the public's access to CBT-I treatment. Few clinicians are trained to deliver this treatment, and insurance reimbursement for treatment services remains problematic.[56] Individuals with CI may have even more limited access to CBT-I, because their functional impairments may make it more difficult for them to visit a clinic for the required number of sessions. Indeed, a recent needs assessment of 26 cancer patients with sleep difficulties indicated that home-based, flexible approaches using technologies such as webcasts, Web sites, and videos would increase the level of participation.[57] Thus, empirically validated self-help CBT-I treatments could play an important role in filling the gap in treatment of CI in particular.

Several previous studies have already documented the efficacy of self-help CBT-I for primary insomnia.[58–61] Two studies thus far have provided self-help CBT-I to CI patients. One study randomized 60 recovering alcoholics to in-person CBT-I or a self-help CBT-I book treatment.[47] Results were comparable across the two treatments and significantly better than controls at post treatment, but the in-person participants demonstrated more clinically significant changes at 6-month follow-up. In 2005 Rybarczyk and colleagues conducted a pilot study that compared the efficacy of a self-help video version of CBT-I to outcomes from a previously published study of classroom CBT-I and a no treatment control group.[39] The self-help CBT-I was not significantly different from classroom CBT on self-report measures of sleep relative to wait-list controls, but the attrition rate was higher (27% vs 19%) and the number of participants who achieved clinically significant change was lower (50% vs 73%). Like the result found for primary insomnia, these findings suggest that self-help treatments for CI are effective but likely to be attenuated relative to therapist-led treatments. Even with these reductions in efficacy, they still may prove to be a preferred first line of treatment due to their accessibility and reduced cost.

Brief behavioral treatments administered by nurses, technicians, and other health professionals may be another form of CBT-I that holds promise for improving access and lowering cost barriers for individuals with CI. CBT-I interventions detailed in **Table 1** typically range from four to eight sessions, with individual sessions lasting 1 hour and group sessions lasting between 90 minutes and 2 hours.[3] However, a recent study examining the dose-response curve of individual CBT-I treatment sessions showed that four sessions delivered over 8 weeks was superior to eight weekly sessions.[62] There have been three recent pilot studies that have tested even briefer interventions for CI. Germaine and colleagues[7] provided a single 90-minute modified CBT-I and nightmare reduction technique to seven adult victims of violent crimes with a diagnosis of PTSD. Participants reported improvements in self-report and sleep diary measures of sleep quality and dream frequency post intervention. Clinically meaningful reductions in daytime PTSD symptom severity were also observed. Hudson and colleagues[63] administered a single-session sleep hygiene intervention that included elements of stimulus control to a convenience sample of 30 HIV-positive women. After 1 week there was a significant improvement in their perception of sleep and a significant change in their actigraphy recordings of 24-hour activity, with more activity and less napping during the day. A third study by Goodie and colleagues[43] provided three brief individualized CBT-I sessions along with a self-help book to 29 primary care patients with insomnia (approximately 58% with chronic medical conditions). At posttreatment assessment, 83% of participants achieved a mean sleep efficiency of more than 85%, compared with only 14% at baseline.

Lastly, in light of the shortage of CBT-I trained psychologists that will likely continue for some time into the future,[56] there is a need to examine the feasibility and efficacy of training nurses and other professionals to administer CBT-I. A recent RCT reviewed later in this article[9] showed that an intervention for cancer patients delivered by oncology nurses, with no expertise or even prior experience in sleep medicine, produced effect sizes that were comparable to interventions delivered by psychologists. In this case the nurses were given brief training by expert psychologists; this serves as a model of how specialists might train and subsequently supervise more available staff to deliver CBT-I. That CBT-I is robust enough to yield results in a variety of cost-effective and more feasible formats testifies to its strong potential for more widespread application. However, ideally these treatments should be offered in a stepped-care continuum that would provide more intensive treatment or treatment delivered by CBT-I trained psychologists when self-help or brief treatments have failed.

CANCER AND COMORBID INSOMNIA

Insomnia is a common and distressing complaint among individuals with cancer, with well-designed studies indicating that between 19% and 30% meet diagnostic criteria for insomnia.[64–68] The variation in the reported insomnia prevalence rates is likely due to the combination of the different types and stages of cancer, assessment of patients at different points in the continuum of cancer treatment, and differences in the level of rigor in the measurement of insomnia symptoms.[65,68] For example, using reliable and valid measures of insomnia in a study of 300 women who underwent radiation therapy for nonmetastatic breast cancer, investigators found a prevalence rate of 19%.[69] As an indication of how distressing insomnia is for cancer patients, studies report that as many as 25% of patients use hypnotic medications despite their contraindications in terms of drug interactions and increasing fatigue.[55]

Although there has been limited research on the etiology of sleep problems in cancer patients,[70] it is hypothesized that insomnia in this population is associated with psychological (anxiety and depression), medical (pain and medication effects), and behavioral (increased napping) factors.[71] Cancer researchers recently have begun to consider insomnia as part of a symptom cluster or a group of interrelated cancer symptoms that commonly occur together, such as depression, fatigue, and pain.[72] The concept of a symptom cluster recognizes that there are complex interrelationships between these groups of symptoms that are not readily explained by unidirectional cause-and-effect models.[71] One recent study analyzed self-report data of insomnia, fatigue, depression, and pain from a sample of 11,445 cancer patients using structural equation modeling.[73] The resulting model found that trouble sleeping was significantly increased as a consequence of depressed mood and recent chemotherapy (within prior 30 days). Increased trouble sleeping led to increased pain and fatigue in patients with cancer. These results have implications for improvement in daytime functioning as an outcome of improved sleep, as described later.

Given the prevalence of disturbed sleep and the quality of life implications in this population, cancer patients have been by far the largest target of studies of CBT-I for CI,[9,10,32,35,40,48,74] with four of these studies being RCTs. These seven studies have shown significant outcomes on a wide array of measures and have also had some of the largest effect sizes in the CI literature. The fact that four of the seven studies have been RCTs further strengthens the importance of these findings.

In 1983 the first experimental study of any kind testing a behavioral treatment for CI, an RCT, remarkably, compared relaxation training to a control condition for pain patients with CI.[32] The results showed significant changes in overall sleep report compared with controls at post treatment. Following a series of nonrandomized studies supporting CBT-I for insomnia in cancer patients,[40,48,74] three additional RCTs were conducted. Savard and Dirksen[35] randomized 57 women with insomnia caused or aggravated by breast cancer to CBT-I (including fatigue management strategies) or a wait-list control group. Compared with controls, CBT-I recipients had significantly better subjective sleep and a reduction in nights when they used medication at both posttreatment and 12-month follow-up. Esptein and Dirksen[10] randomized a group of 72 breast cancer survivors to a CBT-I condition or a sleep hygiene and education only treatment condition. These investigators found within-group effects for self-report and sleep efficiency, but only minor treatment differences between multicomponent and single-component treatment. Espie and colleagues[9] randomized 150 patients who completed active therapy for breast, prostate, colorectal, or gynecologic cancer to CBT-I or treatment as usual, and found substantial effects for both diary and actigraphy sleep measures at posttreatment and 6-month follow-up.

Due to possible reciprocal effects within symptom clusters in cancer patients, effective treatment of insomnia should have implications for the reduction or prevention of other interrelated cancer symptoms such as depression, pain, and fatigue. In fact, the most consistent daytime functioning effects from CBT-I for CI, especially among the more rigorous RCT studies, have been found in cancer patients.[3] The 2008 RCT by Espie and colleagues showed improvements relative to controls in an impressive five of seven quality of life outcome measures.[9] The 2003 study by Quesnel and colleagues demonstrated that cancer patients receiving CBT-I showed improvements in mood, general and physical fatigue, and global and cognitive dimensions of quality of life.[48] Finally, the 2005 study by Savard and colleagues showed that cancer patients in the treatment group had lower depression and anxiety as well as greater global quality of life compared with controls.[35] The collective findings make a strong case for targeting cancer patients as a critical need group for the dissemination of accessible CBT-I interventions.

DEPRESSION AND COMORBID INSOMNIA

Depression is one of the most prevalent comorbid disorders that occurs with insomnia. Approximately 60% to 80% of patients presenting with major depression report significant symptoms of insomnia as well. In contrast, 35% to 47% of those with insomnia report significant symptoms of depression.[13,75,76] Odds ratios for patients with major depressive disorder experiencing mild to severe insomnia range from 2.3 to 8.2, respectively.[77] Insomnia is one of the most common symptoms of depression; however, studies have suggested that it may not only be a symptom but also a risk factor for onset of depression, decreased response to treatments for depression, and depression symptom relapse.[78] In recent studies, insomnia is thought of as less of a correlate of depression but a separate disease process that has a reciprocal relationship with depressive symptoms. In some situations insomnia precedes depression and in other situations the opposite is true. The two may perpetuate and exacerbate one another rather than be linked as cause and effect, suggesting that the relationship between depression and insomnia may be too complex to determine causality.[2,79]

Etiologic theories of insomnia are rooted in the diathesis-stress model, which suggests that a predisposition coupled with an environmental stressor may result in maladaptive behavior patterns that lead to symptoms of disturbed sleep. This model can help us to understand depression as both a precursor to and consequence of insomnia. Depression symptoms may develop as a result of the insomnia that follows a particularly stressful life event, but depression can also function as a stressor in itself.[80] Behavioral treatments to treat symptoms of insomnia have the potential to also improve symptoms of depression, interrupting the perpetuating cycle of symptoms associated with these comorbid disorders.

The findings of two recent studies provide strong initial support for the efficacy of treating insomnia in the context of depression. A 2007 pilot study provided 6 sessions of CBT-I to a group of individuals with mild depression.[6] There were no additional treatments provided for the depression. Among the 8 participants who completed treatment, 100% achieved normal sleep scores on self-report and 87.5% obtained scores in the normal range on a depression inventory. These gains were maintained at 3-month follow-up. A 2008 randomized clinical trial was the first to test a treatment combination of pharmacologic treatment for depression and behavioral treatment for insomnia.[8] Thirty individuals with major depressive disorder and clinically significant insomnia were randomly assigned to seven sessions of CBT-I and escitalopram, or seven sessions of a control treatment (quasi-desensitization) and escitalopram. Consistent with the hypothesis, adjunctive CBT-I led to remission of insomnia in 50% of the active treatment participants versus 7.7% remission in the control group. More notably, the CBT-I treatment also synergized the medication treatment of depression, resulting in almost double the rate of remission from depression compared with controls (61.5% vs 33.3%). If future studies replicate these important findings, in the near future simultaneous treatment of depression and insomnia may become the standard of care.

CHRONIC PAIN AND COMORBID INSOMNIA

Insomnia is known to frequently accompany chronic pain conditions, with between 50% and 88% of chronic pain sufferers reporting significant sleep disturbance.[4] Arthritis-related pain is the most common factor predicting sleep disturbance in the general population,[81] and chronic low-back pain, the most common cause of pain, and fibromyalgia[82] are also strongly associated with CI.[83] It has been established that pain interferes with sleep,[84] and more recent research demonstrates that disturbed sleep lowers pain threshold.[85–87] One study showed a relationship between episodes of exacerbated pain and poor sleep at night in individuals with a variety of chronic musculoskeletal pain conditions.[88] Reciprocal effects whereby poor sleep worsens pain and vice versa in clinical populations are logical and have been supported by studies of fibromyalgia patients,[82] burn patients,[89] and osteoarthritis patients.[90]

The apparent reciprocal nature of pain and sleep makes a strong case for applying CBT-I to pain patients to simultaneously address these related symptoms. Therefore, it is not surprising that the first experimental study of the CBT-I treatment package for CI, in 1989, was conducted with a group of three chronic pain patients.[91] In this multiple baseline study, three subjects who received CBT-I showed improvements on polysomnography and self-report measures of sleep that were well maintained at

follow-up. However, another 11 years passed before the next study, an RCT, compared CBT-I to a wait-list control condition in a group of 60 chronic pain patients.[34] Sleep improvements were found for both self-report and actigraphy relative to controls, and these improvements were largely maintained at 3-month follow-up. Although not included in **Table 1** due to the lack of methodological details contained in a brief report, a third study is worth mentioning because it provided treatment to a group of 70 children with migraine headaches and CI.[92] Subjects randomized to a sleep hygiene treatment had reductions in the frequency and duration of their migraines compared with a treatment-as-usual control group. A next step in research is to test a combination of established behavioral treatments for pain with CBT-I to determine whether there may be a synergistic effect for both treatments, as found in the study by Manber and colleagues[8] for depression and CI.

SUMMARY

There is now strong empirical support for viewing CI as a functional equivalent to primary insomnia occurring in an otherwise healthy individual. In both cases CBT-I should be viewed as a highly efficacious first line of treatment. In addition, when psychiatric conditions are present the benefits from the alleviation of CI may translate into improvements in the coexisting condition and functional status in both medical and psychiatric comorbid conditions, especially among individuals with cancer, depression, and chronic pain. Furthermore, self-help, abbreviated, and nonexpert delivered methods of treatment seem to be nearly as efficacious, and warrant further investigation. These less expensive and more accessible interventions may serve as a first step in a stepped-care model of CI treatment. Additional research using RCT methodologies is needed, with studies addressing CI occurring in the context of specific psychiatric conditions yet to be studied (eg, anxiety disorders, bipolar disorder). Methodological improvements in objective assessment of CI are also needed to further support and elucidate the consistent and large effects that are found for self-report measures of sleep.

ACKNOWLEDGEMENT

Preparation of this article was supported in part by National Institute of Aging grant AG017491 awarded to the first author.

REFERENCES

1. Zorick FJ, Walsh JK. Evaluation and management of insomnia: an overview. In: Kryger MH, Roth T, Dement WC, editors. Principles and practices of sleep medicine. 3rd edition. Philadelphia: WB Saunders Company; 2000. p. 615–23.

2. National Institutes of Health. National Institutes of Health State of the Science Conference statement on manifestations and management of chronic insomnia in adults, June 13–15. Sleep 2005;28:1049–57.

3. Lichstein KL, Rybarczyk B, Dillon HR. Cognitive-behavior therapy for comorbid and late-life insomnia, in press.

4. Smith MT, Huang MI, Manber R. Cognitive behavior therapy for chronic insomnia occurring within the context of medical and psychiatric disorders. Clin Psychol Rev 2005;25(5):559–92.

5. Stepanski EJ, Rybarczyk B. Emerging research on the treatment and etiology of secondary or comorbid insomnia. Sleep Med Rev 2006;10:7–18.

6. Taylor DJ, Lichstein KL, Weinstock J, et al. A pilot study of cognitive-behavioral therapy of insomnia in people with mild depression. Behav Ther 2007; 38:49–57.

7. Germaine AM, Shear K, Hall M, et al. Effects of a brief behavioral treatment for PTSD-related sleep disturbances: a pilot study. Behav Res Ther 2007;45: 627–32.

8. Manber R, Edinger JD, Gress JL. Cognitive behavioral therapy for insomnia enhances depression outcome in patients with comorbid major depressive disorder and insomnia. Sleep 2008;31(4): 489–95.

9. Espie CA, Fleming L, Cassidy J, et al. Randomized controlled clinical effectiveness trial of cognitive behavior therapy compared with treatment as usual for persistent insomnia in patients with cancer. J Clin Oncol 2008;26(28):4651–8.

10. Epstein DR, Dirksen SR. Randomized trial of a cognitive-behavioral intervention for insomnia in breast cancer survivors. Oncol Nurs Forum 2007;34(5): E51–9.

11. Murtagh DR, Greenwood KM. Identifying effective psychological treatments for insomnia: a meta-analysis. J Consult Clin Psychol 1995;63:79–89.

12. Morin CM, Culbert JP, Schwartz SM. Nonpharmacological interventions for insomnia: a meta-analysis of treatment efficacy. Am J Psychiatry 1994;151: 1172–80.

13. Buysse D, Reynolds C, Kupfer D, et al. Effects of diagnosis on treatment recommendations in chronic insomnia—a report from the APA/NIMH DSM-IV field trial. Sleep 1997;20:542–52.

14. Chesson AL, Andersin WM, Littner M, et al. Practice parameters for the nonpharmacologic treatment of chronic insomnia. Sleep 1999;22:1128–33.

15. Ohayon MM. Epidemiology of insomnia what we know and what we still need to learn. Sleep Med Rev 2002;6:97–111.

16. Buysse D, Reynolds C, Kupfer D, et al. Clinical diagnoses in 216 insomnia patients using the international classification of sleep disorders (ICSD), DSM-IV, and ICD-10 categories: a report from the APA/NIMH DSM-IV field trial. Sleep 1994;17:630–7.

17. Spielman AJ, Caruso L, Glovinsky P. A behavioral perspective on insomnia. Psychiatr Clin North Am 1987;10:541–53.

18. Griffiths MF, Peerson A. Risk factors for chronic insomnia following hospitalization. J Adv Nurs 2005;49(3):245–53.

19. Smith MT, Klick B, Kozachik S, et al. Sleep onset insomnia symptoms during hospitalization for major burn injury predict chronic pain. Pain 2008;138: 497–506.

20. Stepanski EJ. The effect of sleep fragmentation on daytime function. Sleep 2002;25(3):268–76.

21. Bonnet MH, Arand D. 24-hour metabolic rate in insomniacs and matched normal sleepers. Sleep 1995;18:581–8.

22. Shaver JL, Johnston SK, Lentz MJ, et al. Stress exposure, psychological distress, and physiological stress activation in midlife women with insomnia. Psychosom Med 2002;64:793–802.

23. Vgontzas AN, Chrousos GP. Sleep, the hypothalamic-pituitary-adrenal axis, and cytokines: multiple interactions and disturbances in sleep disorders. Endocrinol Metab Clin North Am 2002;31(1):15–36.

24. Stepanski E, Zorick F, Roehrs T, et al. Daytime alertness in patients with chronic insomnia compared with asymptomatic control subjects. Sleep 1988; 11:54–60.

25. Stepanski E, Glinn M, Zorick F, et al. Heart rate changes in chronic insomnia. Stress Med 1994;10: 261–6.

26. Perlis ML, Merica H, Smith MT, et al. Beta EEG in insomnia. Sleep Med Rev 2001;5:364–75.

27. Bonnet MH, Arand D. Heart rate variability in insomniacs and matched normal sleepers. Psychosom Med 1998;60:610–5.

28. Vgontzas AN, Zoumakis M, Bixler EO, et al. Impaired nighttime sleep in healthy old versus young adults is associated with elevated plasma interleukin-6 and cortisol levels: physiologic and therapeutic implications. J Clin Endocrinol Metab 2003;88:2087–95.

29. Mallon L, Broman JE, Hetta J. Sleep complaints predict coronary disease mortality in males: a 12-year follow-up study of a middle-aged Swedish population. J Intern Med 2002;251:207–16.

30. Dreher HM. The effect of caffeine reduction on sleep quality and well being in persons with HIV. J Psychosom Res 2003;54:191–8.

31. Edinger JD, Fins AI, Sullivan RJ, et al. Comparison of cognitive-behavioral therapy and clonazepam for

treating periodic limb movement disorder. Sleep 1996;19(5):442–4.

32. Cannici J, Malcolm R, Peek LA. Treatment of insomnia in cancer patients using muscle relaxation training. J Behav Ther Exp Psychiatry 1983;14(3): 251–6.

33. Greeff AP, Conradie WS. Use of progressive relaxation training for chronic alcoholics with insomnia. Psychol Rep 1998;82:407–12.

34. Currie SR, Wilson KG, Pontefract AJ. Cognitive-behavioral treatment of insomnia secondary to chronic pain. J Consult Clin Psychol 2000;68(3):407–16.

35. Savard J, Simard S, Ivers H, et al. Randomized study on the efficacy of cognitive-behavioral therapy for insomnia secondary to breast cancer, part I: sleep and psychological effects. J Clin Oncol 2005;23:6083–96.

36. McCurry SM, Gibbons LE, Logsdon RG. Nighttime insomnia treatment and education for Alzheimer's disease: a randomized, controlled trial. J Am Geriatr Soc 2005;53:793–802.

37. Lichstein KL, Wilson NM, Johnson CT. Psychological treatment of secondary insomnia. Psychol Aging 2000;15(2):232–40.

38. Perlis ML, Sharpe M, Smith MT, et al. Behavioral treatment of insomnia: treatment outcome and the relevance of medical and psychiatric morbidity. J Behav Med 2001;24:281–96.

39. Rybarczyk B, Lopez M, Schelble K, et al. Home-based video CBT for comorbid geriatric insomnia: a pilot study using secondary data analyses. Behav Sleep Med 2005;3:158–75.

40. Simiet R, Deck R, Conta-Marx B. Sleep management training for cancer patients with insomnia. Support Care Cancer 2004;12:176–83.

41. Rybarczyk B, Stepanski E, Fogg L, et al. A placebo-controlled test of cognitive-behavioral therapy for comorbid insomnia in older adults. J Consult Clin Psychol 2005;73:1164–74.

42. Edinger JD, Wohlgemuth WK, Krystal AD. Behavioral insomnia therapy for fibromyalgia patients: a randomized clinical trial. Arch Intern Med 2005; 165(21):2527–35.

43. Goodie JL, Isler WC, Hunter C, et al. Using behavioral health consultants to treat insomnia in primary care: a clinical case series. J Clin Psychol 2009; 65(3):294–304.

44. Krakow B, Johnston L, Melendez D, et al. An open-label trial of evidence-based cognitive behavioral therapy for nightmares and insomnia in crime victims with PTSD. Am J Psychiatry 2001;158: 2043–7.

45. DeViva JC, Zayfert C, Pigeon WR, et al. Treatment of residual insomnia after CBT for PTSD: case studies. J Trauma Stress 2005;18(2):155–9.

46. Dopke CA, Lehner RK, Wells AM. Cognitive-behavioral group therapy for insomnia in individuals with serious mental illnesses: a preliminary evaluation. Psychiatr Rehabil J 2004;27(3):234–42.

47. Currie SR, Clark S, Hodgins DC, et al. Randomized controlled trial of brief cognitive-behavioral interventions for insomnia in recovering alcoholics. Addiction 2004;99:1121–32.

48. Quesnel C, Savard J, Simard S, et al. Efficacy of cognitive-behavioral therapy for insomnia in women in treatment for nonmetastatic breast cancer. J Consult Clin Psychol 2003;71:189–200.

49. Rybarczyk B, Lopez M, Benson R, et al. Efficacy of two behavioral treatment programs for comorbid geriatric insomnia. Psychol Aging 2002;17:288–98.

50. Sivertsen B, Omvik S, Havik OE, et al. A comparison of actigraphy and polysomnography in older adults treated for chronic primary insomnia. Sleep 2006; 29:1353–8.

51. Morin CM, Colecchi C, Stone J, et al. Behavioral and pharmacological therapies for late-life insomnia: a randomized controlled trial. JAMA 1999;281:991–9.

52. Sivertsen B, Omvik S, Pallesen S, et al. Cognitive behavioral therapy vs zopiclone for treatment of chronic primary insomnia in older adults: a randomized controlled trial. JAMA 2006;295:2851–8.

53. Allain H, Bentué-Ferrer D, Tarral A, et al. Effects on postural oscillation and memory functions of a single dose of zolpidem 5 mg, zopiclone 3.75 mg and lormetazepam 1 mg in elderly healthy subjects. A randomized, cross-over, double-blind study versus placebo. Eur J Clin Pharmacol 2003;59(3):179–88.

54. Vermeeren A. Residual effects of hypnotics: epidemiology and clinical implications. CNS Drugs 2004; 18(5):297–328.

55. Curt GA. Fatigue in cancer. BMJ 2001;322:1560.

56. Perlis ML, Smith MT. How can we make CBT-I and other BSM services widely available? J Clin Sleep Med 2008;4(1):11–3.

57. Davidson JR, Feldman-Stewart D, Brennenstuhl S, et al. How to provide insomnia interventions to people with cancer: insights from patients. Psychooncology 2007;16(11):1028–38.

58. Riedel BW, Lichstein KL, Dwyer WO. Sleep compression and sleep education for older insomniacs: self-help versus therapist guidance. Psychol Aging 1995;10:54–63.

59. Mimeault V, Morin CM. Self-help treatment for insomnia: bibliotherapy with and without professional guidance. J Consult Clin Psychol 1999; 67(4):511–9.

60. Morin CM, Beaulieu-Bonneau S, LeBlanc M, et al. Self-help treatment for insomnia: a randomized controlled trial. Sleep 2005;28(10):1319–27.

61. Ström L, Pettersson R, Andersson G. Internet-based treatment for insomnia: a controlled evaluation. J Consult Clin Psychol 2004;72(1):113–20.

62. Edinger JD, Wohlgemuth WK, Radtke RA, et al. Dose-response effects of cognitive-behavioral

insomnia therapy: a randomized clinical trial. Sleep 2007;30(2):203–12.

63. Hudson AL, Portillo CJ, Lee KA. Sleep disturbances in women with HIV or AIDS: efficacy of a tailored sleep promotion intervention. Nurs Res 2008;57(5): 360–6.

64. Cleeland CS, Mendoza TR, Wang XS, et al. Assessing symptom distress in cancer patients: the M.D. Anderson Symptom Inventory. Cancer 2000;89(7): 1634–46.

65. Davidson JR, MacLean AW, Brundage MD, et al. Sleep disturbance in cancer patients. Soc Sci Med 2002;54(9):1309–21.

66. Fortner BV, Stepanski EJ, Wang SC, et al. Sleep and quality of life in breast cancer patients. J Pain Symptom Manage 2002;24(5):471–80.

67. Hewitt M, Greenfield S, Stovall E. Committee on cancer survivorship: improving care and quality of life IoMaNRC. From cancer patient to cancer survivor. Lost in transition. Washington, DC: National Academic Press; 2006.

68. Koopman C, Nouriani B, Erickson V, et al. Sleep disturbances in women with metastatic breast cancer. Breast J 2002;8(6):362–70.

69. Savard J, Simard S, Blanchet JB, et al. Prevalence, clinical characteristics, and risk factors for insomnia in the context of breast cancer. Sleep 2001;24(5): 583–90.

70. Berger AM, Sankaranarayanan J, Watanabe-Galloway S. Current methodological approaches to the study of sleep disturbances and quality of life in adults with cancer: a systematic review. Psychooncology 2007;16(5):401–20.

71. Stepanski EJ, Burgess HJ. Sleep and cancer. Sleep Med Clin 2007;2:67–75.

72. Miaskowski C, Dodd M, Lee K. Symptom clusters: the new frontier in symptom management research. J Natl Cancer Inst Monogr 2004;32:17–21.

73. Stepanski EJ, Walker MS, Schwartzberg LS, et al. The relation of trouble sleeping, depressed mood, pain, and fatigue in patients with cancer. J Clin Sleep Med 2009;5:132–6.

74. Davidson JR, Waisberg JL, Brundage MD, et al. Nonpharmacologic group treatment of insomnia: a preliminary study with cancer survivors. Psychoon cology 2001;10(5):389–97.

75. Coleman RM, Roffwarg HP, Kennedy SJ, et al. Sleep-wake disorders based on a polysomnographic diagnosis. A national cooperative study. JAMA 1982;247:997–1003.

76. McCall WV, Reboussin BA, Cohen W. Subjective measurement of insomnia and quality of life in depressed inpatients. J Sleep Res 2000;9:43–8.

77. Katz DA, McHorney CA. Clinical correlates of insomnia in patients with chronic illness. Arch Intern Med 1998;158:1099–107.

78. Perlis ML, Giles DE, Buysse DJ, et al. Self-reported sleep disturbance as a prodromal symptom in recurrent depression. J Affect Disord 1997;42:209–12.

79. Turek FW. Insomnia and depression: if it looks and walks like a duck. Sleep 2005;28:1362–3.

80. Benca R. Mood disorders. In: Kryger MH, Roth T, Dement WC, editors. Principles and practices of sleep medicine. 3rd edition. Philadelphia: W.B. Saunders; 2000. p. 1140–57.

81. Moffitt PF, Kalucy EC, Kalucy RS, et al. Sleep difficulties, pain and other correlates. J Intern Med 1001; 230(3):245–9.

82. Affleck G, Urrows S, Tennen H, et al. Sequential daily relations of sleep, pain intensity, and attention to pain among women with fibromyalgia. Pain 1996;68:363–8.

83. Rives PA, Douglass AB. Evaluation and treatment of low back pain in family practice. J Am Board Fam Pract 2004;17:S23–31.

84. Smith MT, Haythornthwaite JA. How do sleep disturbances and chronic pain inter-relate? Insights from the longitudinal and cognitive-behavioral clinical trials. Sleep Med Rev 2004;8(2):119–32.

85. Haack M, Sanchez E, Mullington JM. Elevated inflammatory markers in response to prolonged sleep restriction are associated with increased pain experience in healthy volunteers. Sleep 2007; 30(9):1145–52.

86. Smith MT, Edwards RR, McCann UD, et al. The effects of sleep deprivation on pain inhibition and spontaneous pain in women. Sleep 2007;30(4):494–505.

87. Roehrs T, Hyde M, Blaisdell B, et al. Sleep loss and REM sleep loss are hyperalgesic. Sleep 2006;29(2): 145–51.

88. Wilson KG, Watson ST, Currie SR. Daily diary and ambulatory activity monitoring of sleep in patients with insomnia associated with chronic musculoskeletal pain. Pain 1998;75:75–84.

89. Raymond I, Nielsen TA, Lavigne G, et al. Quality of sleep and its daily relationship to pain intensity in hospitalized adult burn patients. Pain 2001;92(3):381–8.

90. Moldofsky H, Lue FA, Saskin P. Sleep and morning pain in primary osteoarthritis. J Rheumatol 1987; 14(1):124–8.

91. Morin CM, Kowatch RA, Wade JB. Behavioral management of sleep disturbances secondary to chronic pain. J Behav Ther Exp Psychiatry 1989; 20:295–302.

92. Bruni O, Galli F, Guidetti V. Sleep hygiene and migraine in children and adolescents. Cephalalgia 1999;19(Suppl 25):57–9.

Management of Hypnotic Discontinuation in Chronic Insomnia

Lynda Bélanger, PhD[a,b],*, Geneviève Belleville, PhD[c,d],
Charles M. Morin, PhD[a,b]

KEYWORDS

- Insomnia • Benzodiazepines • Hypnotic medications
- Discontinuation • Stepped-care approach • Sleep disorder

Pharmacologic approaches are the most widely used treatment options for the management of chronic insomnia.[1,2] Hypnotic medications are indicated and efficacious for treating situational insomnia.[3] However, despite clear guidelines suggesting that hypnotic drug use should be time limited,[3] a considerable proportion of individuals with insomnia use hypnotics on a nightly basis for prolonged periods of time, often reaching many years. Furthermore, many individuals will continue reporting significant sleep disturbances despite an appropriate therapeutic use of hypnotic medications.[4] In clinical practice, clinicians treating patients with chronic complaints of sleep difficulties are often faced with the dilemma of hypnotic discontinuation versus continued prescription. Although long-term use of hypnotics for the management of chronic insomnia remains controversial, information regarding hypnotic discontinuation is still scarce.

This article discusses different aspects of long-term hypnotic use in chronic insomnia, with a focus on the management of hypnotic withdrawal. Issues such as preoccupation with long-term use, factors associated with the development of hypnotic-dependent insomnia, and step-by-step treatment strategies to help discontinuation of hypnotic use are presented.

LONG-TERM HYPNOTIC USE
Preoccupation with Long-term Use

Chronic insomnia is consistently associated with significant reduction in the quality of life, higher risk of depression, and increased use of health care services.[5] Different drug classes are routinely used for the management of insomnia. These include benzodiazepine receptor agonists (BzRAs), selective melatonin receptor agonists, and sedating antidepressants. This article focuses on BzRA hypnotics only. This drug class includes 2 groups of prescription hypnotics: the classical benzodiazepines (BZDs; eg, temazepam, triazolam, flurazepam, quazepam, estazolam) and the more recently introduced drugs that have a non-BZD structure but act at the BZD receptor sites (eg, zaleplon, zolpidem, eszopiclone). Although classical BZDs have for many years been the drug class of choice for the treatment of insomnia, non-BZD hypnotics are now the indicated drug class

[a] Université Laval, École de Psychologie, 2325, Rue des Bibliothèques, Québec, QC G1V 0A6, Canada
[b] Centre de Recherche Université Laval/Robert-Giffard, Québec, QC G1J 2G3, Canada
[c] Département de Psychologie, Université du Québec à Montréal, CP 8888, Succ Centre-Ville, Montréal, QC H3P 3C8, Canada
[d] Centre de Recherche Fernand-Seguin, Hôpital Louis-H.-Lafontaine, 7401, Rue Hochelaga, Montréal, QC H1N 3M5, Canada
* Corresponding author. Université Laval, École de Psychologie, 2325, Rue des Bibliothèques, Québec, QC, Canada.
E-mail address: lynda.belanger@psy.ulaval.ca (L. Bélanger).

Sleep Med Clin 4 (2009) 583–592
doi:10.1016/j.jsmc.2009.07.011

for insomnia pharmacotherapy.[6] The main advantages that newer non-BZDs present over the traditional BZDs are their faster elimination rate and relative α-1 binding selectivity, which significantly decrease some of the side effects associated with the classical BZDs.[7] However, they are not free from side effects or adverse effects and, like their predecessors, have been associated with risks of dependence, higher risks of accidents and falls, and cognitive disturbances, which again calls for increased caution when they are prescribed to some specific groups of patients.[7–10] Furthermore, the risks associated with their prolonged daily use are still not very well documented, and well-designed studies to examine those risks are warranted. There is also very limited evidence in the literature regarding their sustained long-term efficacy over several years.[11–13] Another important limitation associated with hypnotic use for chronic insomnia is that treatment cessation is often associated with a return of sleep difficulties or with rebound insomnia, an exacerbation of the original insomnia severity. Recrudescence of insomnia symptoms after hypnotic discontinuation has been hypothesized to play a role in the development of hypnotic-dependent insomnia.[14] For these reasons, long-term use of hypnotics for the management of insomnia remains controversial.[3,15]

Factors Associated with the Development of Hypnotic-dependent Insomnia

Approximately 5% to 7% of the adult population uses prescribed sleep-promoting medications during the course of a year.[1,2,16] For most people, medication is used for a limited period of time (as in acute stress). For many patients, however, the pattern of use is occasional but recurrent and for others, medication is used on a regular and long-term basis. In most cases, sleep medication is initiated during acute episodes of insomnia that results from psychological stress, medical illness, or important schedule changes associated with jet lag or shift work. It may also be initiated in the context of chronic insomnia, when a person can no longer cope with the daytime impairments produced by recurring sleep disturbances.

Although the initial intent for both patients and prescribing physicians is to use medication for the shortest possible duration (ie, a few nights), some patients continue using it over prolonged periods of time, either because of persistent sleep disturbances or, on a prophylactic basis, in an attempt to prevent insomnia. Several psychological, behavioral, and physiologic factors contribute to maintain this pattern of habitual and long-term use.

With nightly use, tolerance is likely to develop with most hypnotic drugs. To maintain efficacy, it is sometimes necessary to increase dosage, but when the maximum safe dosage is reached, the person is caught in a vicious cycle. Although the medication may have lost its hypnotic properties, attempts at discontinuing it is likely to produce withdrawal symptoms, including rebound insomnia. Rebound insomnia is usually temporary but may persist for several nights in some patients. In any case, the experience of rebound insomnia heightens the patient's anticipatory anxiety and reinforces the belief that he or she cannot sleep without medication. This chain reaction is quite powerful in prompting the patient to resume medication use, and hence the vicious cycle of hypnotic-dependent insomnia is perpetuated.

Conditioning factors are also involved in long-term hypnotic use. For instance, by alleviating an aversive state (ie, sleeplessness), hypnotic drugs quickly acquire powerful reinforcing properties; as such, the pill-taking behavior becomes negatively reinforced. Although sleep medications are usually prescribed on an "as needed" basis to prevent tolerance, this intermittent schedule can also be quite powerful in maintaining the pill-taking behavior. A form of reverse sleep state misperception can also perpetuate hypnotic use. In general, unmedicated insomniacs tend to overestimate the time spent awake at night and underestimate total sleep time; conversely, medicated insomniacs (with BZD hypnotics) have a reversed sleep state misperception in that they overestimate sleep time and underestimate wake time while on medication and, upon withdrawal, become acutely aware of their sleep disturbances, a phenomenon that might very well be attributed to the amnestic properties of BZDs.[17] This might also explain why so many individuals continue using BZDs despite objective evidence that their sleep is impaired.[18]

In most cases of long-term hypnotic use, patients do not abuse their medications, in the sense of escalating and exceeding the recommended dosages; rather, they remain on the same therapeutic dose without escalation but continue using it for much longer periods than was initially intended and are unable to discontinue use. This self-contained and habitual pattern of drug use is likely to lead to dependency, although this type of dependency is often more psychological than physiological.

Although there is no specific profile that characterizes long-term hypnotic users, such use is more common among older adults, women, and persons with more severe insomnia, higher psychological distress, and more health problems.[10,19,20] Lack of standard monitoring and follow-up of patients may also contribute to long-term use. On the other hand, some patients may place undue pressure on their family physicians requesting sleep medications. Prescribing medication is certainly less time consuming,[20] at least in the short term, than providing behavioral recommendations for insomnia.

HYPNOTIC DISCONTINUATION

Side effects and risks associated with long-term use are often major reasons for encouraging patients to discontinue use despite their perception of continued efficacy. Enduring insomnia symptoms in spite of appropriate therapeutic use may also warrant discontinuation and the need to seek other types of treatment. Other reasons may come from the patients themselves. By discontinuing hypnotic use, some patients report that they want to recover a more natural sleep, others want to feel less dependent on hypnotics or simply feel that they have been using hypnotics for too long and fear long-term effects. On the other hand, risks and benefits associated with long-term hypnotic use need to be weighted against those associated with untreated or self-treated insomnia[6] and availability of nonpharmacologic approaches.

Discontinuing hypnotic medications can pose quite a challenge to some individuals, especially for long-term users.[17,21,22] Several physiologic (withdrawal symptoms) and psychological factors (anticipatory anxiety, fear of rebound insomnia, personality) have been shown to influence discontinuation.[9,23,24] However, it remains difficult to predict who will encounter withdrawal problems, and factors predicting relapse are still poorly understood.

Difficulties encountered during hypnotic withdrawal and a high relapse rate after discontinuation have prompted the development of clinical treatment strategies to help patients discontinue long-term use of hypnotics. These interventions vary in their format and the degree of specialized care that the patients require, ranging from advice given during routine medical consultations to formal cognitive behavior therapy (CBT) delivered in the context of weekly therapy sessions by behavioral sleep medicine specialists.

Stepped-care Approach to Hypnotic Discontinuation

Russell and Lader[25] have proposed a stepped-care approach to manage discontinuation of long-term therapeutic use of BZDs (taken as anxiolytics or hypnotics). This approach tailors the amount of intervention according to patients' needs. According to this model, the first step is to give simple advice in the form of a letter or meeting to a large group of individuals regarding medication discontinuation and, if this fails, to gradually augment treatment from formal supervised medication tapering to specialized care, including different augmentation strategies such as CBT. Results of studies that have examined the outcome of this first-step intervention suggest that a simple information letter may be sufficient for some patients in helping them stop their hypnotic use. For example, in their study examining BZD taper with or without group CBT, Voshaar and colleagues[26] reported that a significant portion (14%; 285/2004) of the sample, who had received a personalized letter from their family physician advising them to discontinue BZD use, effectively discontinued use without more formal help. Using a similar first-step strategy, Gorgels and colleagues[27] observed a similar proportion of individuals in their sample who discontinued BZD use (15%–28%) after having been advised to do so by their family physician.

For those who may need more intensive and structured guidance in discontinuing their medication, a next step may be to implement a systematic supervised taper alone program. Many individuals, who had previously unsuccessfully attempted to stop the use of hypnotics, seem to benefit from a supervised, structured, and goal-oriented approach.[26,27] In a study comparing a taper alone program to taper combined with CBT for insomnia,[28] the proportion of participants who stopped their hypnotic use was greater in the group receiving the combined intervention (85%); however, a significant proportion of participants (48%) succeeded in discontinuing hypnotic use in the taper alone program group. Furthermore, when examining long-term outcome after discontinuation, those participants fared as well regarding abstinence as those who received the combined intervention.[29]

Systematic Discontinuation Procedures

There is clear evidence that hypnotic drugs should be discontinued gradually because abrupt discontinuation is associated with higher risks of withdrawal symptoms and health complications.[30,31] However, there are no empirically validated guidelines regarding the optimal rate of tapering. A regimen that has been frequently used in hypnotic reduction studies is to decrease initial dosage by 25% slices weekly or every other week until the smallest minimal dosage is reached.[23,28,32] It is important to keep in mind that taper pace may need to be adjusted according to the presence of withdrawal symptoms and anticipatory anxiety; it can also be slowed if the person finds it too difficult to cope or feels unable to meet the reduction goal.[28,33] Nevertheless, taper duration should be time limited as much as possible, to mobilize the person's efforts over a restricted period.[34] Ideally, withdrawal should be supervised by a health care professional, and regular follow-ups should be scheduled during discontinuation. The taper process should be carefully planned with the patient, and it should be individualized to take into account the type of hypnotic used; dosage; frequency and length of use; and psychological factors, such as motivation, anxiety level, and anticipations.[24,33,35–37] A step-by-step hypnotic discontinuation program and taper schedule is proposed in **Table 1**.

According to this procedure, the first step is to carefully plan the discontinuation strategy with the patient and to set clear reduction goals. For individuals using more than 1 hypnotic drug, the first step is to stabilize use on 1 compound only, preferably the drug with the longer half-life. Another strategy that has been used in withdrawal studies is to switch the original short-acting drug to a longer-acting drug (eg, diazepam) to minimize

withdrawal symptoms. However, there is little evidence in the literature to show that this strategy is associated with better outcomes. Broad anchor points can be set a priori, for example, to reduce initial dosage by 25% at the second week, 50% by the fourth week, and 100% by the tenth week. At the end of taper, when the smallest dosage is reached, medication-free nights are gradually introduced. At first, these "drug-holidays" can be planned on nights when the person feels it will be easier for him or her to refrain from taking sleep medication (eg, a weekend night, when there is no obligation the following day). Then, preselected nights when the hypnotic will be used regardless of whether the person feels they need it or not will be introduced. This last step may prevent the use of a medication on more "difficult" nights and, at the opposite, medication may be used on a night when there is no need for it. This strategy is used to weaken the association between lying in bed not sleeping and the pill-taking behavior.[21] An example of this taper strategy is illustrated in **Fig. 1**. Some individuals may apprehend the final step of complete cessation and worry over the potential consequences of hypnotic withdrawal on their sleep. It may then be useful to remind them that

Table 1
Step-by-step hypnotic discontinuation program in long-term users

Steps to Taper Hypnotic Medications	Procedure
Plan the whole process: Physician and patient plan the discontinuation process over the following weeks in a collaborative fashion.	Assess regular daily dosage used. Stabilize dosage if needed. When patients use more than 1 hypnotic, stabilize dosage on only 1 drug (1–2 wk). Estimate total number of weeks required to complete withdrawal if medication is decreased by 25% every other week. A written plan can be given out to the patient as a worksheet to increase adherence.
Gradual taper	Decrease daily intake by 25% of initial dosage for 2 weeks. Repeat this step, until the smallest dosage is reached.
Hypnotic-free nights are gradually introduced	In the first week, it may be best to preselect nights associated with apprehension regarding next day's functioning. Increase number of those hypnotic-free nights in the second week.
Use on predetermined nights	Preselect nights regardless of next day's activities or anticipations. Strongly encourage adherence to the initial plan; give rationale.
Complete discontinuation. Plan follow-ups to assess maintenance and prevent relapse	Assess patient's anxiety regarding complete cessation and go over coping strategies. Remind the patient that the minimal dosage used in the last weeks likely had few objective effects on his/her sleep.

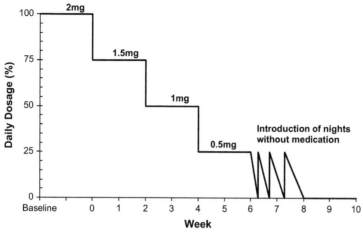

Fig. 1. Individualized taper program (eg, lorazepam, 2 mg).

the very small quantity of medication used in the final weeks of discontinuation was probably producing very little benefit on their sleep. Such apprehensions and worry about complete cessation should be addressed directly, because they may very well contribute to residual sleep disturbances after hypnotic discontinuation.[19,21]

Use of CBT During Hypnotic Discontinuation

There is now solid evidence that CBT is efficacious for treating insomnia and produces sustained benefits over time. For many individuals, CBT is recognized as the treatment of choice.[3,38] CBT for insomnia is often necessary to help long-term hypnotic users learn new skills to manage their sleep difficulties. The goals of using CBT during hypnotic discontinuation are twofold: to help reduce hypnotic use per se and to improve sleep during and after withdrawal. CBT for insomnia is a multidimensional, time-limited, and sleep-focused approach, which includes several strategies that target maintenance factors of insomnia. Strategies most commonly used are summarized in **Table 2**.

The benefits of using cognitive and behavioral interventions to facilitate hypnotic taper and to help maintain abstinence among individuals with insomnia are supported by empiric evidence.[19,26,28,32,39–45] Lichstein and colleagues[39] showed that progressive relaxation during supervised gradual medication withdrawal leads to significant hypnotic reduction and that participants who received relaxation training reported higher sleep quality and efficiency and reduced withdrawal symptoms compared with those who did not. Baillargeon and colleagues[40] compared 2 systematic taper programs; 1 was combined with

multicomponent CBT, and the other was not. Results showed that a greater proportion of participants had completely discontinued hypnotic medication in the group with CBT (77% vs 38%). A study by Morin and colleagues[28] showed similar results, with a greater proportion of drug-free participants in the group that received a systematic hypnotic taper program combined with CBT compared with the group that received the taper alone (85% vs 48%). The results of this study also showed greater subjective sleep improvements in participants who discontinued sleep medication while undergoing CBT. Zavesicka and colleagues[32] have specifically examined the effect of discontinuing sleep medications during CBT on sleep quality and have shown that long-term hypnotic users may benefit to the same extent from this intervention, and maybe even more, than people with insomnia who did not use hypnotics. Their results showed that long-term users discontinuing hypnotic use showed greater sleep efficiency improvements after CBT compared with those who had received the same treatment, but had not previously resorted to pharmacologic sleep aids. However, the study did not include a follow-up of participants and thus does not provide information about long-term outcomes.

Some of the studies examining the usefulness and efficacy of CBT for insomnia have included hypnotic users in their sample, without addressing hypnotic discontinuation per se or providing a structured taper program. Nevertheless, several of these studies report significant reductions in hypnotic dosage, frequency of use, or both.[19,46,47] Morgan and colleagues[19] examined the effect of CBT on hypnotic reduction without pairing it with a systematic taper intervention. Their results showed that CBT alone helps reduce hypnotic use and improves

Table 2
CBT for insomnia

Component	Aim	Strategy
Sleep restriction	Consolidate sleep on a shorter period of time	Curtail time in bed to actual sleep time.
Stimulus control	Rebuild the association between the bed and bedroom and sleep	Go to bed only when sleepy. Use the bed and bedroom only for sleep and sex. Get out of bed and bedroom if unable to fall asleep within 20 min. Rise at the same time every morning regardless of the amount of sleep obtained the previous night. Avoid napping.
Cognitive therapy	Reduce cognitive activation at bedtime and during nocturnal awakenings Improve the management of daytime consequences of insomnia	Identify and challenge beliefs and attitudes that exacerbate insomnia, such as unrealistic expectations about sleep requirement, dramatization of the consequences of insomnia, erroneous beliefs about strategies to promote sleep, etc.
Sleep hygiene education	Reduce the impact of lifestyle and environmental factors on sleep disturbances	Review sleep hygiene principles about the effects of exercise, caffeine, alcohol, and environmental factors on sleep.

sleep quality, although the proportion of participants who no longer used hypnotics after 6 months was lesser (33%) than that reported in the previously cited studies. The authors suggested that this may in part be because of the fact that participants had not received explicit instructions to discontinue hypnotic use. Nevertheless, it is noteworthy that a third of the sample discontinued sleep medications after having learned new ways to manage their sleep difficulties, without having been directly advised to do so. In their comparative study, Morin and colleagues[28] had included a control group that received CBT, and the participants did not receive any formal guidelines or recommendations to discontinue medication. Participants who expressed the wish to stop hypnotic use during the study were invited to consult their family physician. Results in this group showed that 54% of the sample had discontinued use by the end of the study. However, information as to which procedure they followed or how much intervention they received regarding medication discontinuation was not systematically collected, thus limiting the possibility to further interpret these data.

Long-term outcomes after discontinuation were later analyzed in this sample,[29] and the results showed that the participants from this group who had stopped their hypnotic use had significantly higher relapse rates than participants who had received the supervised taper program, either alone or combined with CBT. Soeffing and colleagues[4] examined insomnia treatment in older adults who were long-term users of hypnotic medications and showed that even when patients kept their hypnotic use stable throughout the intervention, CBT was also associated with significant sleep improvements.

An important issue that often arises in clinical practice is about when to implement CBT in the context of hypnotic discontinuation. Should CBT be initiated before, at the same time, at any step during, or after hypnotic discontinuation? Most discontinuation studies have implemented CBT and hypnotic discontinuation concurrently. In the studies conducted by Morin and colleagues[28] and Belleville and colleagues,[42] the first intervention week included 2 appointments: a consultation with a physician (when the first reduction goal was set and instruction was given to start taper the same night) and the first CBT session (either therapist-guided[28] or via self-help brochure,[42] when information on sleep was provided and sleep restriction was introduced). At week 2, the second reduction goal was set, and session 2 of CBT, introducing stimulus control strategies, was provided. At week 3, the third reduction goal was set while the third session of CBT was provided, and so on. This strategy has the advantage of introducing new CBT strategies to manage sleep while patients are progressively letting go of their hypnotics. However, a potential drawback of this combined strategy is the considerable amount of information and recommendations given to patients at the same time. In the study comparing hypnotic discontinuation with and without self-help CBT,[42] 5 participants in the CBT group dropped out of the program. They all reported that hypnotic discontinuation and CBT guidelines were too difficult to follow. It is possible, however, that these patients needed direct therapist guidance. For some patients, it may be easier to introduce CBT before tapering or, on the contrary, begin taper for a few weeks, and then introduce CBT if sleep difficulties occur. In a small pilot study, Espie and colleagues[48] had found that patients who were withdrawn from medication early on in the behavioral treatment achieved better sleep outcomes than those withdrawn after the behavioral intervention.

In some cases, even if more clinical attention than a supervised taper program alone seems warranted, it may not be necessary to implement a full course of CBT (including 8–10 weekly sessions) delivered by a sleep specialist. It is possible that hypnotic discontinuation programs may be successful with fewer consultation visits (eg, at week 1 and week 4) and a self-help format of CBT. In such a context, brief weekly (15–20 minutes) phone contacts with a therapist to discuss sleep difficulties and to implement CBT strategies could be provided. This type of minimal intervention was examined, and it led to complete discontinuation of hypnotic use for two-thirds of participants posttreatment and for about half at the 6-month follow-up.[42] A secondary analysis of these data indicated that individuals experiencing worsening insomnia, more withdrawal symptoms and psychological distress (eg, anxiety or depressive symptoms), and lower self-efficacy (ie, confidence in one's own ability to stop medication) during and after the discontinuation program were less likely to be drug-free at the end of the intervention and 6 months after.[35] These might be indications that more intensive and individualized therapeutic supervision may be warranted for these individuals.

Using a more intensive program (ie, 10 weekly medical consultations with or without 10 weekly 90-minute CBT group sessions) led to an average interval of 2.6- and 18.6-month interval before relapse, ie, resuming regular use of hypnotics after the end of treatment, for individuals tapering their hypnotics with and without CBT.[29] Once again, higher insomnia severity and psychological distress were associated with shorter interval to relapse. These observations led to the suggestion that booster sessions might prove useful in preventing relapse, but this is yet to be empirically tested.

Clinical and Practical Considerations

Hypnotic discontinuation may require a good deal of adaptation for some patients, especially for long-term users with residual persistent insomnia symptoms, who therefore need to learn new ways of managing their sleep difficulties. Aspects such as readiness to change and motivation,[35] self-efficacy in being able to discontinue use or comply with the taper program,[33] and anticipations[22,28,33] are important factors to assess before withdrawal. The person needs to be willing and ready to change his or her habitual way of coping with insomnia, and motivation should be intrinsic rather than a result of pressure from a spouse or other family member. The latter is more likely to be associated with failure. Timing is also important; discontinuation of hypnotics in periods of acute stress or major life changes may be more difficult, and waiting for a better timing may be preferred. It is also important to define realistic goals for each individual; complete abstinence may not be desirable for all patients. For example, patients with very high anxiety levels may wish to discontinue their medication, but their quality of life may be significantly reduced if their sleep worsens with drug discontinuation. Finally, contraindications to hypnotic withdrawal need to be very carefully assessed. In patients with complex mental health problems (eg, schizophrenia, bipolar disorder) or a history of recurring depressive episodes or seizures, hypnotic discontinuation may provoke a relapse of the psychiatric problem and even worsen the patient's condition.

SUMMARY AND FUTURE DIRECTIONS

Observations stemming from different withdrawal studies suggest that a stepped-care approach to hypnotic discontinuation may be useful and cost-effective. In such an approach, long-term users would be first advised by their family practitioners on how to discontinue hypnotic use. If tapering off is not possible or if they experience a worsening of sleep or psychological distress in doing so, enrollment in a program with systematic interventions but minimal guidance, such as a self-help approach, could be the next step. If this intervention appears to be insufficient to alleviate insomnia symptoms and distress, then patients could be referred to a behavioral sleep medicine specialist who would implement more intensive CBT involving weekly individual consultations. At the end of treatment, a booster session could be planned to monitor and prevent relapse. A meta-analysis examining the success rate of different discontinuation strategies provides some evidence for the efficacy of stepped-care approaches to medication discontinuation.[49] Evidence suggests that a stepped-care approach, in which the amount of intervention is progressively increased according to the needs of patients and according to their autonomy and distress levels in tapering off their medication, may be an interesting way to manage hypnotic discontinuation. However, much research remains necessary to tailor withdrawal programs according to patients' needs. At this time, factors such as treatment characteristics or individual characteristics of those who could most benefit from one or the other strategy, or a combination of those, remain poorly understood.

Current evidence suggests that CBT may be a useful adjunct to systematic hypnotic discontinuation programs. Whether or not it helps to reduce hypnotic use per se is still unclear. It could depend on themes and strategies discussed, but consistent favorable effects of CBT on sleep quality have been repeatedly reported. Guidelines as to when and how to implement CBT during hypnotic taper are still scarce. Most programs start and run both hypnotic taper and CBT at the same time. Evidence regarding optimal sequencing of these interventions is very limited, and future studies examining which combination is associated with better outcomes are necessary.

In summary, although the original intent is to prescribe hypnotics on a short-time basis, some patients will use them for much longer periods than was initially intended and may be unable to discontinue their medication by themselves. Structured taper programs with or without augmentation strategies such as CBT appear promising in facilitating discontinuation.

REFERENCES

1. Roehrs T, Roth T. Hypnotics prescription patterns in a large managed-care population. Sleep Med 2004; 5(5):463–6.

2. Walsh JK. Pharmacologic management of insomnia. J Clin Psychiatry 2004;65(Suppl 16):41–5.

3. National Institutes of Health. National Institutes of Health state of the science conference statement on manifestations and management of chronic insomnia in adults, June 13–15, 2005. Sleep 2005; 28(9):1049–57.

4. Soeffing JP, Lichstein KL, Nau S, et al. Psychological treatment of insomnia in hypnotic-dependent older adults. Sleep Med 2008;9:165–71.

5. Simon GE, VonKorff M. Prevalence, burden, and treatment of insomnia in primary care. Am J Psychiatry 1997;154(10):1417–23.

6. Roehrs TA, Roth T. Safety of insomnia pharmacotherapy. Sleep Med Clin 2006;1(3):399–407.

7. Ebert B, Wafford KA, Deacon S. Treating insomnia: current and investigational pharmacological approaches. Pharmacol Ther 2006;112(3):612–29.

8. Glass J, Lanctot KL, Herrmann N, et al. Sedative hypnotics in older people with insomnia: meta-analysis of risks and benefits [abstract]. BMJ 2005; 331(7526):1169.

9. Roth T, Roehrs TA, Vogel GW, et al. Evaluation of hypnotic medications. In: Prien RF, Robinson DS, editors. Clinical evaluation of psychotropic drugs: principles and guidelines. New York: Raven; 1994. p. 579–92.

10. Taylor S, McCracken CF, Wilson KC, et al. Extent and appropriateness of benzodiazepine use. Results from an elderly urban community. Br J Psychiatry 1998;173:433–8.

11. Walsh JK, Krystal AD, Amato DA, et al. Nightly treatment of primary insomnia with eszopiclone for six months: effect on sleep, quality of life, and work limitations. Sleep 2007;30(8):959–68.

12. Dundar Y, Dodd S, Strobl J, et al. Comparative efficacy of newer hypnotic drugs for the short-term management of insomnia: a systematic review and meta-analysis. Hum Psychopharmacol 2004;19(5): 305–22.

13. Riemann D, Perlis ML. The treatments of chronic insomnia: a review of benzodiazepine receptor agonists and psychological and behavioral therapies. Sleep Med Rev 2009;13(3):205–14.

14. Morin CM. Insomnia: psychological assessment and management. New York: Guilford Press; 1993.

15. Stepanski EJ. Hypnotics should not be considered for the initial treatment of chronic insomnia. J Clin Sleep Med 2005;1(2):125–8.

16. Morin CM, LeBlanc M, Daley M, et al. Epidemiology of insomnia: prevalence, self-help treatments, consultations, and determinants of help-seeking behaviors. Sleep Med 2006;7(2):123–30.

17. Schneider-Helmert D. Why low-dose benzodiazepine-dependent insomniacs can't escape their sleeping pills. Acta Psychiatr Scand 1988;78(6): 706–11.

18. Bastien CH, LeBlanc M, Carrier J, et al. Sleep EEG power spectra, insomnia, and chronic use of benzodiazepines. Sleep 2003;26(3):313–7.

19. Morgan K, Dixon S, Mathers N, et al. Psychological treatment for insomnia in the management of long-term hypnotic drug use: a pragmatic randomised controlled trial. Br J Gen Pract 2003; 53(497):923–8.

20. Brentsen P, Hensig G, McKenzie L, et al. Prescribing benzodiazepines: a critical incident study of a physician dilemma. Soc Sci Med 1999;49:459–67.

21. Morin CM, Baillargeon L, Bastien C. Discontinuation of sleep medications. In: Lichstein LK, Morin CM, editors. Treatment of late-life insomnia. Thousand Oak (CA): Sage Publications; 2000. p. 271–96.

22. Kan CC, Breteler MH, Zitman FG. High prevalence of benzodiazepine dependence in out-patient users, based on the DSM-III-R and ICD-10 criteria. Acta Psychiatr Scand 1997;96(2):85–93.

23. O'Connor KP, Marchand A, Belanger L, et al. Psychological distress and adaptational problems associated with benzodiazepine withdrawal and outcome: a replication. Addict Behav 2004;29(3): 583–93.

24. Voshaar RC, Gorgels WJ, Mol AJ, et al. Predictors of long-term benzodiazepine abstinence in participants of a randomized controlled benzodiazepine withdrawal program. Can J Psychiatry 2006;51(7): 445–52.

25. Russell VJ, Lader MH. Guidelines for the prevention and treatment of benzodiazepine dependence. London: Mental Health Fondation; 1993.

26. Voshaar RC, Gorgels WJ, Mol AJ, et al. Tapering off long-term benzodiazepine use with or without group cognitive-behavioural therapy: three-condition, randomised controlled trial. Br J Psychiatry 2003; 182:498–504.

27. Gorgels WJ, Oude Voshaar RC, Mol AJ, et al. Discontinuation of long-term benzodiazepine use by sending a letter to users in family practice: a prospective controlled intervention study. Drug Alcohol Depend 2005;78(1):49–56.

28. Morin CM, Bastien C, Guay B, et al. Randomized clinical trial of supervised tapering and cognitive behavior therapy to facilitate benzodiazepine discontinuation in older adults with chronic insomnia. Am J Psychiatry 2004;161(2):332–42.

29. Morin CM, Belanger L, Bastien C, et al. Long-term outcome after discontinuation of benzodiazepines for insomnia: a survival analysis of relapse. Behav Res Ther 2005;43(1):1–14.

30. Rickels K, Schweizer E, Case WG, et al. Long-term therapeutic use of benzodiazepines. I. Effects of abrupt discontinuation. Arch Gen Psychiatry 1990; 47(10):899–907.

31. Soldatos CR, Dikeos DG, Whitehead A. Tolerance and rebound insomnia with rapidly eliminated hypnotics: a meta-analysis of sleep laboratory studies. Int Clin Psychopharmacol 1999;14(5): 287–303.

32. Zavesicka L, Brunovsky M, Matousek M, et al. Discontinuation of hypnotics during cognitive behavioural therapy for insomnia. BMC Psychiatry 2008;8:80.

33. Belanger L, Morin CM, Bastien C, et al. Self-efficacy and compliance with benzodiazepine taper in older adults with chronic insomnia. Health Psychol 2005; 24(3):281–7.

34. Lader M, Tylee A, Donoghue J. Withdrawing benzodiazepines in primary care. CNS Drugs 2009;23(1): 19–34.

35. Belleville G, Morin CM. Hypnotic discontinuation in chronic insomnia: impact of psychological distress, readiness to change, and self-efficacy. Health Psychol 2008;27(2):239–48.

36. Holton A, Riley P, Tyrer P. Factors predicting long-term outcome after chronic benzodiazepine therapy. J Affect Disord 1992;24(4):245–52.

37. Schweizer E, Rickels K, De Martinis N, et al. The effect of personality on withdrawal severity and taper outcome in benzodiazepine dependent patients. Psychol Med 1998;28(3):713–20.

38. Morin CM, Bootzin RR, Buysse DJ, et al. Psychological and behavioral treatment of insomnia: update of the recent evidence (1998–2004). Sleep 2006; 29(11):1398–414.

39. Lichstein KL, Peterson BA, Riedel BW, et al. Relaxation to assist sleep medication withdrawal. Behav Modif 1999;23:379–402.

40. Baillargeon L, Landreville P, Verreault R, et al. Discontinuation of benzodiazepines among older insomniac adults treated with cognitive-behavioural therapy combined with gradual tapering: a randomized trial. CMAJ 2003;169(10):1015–20.

41. Baillargeon L, Demers M, Ladouceur R. Stimulus-control: nonpharmacologic treatment for insomnia. Can Fam Physician 1998;44:73–9.

42. Belleville G, Guay C, Guay B, et al. Hypnotic taper with or without self-help treatment: a randomized clinical trial. J Consult Clin Psychol 2007;75(2): 325–35.

43. Morin CM, Colecchi CA, Ling WD, et al. Cognitive behavior therapy to facilitate benzodiazepine discontinuation among hypnotic-dependent patients with insomnia. Behav Ther 1995;26:733–45.

44. Lichstein KL, Johnson RS. Relaxation for insomnia and hypnotic medication use in older women. Psychol Aging 1993;8:103–11.

45. Riedel BW, Lichstein KL, Peterson BA, et al. A comparison of the efficacy of stimulus control for medicated and non-medicated insomniacs. Behav Modif 1998;22:3–28.

46. Backhaus J, Hohagen F, Voderholzer U, et al. Long-term effectiveness of a short-term cognitive-behavioral group treatment for primary insomnia. Eur Arch Psychiatry Clin Neurosci 2001;251:35–41.

47. Verbeek I, Schreuder K, Declerck G. Evaluation of short-term nonpharmacological treatment of insomnia in a clinical setting. J Psychosom Res 1999;47:369–83.

48. Espie CA, Lindsay WR, Brooks DN. Substituting behavioural treatment for drugs in the treatment of insomnia: an exploratory study. J Behav Ther Exp Psychiatry 1988;19(1):51–6.

49. Oude Voshaar RC, Couvee JE, van Balkom AJ, et al. Strategies for discontinuing long-term benzodiazepine use: meta-analysis. Br J Psychiatry 2006;189: 213–20.

Treatment of Late-life Insomnia

Christina S. McCrae, PhD*, Joseph M. Dzierzewski, MS,
Daniel B. Kay, MS

KEYWORDS

- Insomnia - Elderly - Older adults - Geriatric - Sleep

Insomnia, defined as difficulty initiating or maintaining sleep at least 3 nights per week that is accompanied by complaints of sleep-related daytime impairment,[1,2] is the most common sleep disturbance in later life. Although insomnia can occur as an acute disorder (7 days or less), older adults are often afflicted with chronic insomnia (12 months or more[3]). Additionally, insomnia in older individuals is most frequently comorbid in nature, occurring in the context of age-related medical or psychiatric conditions, increased medication usage, or polypharmacy. This article focuses on the conceptualization, assessment, and treatment of late-life insomnia from a behavioral sleep medicine perspective. Evidence for both behavioral and pharmacologic treatment approaches is presented. As is shown, however, late-insomnia's chronic and comorbid nature makes behavioral techniques the preferable treatment approach.

RATES OF LATE-LIFE INSOMNIA

The prevalence and incidence rates of late-life insomnia depend largely on the criteria used in the specific study in question. Epidemiologic surveys in the United States generally do not reference the chronicity of the sleep complaint, do not require daytime impairment in the criteria of insomnia, or fail to screen out insomnia participants with comorbid somatic complaints. Likewise, these studies tend to yield larger prevalence rates (ie, 30%–60%)[4,5] than rates derived from studies that include these more stringent criteria (ie, 12%–25%).[6,7] Regardless of the criteria, prevalence and incidence rates of insomnia significantly increase with age.[4,8] The 1-year incidence rate of insomnia in the 65+ population has been reported to range between 3.1% and 7.3%.[9,10] Importantly, the increased prevalence of late-life insomnia may be at least partially attributable to the finding that remission of insomnia is less common in older individuals than it is in younger individuals.[11] Research suggests that the increased rates of insomnia from mid-life to late-life are seen most prominently among older women, because elderly women present in a medical setting with insomnia complaints more frequently than men.[6,9,12,13] Although aging is associated with increased rates of insomnia, normal aging does not necessitate the onset of insomnia.[12,14] Indeed, when mental and physical comorbidities are controlled, the prevalence of late-life insomnia may be as low as 1% to 7.5%.[4,15] Insomnia leads to and is precipitated by several health complaints,[16] and because insomnia is often comorbid with age-related health problems, determining if aging has a direct or indirect role in the increased prevalence of insomnia has been difficult.

TREATMENT SEEKING

Older adults are more likely to present in a primary care setting (ie, general practice) with sleep complaints than are younger adults.[17,18] This may be caused in large part by the increased comorbidity, chronicity, and severity of late-life insomnia.[9] Indeed, the likelihood of a complaint of insomnia increases when the sleep disturbance is more chronic and severe.[10] In the primary care setting, however, sleep complaints are often

Department of Clinical and Health Psychology, University of Florida, PO Box 100165 (HSC), 101 South Newell Drive, Gainesville, FL 32610–0165, USA
* Corresponding author.
E-mail address: csmccrae@phhp.ufl.edu (C.S. McCrae).

Sleep Med Clin 4 (2009) 593–604
doi:10.1016/j.jsmc.2009.07.006
1556-407X/09/$ – see front matter © 2009 Elsevier Inc. All rights reserved.

poorly assessed, trivialized, or attributed to other mental or physical comorbidities.[19] The recommendation that any comorbid mental and physical health complaint should be the primary aim of treatment in late-life insomnia has been long maintained. Two erroneous assumptions stemming from this perspective must be avoided: that insomnia generally subsides once the comorbidities have been treated, and that the behavioral treatment of insomnia cannot be successful in the presence of serious comorbidities.

First, insomnia generally persists long after comorbidities have subsided. Even when insomnia is preceded by another health condition, cognitive and behavioral factors often emerge to precipitate and perpetuate insomnia. Late-life insomnia presents so commonly with other health complaints that it may more appropriately be thought of as a comorbid condition rather than a secondary complaint (ie, secondary insomnia). At a recent National Institute of Health State-of-the Science Conference, it was recommended that the term "comorbid insomnia" be used in place of secondary insomnia.[20]

Second, cognitive-behavioral treatment for insomnia (CBTi) was effective for late-life insomnia in a study sample of older adults with representative rates of mental and physical comorbidities, suggesting that CBTi need not be postponed until after comorbid conditions have been treated.[21] Additional research is needed to validate or modify CBTi for specific comorbid conditions. Ultimately, late-insomnia (comorbid or in isolation) should be viewed as a disorder that can be effectively treated.[14] Many older adults with insomnia do not receive evidence-based assessment or treatment for their sleep complaints,[22] however, which may contribute to a dramatic difference in the way in which older adults receive treatment for insomnia in the primary care setting compared with younger adults. For example, older adults are more than twice as likely to be prescribed a sedative or hypnotic medication for insomnia as are younger adults.[23] Over the course of a year, roughly 32% of older adults with insomnia[24] and 14% of the total population of adults aged 65 to 79 report using some type of hypnotic drug as a sleep aid.[5] Older women are more likely to be prescribed hypnotic medications for sleep complaints than are older men. Many sleep medications involve risk of tolerance and dependence, and for older adults sleep aids may pose additional risks including polypharmacy, increased side effects, and exacerbation of sleep apnea.[25] In addition, although most sleep medications are not implicated for use beyond 4 to 8 weeks, adults over the age of 65 make up 50%

of people using hypnotic medication for months and even years.[5] Conversely, CBTi has been implicated for the treatment of chronic late-life insomnia and has no known adverse side effects. CBTi is an optimal candidate for the treatment of insomnia complaints in older adults. Although older adults are increasingly seeking care, the availability of professionally delivered CBTi is still relatively sparse.

MODELS OF INSOMNIA

Several models of insomnia have been developed. This section discusses the major models of insomnia in relationship to late-life insomnia. No current model of insomnia adequately captures the myriad factors and variables that may be involved in late-life insomnia, but each has use in understanding late-life insomnia.

Physiologic Sleep Models of Insomnia

Physiologic sleep models of insomnia consider dysfunction in the sleep systems to be the primary source of sleep disturbance. Borbély[26] has developed a theory of sleep that includes two major sleep systems: the circadian and the homeostatic processes. Advanced age is associated with changes in these sleep systems. Amplitude and phase changes are seen in the circadian system,[27,28] and reduced amounts of slow wave activity, sleep fragmentation, and early morning awakening are seen in the homeostatic system.[29,30] Dysregulation of these systems may explain in part the increase rates of insomnia in late-life.

Hyperarousal Models of Insomnia

Physiologic arousal models
Physiologic models posit that the arousal and the sleep systems function independently and that insomnia is caused by dysfunction in the sympathetic arousal system[31] and not an internal dysfunction of the sleep systems themselves. Age-related changes in the arousal system or increased rates of hyperarousal-related heath conditions in late-life, such as chronic pain, may play a central role in the increased rates of insomnia in late-life.

Behavioral models
Behavioral models of insomnia highlight behavioral-environmental interactions that prevent and promote healthy sleep. Lifestyle, living situations, and behavioral changes common in late-life are thought to drive the increased prevalence of late-life insomnia. Behavioral factors that may contribute to increased rates of late-life insomnia

include decreased physical activity, bereavement, napping, spending more time in bed, and delayed or reduced light exposure.[24] Behavioral changes in late-life are observed in both healthy and poor sleeping older adults; these changes should not be thought of as the cause of late-life insomnia.[32] Nonetheless, behavioral changes in late-life may contribute to the overall increased rates of insomnia in this population in conjunction with other factors (ie, age-related health factors).

Cognitive models

Cognitive models focus on mental processes that activate arousal and disrupt sleep. Reduced working memory, processing speed, reaction time, and controlled attention are considered part of normal aging. Additional research is needed to parse out the potential role normal age-related changes in cognitive functioning may play in insomnia in late-life.

ASSESSMENT OF LATE-LIFE INSOMNIA

Late-life insomnia is a complex disorder to assess because it is often comorbid with other mental, physical, and sleep disorders. This section reviews the evidenced-based tools and techniques available for clinicians to assess and diagnose late-life insomnia from the scientist-practitioner approach, which uses the scientific method to inform clinical practice. A three-step process is applied to assessment: (1) clinical data about the patient is obtained (2) a "diagnosis hypothesis" is formulated and tested, and (3) these steps are repeated as needed to rule-in and rule-out differential diagnoses.

Because insomnia is highly comorbid with myriad physical health problems, older adults are more likely to present in a primary care setting with complaints of physical aliments rather than to a sleep center with insomnia complaints.[33,34] Primary care physicians should be aware that cardiopulmonary disease, painful muscle conditions, depression, and prostrate problems commonly predispose individuals to the development of insomnia,[35] and patients are generally not aware of the impact that these health problems may have on their sleep.[34] It is the responsibility of the primary care physician to identify potential markers of sleep disturbance and consider any sleep complaint as an issue for further evaluation.[36] Even partial, or subclinical, symptoms of insomnia can have a profound impact on the patient's health and often proceed the onset of chronic insomnia. Early detection and intervention of insomnia symptoms may prevent or mitigate these negative consequences.[19] Negative

consequences of late-life insomnia include increased risk for falls, poorer health, fatigue, and decreased quality of life. Regrettably, late-life insomnia often goes unnoticed by primary care physicians caring for older adults.[18] Bailes and coworkers[37] suggested that primary care physicians may be aided in identifying those patients who require additional sleep assessment by giving a brief questionnaire, such as the Sleep Symptom Checklist or the Pittsburgh Sleep Quality Index.[38] Patients who endorse insomnia symptoms and who are amenable to further assessment are likely to benefit from referral and further sleep assessment by a sleep specialist. When insomnia and medical problems are combined, patients commonly present with a host of mental health concerns. Insomnia patients may best be served if referred to an integrative health care team that includes a clinical and health psychologist trained to handle the psychologic side of the patient's care. Indeed, with the relatively recent recognition of psychology as a health care profession, psychologists are better able to become integrated into the general health care arena to provide more comprehensive care for patients.[39] This is nowhere more apparent than for clinical and health psychologists with training in behavioral sleep medicine. Ideally, in a collaborative and comprehensive health care system, older adults who present to their primary care doctor with insomnia complaints should routinely be referred to a behavioral sleep specialist to receive assessment and treatment. Currently, there are not enough behavioral sleep specialists to meet the potential demand for their services. Recognition of the need for such services has prompted greater interest in the field of behavioral sleep medicine, however, and as a result growing numbers of psychologists and other health care providers are choosing to specialize in this area.

Step 1: Gathering Data

The major goal in assessing late-life insomnia is first to determine if the disrupted sleep of the patient is related to clinically significant daytime impairment, and second to determine if the sleep disturbance meets criteria for insomnia and is not attributable to another sleep disorder. Doing this requires the clinician to gather data from multiple sources, because daytime dysfunction in older adults may be related to other mental or physical complications yet be wrongly attributed to sleep disturbance by the patient. Moreover, sleep disorders other than insomnia (ie, sleep apnea) are more prevalent among older adults and must be carefully differentiated from insomnia. Finally, age-related changes in sleep can imitate the symptoms of insomnia. Many older adults may present with insomnia complaints but do not require treatment. Discussed next are several sources of data that are useful in assessing and diagnosing late-life insomnia.

Available medical records

As clinical and health psychologists become more integrated in the larger health care system, access to medical records will enhance the clinicians' ability to assess and treatment late-life insomnia. Particular attention should be paid to previous and current medical or psychiatric conditions that cosegregate with late-life insomnia, such as chronic pain, depression, cardiovascular complications, and cancer. In addition, current prescriptions should be reviewed to determine what impact the patient's current medication regimen may have on sleep.

Intake packet

Sending an intake packet to the patient's home before the first visit is recommended to save time and to allow the clinician to gather more detailed information during the initial assessment visit. The introductory packet may include questions concerning patient demographics, such as educational attainment, socioeconomic status, work history, social relationships, medical status and history, sleep-wake patterns, and current medication use. Ideally, this information can be compared with available medical records.

Clinical interview

The clinical interview is an essential element in the assessment of late-life insomnia. During this interview, the clinician is able to ask more in-depth questions than can be obtained from questionnaires and can clarify information obtained from the information packet. In addition, the clinical interview provides an opportunity for the clinician to make behavioral observations about the cognitive, motor, and interpersonal functioning of the patient. Most importantly, the clinical interview can assess specific information about the patient's lifestyle, daily stressors, behavioral patterns, and other factors that may impact sleep. In addition, the patient's perception of sleep and daytime functioning can be obtained.

Informant report

Informant report is a good source of information about the patient's history, particularly information relevant to sleep behaviors of which the patient may not be aware, such as symptoms of restless leg syndrome, snoring, and obstructive sleep apnea.

Psychologic and sleep questionnaires

Higher levels of depression on Beck's Depression Inventory and also anxiety on the State-Trait Anxiety Inventory differentiate older adults with insomnia from older adults without insomnia.[40] Assessing mood during the initial interview through these questionnaires provides information regarding whether older adults are experiencing daytime distress related to their sleep problems. Beck's Depression Inventory-II and the Geriatric Depression Scale have support for use in older adults and may appropriately be used in assessing late-life insomnia.

In addition, several questionnaires aimed at assessing sleep and daytime functions have been useful in identifying people with late-life insomnia including the Pittsburg Sleep Quality Index,[41] the Epworth Sleepiness Scale,[42] and the Dysfunctional Beliefs and Attitudes about Sleep.[43] Because these measures rely heavily on the patient's memory over the past weeks and months, these tools may be ineffective in older adults with memory problems.

Step 2: Formulating and Testing the Diagnosis Hypothesis

From the information obtained from the various sources described, the clinician is prepared to formulate a hypothesis about the patient's sleep problem. Reports of prolonged time to fall asleep, time spent awake in the middle of the night, or early morning awakenings are all indicative of insomnia. Further, a perceived low quality of sleep and the presence of daytime dysfunction (eg, fatigue, concentration problems, and so forth) may also suggest insomnia. When formulating the diagnosis hypothesis, it is imperative to consider alternative diagnoses (ie, another sleep disturbance). The Diagnostic and Statistical Manual of Mental Disorder (4th edition text revision) is a valuable assessment tool that outlines the criteria against which the diagnosis hypothesis is evaluated. The criteria set for the diagnosis of insomnia are difficulty initiating or maintaining sleep for at least 3 nights per week that is accompanied by complaints of sleep-related daytime impairment.[7] With the data gathered from step one, a preliminary diagnosis may be established. The first step is to test the null hypothesis (ie, that the sleep disturbance is not caused by insomnia). To reject the null hypothesis, differential diagnoses (ie, other sleep disorders) must first be ruled out by collecting additional data from sleep diaries, actigraphy, or polysomnography (PSG). A discussion of the use of these tools in assessing insomnia follows. Differential diagnosis is complicated by the fact that insomnia can and often does co-occur with other sleep disorders. As discussed later in Step 3, even when another sleep disorder is diagnosed, it is important to consider whether the insomnia is an independent disorder or is simply a symptom.

Sleep diary

Sleep diaries supplement and confirm the insomnia diagnosis. They are an inexpensive way to obtain data about the daily patterns of the patient's sleep. It is recommended that 2 weeks of sleep diary data be obtained.[14,44] Not only are sleep diaries used to help diagnose late-life insomnia,[41] they can also be used during treatment as a scientific gauge of progress throughout therapy.[17]

Actigraphy

Actigraphy is a relatively recent objective measure used to assess sleep-wake continuity. The clinical use and accuracy of actigraphy compared with PSG in older adults has been validated in several studies.[45,46] The accuracy of actigraphy is particularly low in patents with poor sleep quality and highly impaired sleep, however, and should be interpreted with caution in these patients. Because actigraphy poorly detects wakefulness, it may be more effectively used in the clinical setting in conjunction with other assessment methods.[47] For example, when combined with sleep diaries, actigraphy may be a relatively inexpensive way to assess sleep state misperception, sleep-disordered breathing, or respiratory disorders. Obtaining at least 3 days of actigraphy data is recommended when assessing insomnia.[48] Obtaining several days and weeks of actigraphy may be helpful in assessing the effectiveness of treatment for late-life insomnia.[17]

Polysomnography

PSG is not indicated for the routine assessment of insomnia. This is because of the subjective nature of an insomnia complaint and the high expense and invasiveness of PSG.[49] It is, however, recommended to obtain a differential diagnosis for the other sleep disorders highly comorbid with late-life insomnia, specifically obstructive sleep apnea, sleep-related breathing disorder, periodic leg movements in sleep, and persistent circadian disorders. In the differential diagnosis of obstructive sleep apnea in particular, self-report questions about snoring or gasping for breath are insufficient in making a differential diagnosis, and PSG is required. Because late-life insomnia is highly comorbid with these other sleep disorders, the usefulness of PSG in assessing insomnia may increase with age.[50]

Step 3: Ruling-in and Ruling-out Insomnia

In late-life, insomnia becomes increasingly comorbid not only with other sleep problems but also with mental and physical conditions for which sleep disturbance is a symptom and with medications that induce sleep disturbance. This makes it more difficult to rule-out insomnia when another disorder has been ruled-in. Even when other sleep disorders are diagnosed, insomnia may still be present. For example, 50% of patients diagnosed with sleep-disordered breathing have problematic insomnia symptoms that may be ruled-in as insomnia.[51] Regardless of comorbidities, insomnia should be considered as a potentially independent disorder requiring treatment.

TREATMENT

The treatment of late-life insomnia can be broadly classified into two distinct categories: pharmacologic and behavioral (including cognitive-behavioral). The following sections summarize the empirical evidence for the use of treatments that fall within these domains.

Treatment as Usual

Historically, older adults' complaints of poor sleep were treated with benzodiazepine-receptor agonists, which have been associated with side effects, such as increased risk of confusion and falls.[52] Contemporary non–benzodiazepine-receptor agonists (eg, zolpidem, zaleplom, and eszopicone) were developed to minimize such side effects. Initially, these agents seemed to carry fewer and less severe unwanted side effects (including headache, somnolence, dizziness, bad taste, and decreased balance).[52–54] No differences have been found, however, between the sleep characteristics and number or severity of adverse side effects of older adults treated with benzodiazepine-receptor agonists or non–benzodiazepine-receptor agonists,[53] thereby limiting their use.

Most prescription hypnotic medication clinical trials are funded directly by the manufacturing company, contain few older patients, and have relatively short treatment and follow-up periods. With the exception of eszoplicone, hypnotic medications are not recommended for long-term usage. Given that the oldest patient in these clinical trials was 69 years of age, a recent review of eszoplicone for the treatment of late-life insomnia concluded that there was insufficient evidence to warrant extended use in the elderly.[55] Given the known age-related changes in pharmacodynamics, pharmacokinetics, and drug interactions[54] close monitoring of the elderly patient beginning pharmacotherapy for insomnia is a necessity.

Antidepressant medication (both sedating and nonsedating), although not indicated or approved by the Food and Drug Administration for the treatment of sleep disturbances, is commonly prescribed to improve sleep. Reports of improved sleep following administration of such medication are sparse, particularly in aged patients. Further, the potential of serious adverse events (eg, cognitive impairment, falls, confusion, and exacerbation of occult sleep disorders) suggests antidepressants are a less than optimal alternative to other hypnotic medications and CBTi. Illustrative of this are the results of a randomized, double-blinded controlled trial of paroxetine (an antidepressant selective serotonin reuptake inhibitor) combined with sleep hygiene (a behavioral technique empirically shown to be relatively inert as a stand-alone treatment option) versus placebo in combination with sleep hygiene.[56] Reynolds and colleagues[56] aptly concluded that paroxetine is not effective in the treatment of late-life insomnia.

Hypnotic medication use is very common in older adults. The questionable effectiveness of such medications and the potential for adverse events (including the potential for serious interactions) suggests, however, that alternative treatment modalities are needed. Based on the evidence presented next, CBTi should always be considered a forerunner in the selection of potential treatment options for older adults with insomnia.

Behavioral Sleep Medicine Treatment Approaches

Behavioral sleep medicine specialists use a vast array of techniques all aimed at producing improvements in the sleep of older adults with insomnia. Commonly used techniques include sleep education, sleep hygiene, relaxation training, stimulus control, and sleep restriction or compression. Generally, these techniques are better researched than the aforementioned pharmacotherapies. These techniques are individually detailed next and subsequently followed by a section describing commonly applied combination packages of techniques (CBTi).

Sleep education

Sleep education is comprised of several basic facts related to age-related changes in sleep and sleep need. Sleep education has never been evaluated as a stand-alone treatment modality for late-life insomnia and is used only in adjunct with other commonly used techniques. Further, these basic knowledge principles are not sufficient to engender change independent of other therapeutic techniques. Basic principles of sleep education with older adults are described in **Box 1**.

Sleep hygiene

Sleep hygiene is a set of instructions that aims at eliminating sleep-disruptive behavior from the patient's behavioral repertoire. Common sleep hygiene recommendations are listed in **Box 2**. Limited empirical investigations have investigated the use of sleep hygiene as a stand-alone treatment for late-life insomnia. Several researchers have used sleep hygiene instruction as part of a control or placebo condition,[56–58] clearly indicating the widely held belief that sleep hygiene alone is unlikely to produce meaningful change in the sleep of elderly patients. Additionally, a recent review conducted by McCurry and associates[59] indicated that sleep hygiene alone does not meet the necessary criteria to be considered an evidence-based treatment for late-life insomnia.

Relaxation training

Relaxation includes a variety of strategies all aimed at reducing patient levels of physiologic or cognitive arousal to produce positive changes in the individual's ability to initiate and maintain sleep (**Box 3**). Given older adults greater likelihood to have a concomitant pain disorder, the authors recommend the use of the passive relaxation procedure outlined by Lichstein.[60] The efficacy of relaxation to produce desired changes, however, in isolation in older adults' sleep is questionable. Studies comparing relaxation with other forms of CBTi have universally found minimally positive results, typically inferior to the comparison treatments.[60] This conclusion is highlighted by McCurry and colleagues'[59] finding that relaxation training does not meet the necessary criteria to be considered an evidence-based treatment for late-life insomnia.

Cognitive therapy

Cognitive therapy aims to confront and address sleep-incompatible thoughts and expectations.

Box 1
Common sleep education components for older adults

- Increased prevalence of sleep disturbance
- Increase in sleep-onset latency
- Increase in wake after sleep onset
- Increase in number of nocturnal awakenings
- Increase in hypnotic use
- Increase in napping
- Decreased total sleep time
- Good sleep can be relearned

Box 2
Common sleep hygiene components

- Avoid caffeine after noon
- Avoid exercise within 2 hours of bedtime
- Avoid nicotine within 2 hours of bedtime
- Avoid alcohol within 2 hours of bedtime
- Avoid heavy meals within 2 hours of bedtime

Box 4
Stimulus control instructions

- Go to bed only when tired
- Do not use the bed or bedroom for anything but sleep and sex
- If sleep is not obtained in 15 minutes, leave the bed or bedroom
- Only return to bed on tiredness
- Repeat bullet #3 as necessary
- Wake at the same time every morning
- Avoid daytime napping

This is typically done through the use of such techniques as cognitive restructuring and thought challenging. There is no published research examining the effects of cognitive therapy alone on the sleep complaints of older adults. Accordingly, McCurry and colleagues'[59] review of the literature did not reveal sufficient evidence to suggest cognitive therapy is considered an evidence-based treatment for late-life insomnia, according to American Psychological Association criteria. Cognitive therapy is commonly used in combination with other CBTi techniques, however, to treat insomnia in late-life.

Stimulus control

Stimulus control[61] is a set of techniques that target the patient's learned behavioral association between the bed, the bedroom, and being awake. The instructions are specifically designed to increase the patient's association of the bedroom and the bed to sleeping. The specific instructions (**Box 4**) are intended to limit patient bedroom and bed behavior only to sleep and sex. The effects of stimulus control are generally regarded as positive. It has been suggested that stimulus control is "one of the most effect single-component treatments" for late-life insomnia.[62] This contention is supported by several investigations that report moderate to strong effects of stimulus control on the subjective sleep (sleep-onset latency [SOL] and wake after sleep onset [WASO]) of elders.[63–65] Stimulus control does not meet the necessary criteria, however, to be considered an evidence-based treatment for late-life insomnia, primarily because of a lack of research examining the effect

---

Box 3
Common relaxation practices

- Progressive muscle relaxation
- Passive muscle relaxation
- Autogenic phrases
- Diaphragmatic or deep breathing
- Mental imagery
- Meditation
- Biofeedback

---

of this treatment modality in isolation from other forms of CBTi.[59]

Sleep may initially worsen. This should be expected, but may result in a sleep debt that may facilitate later positive changes.

Sleep restriction and compression

Sleep restriction and sleep compression are similar techniques used to reduce the amount of unwanted awake time the patient experiences during the course of the night by matching the prescribed sleep time to actual time spent asleep (see **Table 1** for detailed instructions). One of the main goals of restriction and compression practices is to provide the patient with a long, continuous block of sleep that is relatively uninterrupted and of good quality. The mechanisms by which these techniques are believed to work are through a reduction of the association between the bed, the bedroom, and being awake and through building a sleep debt that may subsequently aid in improving sleep. The main distinction between the two alternative strategies is that sleep restriction sharply reduces the amount of time the patient spends in bed and then gradually increases this time, if indicated, while sleep compression is conducted by slow and gradual reduction of time spent in bed. Both sleep restriction and compression are regarded as highly efficacious treatments for late-life insomnia. Typical improvements are seen in the self-reported SOL and WASO of older patients. This point is illustrated by the generally positive findings from several studies using one of these two techniques.[45,66–68] Sleep restriction and sleep compression fulfill the American Psychological Association's requirements to be considered an evidence-based treatment for late-life insomnia.[59]

Combination treatments

Using a combination of the previously described techniques, clinicians have developed multicomponent treatment approaches to the treatment of late-life insomnia. These multicomponent treatment approaches are typically referred to as

Table 1	
Sleep restriction and compression instructions	
Sleep Restriction	**Sleep Compression**
Calculate average TIB and TST for the previous 1–2 wk	Calculate average TIB and TWT for the previous 1–2 wk
If average SE >90%, increase TIB by 30 min[a]	Divide TWT by number of proposed treatment sessions
If average SE <85%, decrease TIB by 30 min[a]	Reduce TIB slowly by above calculated increment
Retire at same time every night, wake at the same time every morning	Wake at the same time every morning
Avoid daytime napping	Avoid daytime napping

Abbreviations: SE, sleep efficiency; TIB, time in bed; TST, total sleep time; TWT, total wake time.
[a] If SE is between 85% and 90% do not adjust TIB.

CBTi. Typical treatment packages include use of two or more of the previously described techniques. One of the most common combinations is sleep education, relaxation training, stimulus control, and sleep restriction (sometimes also including cognitive therapy). Such multicomponent treatment packages have been empirically shown to provide improvements in the subjective experience of sleep (SOL, WASO, and sleep quality rating) in older adults with insomnia.[57,64,69] Multicomponent treatment packages fulfill the American Psychological Association's requirements to be considered an evidence-based treatment for late-life insomnia.[59]

Treatment as Usual Versus Behavioral Sleep Medicine Treatment Approaches

The previous reviews of pharmacotherapy and psychotherapy for the treatment of late-life insomnia suggest drastically different outcomes. How these two treatment modalities fair when in direct comparison with one another, however, is a scantly investigated area. Direct comparison of multicomponent CBTi, zopiclone, and a placebo resulted in CBTi producing objective and subjective improvements in sleep, whereas the placebo and zopiclone conditions did not differ from each other.[47] Comparison of multicomponent CBTi, temazepam, combined CBTi and temazepam, and placebo revealed that CBTi, temazepam, and combined CBTi and temazepam were roughly equally capable of producing positive change at 8 weeks. CBTi was rated as the most favorable treatment condition, however, and produced the most sustainable long-term changes, as measured at 24-month follow-up.[70] It seems warranted to conclude that behavioral sleep medicine approaches to the treatment of insomnia in late-life are preferable to hypnotic medications.

Innovative Behavioral Sleep Medicine Approaches With Older Adults

Behavioral sleep medicine is an ever evolving field. New treatment approaches are consistently introduced in the field. Several of these newer approaches are particularly promising when used with older adults and are briefly described next.

Short-term treatment
Multicomponent CBTi is typically delivered in 6 to 10, hour-long sessions spaced approximately 1 week apart. To produce more primary care friendly versions of CBTi, however, several recent investigations have suggested that CBTi can be effectively delivered in a much reduced timeframe. Specifically, investigators have documented the successful implementation of CBTi for older adults in as little as four 30-minute sessions[64]; one 45-minute session (with one 30-minute booster session)[69]; two 25-minute sessions[57]; and two 50-minute sessions (with two 30-minute phone sessions).[58] A recent review of short-term treatment approaches supports their promise for delivering effective CBTi[71] to older individuals.

Group treatment
Multicomponent CBTi is also typically delivered in individual, hour-long sessions. An alternative, however, to the time-consuming practice of individual sessions may be the use of a group therapy format. Several investigations have successfully implemented CBTi in small group settings, although typically in a mixed age range. At least one investigation, however, has successfully implemented CBTi for older adults in groups of four to six patients.[72] A review of group treatment approaches suggests it too holds promises for delivering effective CBTi.[71] McCrae and colleagues[71] have suggested, however, a need to investigate the additive benefit of capitalizing

on group factors rather than simply applying individual CBTi to multiple individuals at once.

Exercise as a treatment

The use of exercise as a potential treatment for late-life insomnia is intriguing, especially given exercise's positive influence on mood (for review see[73]), cognitive functioning (for review see[74]), and independence (for review see[75]) in late-life. To date, several clinical trials have treated older adults with a moderate sleep complaint through exercise.[76,77] All of these trials have produced impressive reductions in SOL and gains in total sleep time. It seems that exercise may be a useful treatment modality for late-life insomnia. Further research is needed to confirm this conclusion.

Treatment of Special Populations of Older Adults

Older adults are at an increased risk for several health-related disorders, making the diagnosis and treatment of primary and solitary insomnia increasingly unlikely with this patient population. Specifically, the next section provides a review of the literature that examines the treatment of insomnia in dementia patients and caregivers, comorbid insomnia in late-life, and hypnotic-dependent insomnia in older adults.

Dementia patients and dementia caregivers

Older patients with dementia often have an accompanying sleep disturbance. This sleep disturbance is typically treated with pharmaco-therapy; however, the efficacy of such practices has been questioned.[78] It seems more appropriate to adapt commonly used CBTi practices to be used with dementia patients. This adaptation may take the shape of training caregivers to implement CBTi with dementia patients.[79] Attention should also be paid, however, to the sleep of the caregiver. Caregivers frequently complain of poor sleep, and CBTi (including exercise) has been suggested as frontline treatment option.[80] Additional research is still needed in this arena.

Comorbid insomnia

Comorbid insomnia includes any case of insomnia that does not occur in solitary. As such, comorbid insomnia is very common and can occur in conjunction with medical (eg, pain, arthritis, cancer, and so forth) or psychologic (eg, depression, anxiety, bereavement, and so forth) conditions. Insomnia of older adults experiencing concomitant medical conditions has been shown to be responsive to CBTi practices.[81] Furthermore, some researchers have not used the typical medical and psychologic exclusion criteria used in treatment studies and have still reported CBTi to be an effective treatment of late-life sleep disturbances.[64,69] In the context of normal age-related medical comorbidities, CBTi seems efficacious in treating insomnia. Lastly, a study comparing the responsiveness of older adults with either comorbid medical or psychologic disturbances to CBTi found no distinctions between the groups. Both responded equally well.[21] In general, it seems that insomnia comorbid with another condition (either medical or psychologic in nature) responds well to CBTi.

Hypnotic-dependent insomnia

Given physicians' propensity to prescribe hypnotic medication and the lack of long-term improvements associated with such medication, hypnotically dependent insomnia in late-life may be quite common. Hypnotic-dependent insomnia is a condition in which an individual continues to experience insomnia symptoms during the course of hypnotic medication use. Sleep may actually worsen on halting medication use; individuals find themselves unable to stop taking their prescription medication but continuing to sleep poorly. CBTi has been shown effective in improving the sleep of hypnotically dependent older adults with insomnia, without medication termination.[82] Additionally, CBTi has been used as an adjunct to traditional medical tapering procedures. When used in this manner, CBTi plus tapering produces much higher rates of hypnotic abstinence at 12-month follow-up[83] and reductions in insomnia symptoms.[84] It seems CBTi should be an integral component of hypnotic withdrawal programs for older adults.

SUMMARY

A variety of factors (sleep architecture changes, medications, comorbidities, chronicity) contribute to the high prevalence of insomnia in later life. Comorbidities seem to play a particularly important role, because when they are controlled for, the prevalence of late-life insomnia drops considerably. Understanding the role of late-life insomnia's multifactorial nature, particularly the role of comorbidities, is important for accurate and effective assessment, diagnosis, and treatment. Older adults are likely to seek treatment for insomnia in primary care settings, and several proved tools are available to help improve the detection of insomnia in such settings. Both pharmacologic and behavioral treatment approaches have demonstrated use. Late-insomnia's chronic and comorbid nature, however, make behavioral techniques the preferable treatment approach.

REFERENCES

1. World Health Organization. The international classification of diseases, 10th revision, Geneva: ICD-10, 1992.
2. American Academy of Sleep Medicine. International classification of sleep disorders. 2nd edition. Diagnostic and coding manual. Westchester (IL); 2005.
3. McCrae CS, Wilson NM, Lichstein KL, et al. Young old and old old poor sleepers with and without insomnia complaints. J Psychosom Res 2003;54(1):11–9.
4. Foley DJ, Monjan AA, Brown SL, et al. Sleep complaints among elderly persons: an epidemiologic study of three communities. Sleep 1995; 18(6):425–32.
5. Mellinger GD, Balter MB, Uhlenhuth EH. Insomnia and its treatment: prevalence and correlates. Arch Gen Psychiatry 1985;42(3):225–32.
6. Bliwise DL, King AC, Harris RB, et al. Prevalence of self-reported poor sleep in a healthy population aged 50–65. Soc Sci Med 1992;34(1):49–55.
7. American Psychiatric Association. Diagnostic and statistical manual of mental disorders. Arlington (VA); 1994.
8. Morin CM, Mimeault V, Gagne A. Nonpharmacological treatment of late-life insomnia. J Psychosom Res 1999;46(2):103–16.
9. Morgan K, Clarke D. Risk factors for late-life insomnia in a representative general practice sample. Br J Gen Pract 1997;47(416):166–9.
10. Rajput V, Bromley SM. Chronic insomnia: a practical review. Am Fam Physician 1999;60(5):1431–8 [discussion: 1441–2].
11. Dodge R, Cline MG, Quan SF. The natural history of insomnia and its relationship to respiratory symptoms. Arch Intern Med 1995;155(16):1797–800.
12. Vitiello MV, Larsen LH, Moe KE. Age-related sleep change: gender and estrogen effects on the subjective-objective sleep quality relationships of healthy, noncomplaining older men and women. J Psychosom Res 2004;56(5):503–10.
13. Ohayon MM. Epidemiology of insomnia: what we know and what we still need to learn. Sleep Med Rev 2002;6(2):97–111.
14. Rajput V, Bromley SM. Chronic insomnia: a practical review. Am Fam Physician 1999;60(5):1431–8 [discussion: 1441–2].
15. Vitiello MV, Moe KE, Prinz PN. Sleep complaints cosegregate with illness in older adults: clinical research informed by and informing epidemiological studies of sleep. J Psychosom Res 2002;53(1):555–9.
16. Foley D, Ancoli-Israel S, Britz P, et al. Sleep disturbances and chronic disease in older adults: results of the 2003 National Sleep Foundation Sleep in America Survey. J Psychosom Res 2004;56(5):497–502.
17. Brooks III JO, Friedman L, Bliwise DL, et al. Use of the wrist actigraph to study insomnia in older adults. Sleep 1993;16(2):151–5.
18. Hohagen F, Kappler C, Schramm E, et al. Prevalence of insomnia in elderly general practice attenders and the current treatment modalities. Acta Psychiatr Scand 1994;90(2):102–8.
19. Katz DA, McHorney CA. Clinical correlates of insomnia in patients with chronic illness. Arch Intern Med 1998;158(10):1099–107.
20. National Institutes of Health. National Institutes of Health State of the Science Conference Statement. Sleep 2005;28(9):1049–57.
21. Lichstein KL, Wilson NM, Johnson CT. Psychological treatment of secondary insomnia. Psychol Aging 2000;15(2):232–40.
22. Ozminkowski RJ, Wang S, Walsh JK. The direct and indirect costs of untreated insomnia in adults in the United States. Sleep 2007;30(3):263–73.
23. Roth T, Roehrs TA. Issues in the use of benzodiazepine therapy. J Clin Psychiatry 1992;53(Suppl):14–8.
24. Morgan K, Clarke D. Longitudinal trends in late-life insomnia: implications for prescribing. Age Ageing 1997;26(3):179–84.
25. Roth T, Zorick F, Wittig R, et al. Pharmacological and medical considerations in hypnotic use. Sleep 1982; 5(Suppl 1):S46–52.
26. Borbely AA. A two process model of sleep regulation. Hum Neurobiol 1982;1(3):195–204.
27. Weitzman ED, Moline ML, Czeisler CA, et al. Chronobiology of aging: temperature, sleep-wake rhythms and entrainment. Neurobiol Aging 1982;3(4):299–309.
28. Czeisler CA, Dumont M, Duffy JF, et al. Association of sleep-wake habits in older people with changes in output of circadian pacemaker. Lancet 1992; 340(8825):933–6.
29. Ohayon MM, Carskadon MA, Guilleminault C, et al. Meta-analysis of quantitative sleep parameters from childhood to old age in healthy individuals: developing normative sleep values across the human lifespan. Sleep 2004;27(7):1255–73.
30. Van Cauter E, Leproult R, Plat L. Age-related changes in slow wave sleep and REM sleep and relationship with growth hormone and cortisol levels in healthy men. JAMA 2000;284(7):861–8.
31. Bonnet MH, Arand DL. Hyperarousal and insomnia. Sleep Med Rev 1997;1(2):97–108.
32. Fichten CS, Creti L, Amsel R, et al. Poor sleepers who do not complain of insomnia: myths and realities about psychological and lifestyle characteristics of older good and poor sleepers. J Behav Med 1995;18(2):189–223.
33. Doghramji PP. Detection of insomnia in primary care. J Clin Psychiatry 2001;62(Suppl 10):18–26.
34. Doghramji K. Assessment of excessive sleepiness and insomnia as they relate to circadian rhythm sleep disorders. J Clin Psychiatry 2004;65(Suppl 16):17–22.
35. Doghramji PP. Recognizing sleep disorders in a primary care setting. J Clin Psychiatry 2004; 65(Suppl 16):23–6.

36. Ancoli-Israel S, Cooke JR. Prevalence and comorbidity of insomnia and effect on functioning in elderly populations. J Am Geriatr Soc 2005;53(Suppl 7): S264–71.

37. Bailes S, Baltzan M, Rizzo D, et al. A diagnostic symptom profile for sleep disorder in primary care patients. J Psychosom Res 2008;64(4):427–33.

38. Smyth CA. Evaluating sleep quality in older adults: the Pittsburgh Sleep Quality Index can be used to detect sleep disturbances or deficits. Am J Nurs 2008;108(5):42–50 [quiz 50–1].

39. Brown RT, Freeman WS, Brown RA, et al. The role of psychology in health care delivery. Prof Psychol Res Pract 2002;33(6):536–45.

40. Morin CM, Gramling SE. Sleep patterns and aging: comparison of older adults with and without insomnia complaints. Psychol Aging 1989;4(3): 290–4.

41. Petit L, Azad N, Byszewski A, et al. Non-pharmacological management of primary and secondary insomnia among older people: review of assessment tools and treatments. Age Ageing 2003;32(1):19–25.

42. Sanford SD, Lichstein KL, Durrence HH, et al. The influence of age, gender, ethnicity, and insomnia on Epworth sleepiness scores: a normative US population. Sleep Med 2006;7(4):319–26.

43. Morin CM, Stone J, Trinkle D, et al. Dysfunctional beliefs and attitudes about sleep among older adults with and without insomnia complaints. Psychol Aging 1993;8(3):463–7.

44. Wohlgemuth WK, Edinger JD, Fins AI, et al. How many nights are enough? The short-term stability of sleep parameters in elderly insomniacs and normal sleepers. Psychophysiology 1999;36(2): 233–44.

45. Friedman L, Benson K, Noda A, et al. An actigraphic comparison of sleep restriction and sleep hygiene treatments for insomnia in older adults. J Geriatr Psychiatry Neurol 2000;13(1):17–27.

46. McCrae CS, Rowe MA, Dautovich ND, et al. Sleep hygiene practices in two community dwelling samples of older adults. Sleep 2006;29(12): 1551–60.

47. Sivertsen B, Omvik S, Pallesen S, et al. Cognitive behavioral therapy vs zopiclone for treatment of chronic primary insomnia in older adults: a randomized controlled trial. JAMA 2006;295(24):2851–8.

48. Morgenthaler T, Alessi C, Friedman L, et al. Practice parameters for the use of actigraphy in the assessment of sleep and sleep disorders: an update for 2007. Sleep 2007;30(4):519–29.

49. American Sleep Disorders Association. Practice parameters for the treatment of snoring and obstructive sleep apnea with oral appliances. Sleep 1995; 18(6):511–3.

50. Lichstein KL, Stone KC, Nau SD, et al. Insomnia in the elderly. Sleep Med Clin 2006;1(2):221–30.

51. Krakow B, Melendrez D, Ferreira E, et al. Prevalence of insomnia symptoms in patients with sleep-disordered breathing. Chest 2001;120(6):1923–9.

52. Antai-Otong D. Risks and benefits of non-benzodiazepine receptor agonists in the treatment of acute primary insomnia in older adults. Perspect Psychiatr Care 2006;42(3):196–200.

53. Bain KT. Management of chronic insomnia in elderly persons. Am J Geriatr Pharmacother 2006;4(2): 168–92.

54. Dolder C, Nelson M, McKinsey J. Use of non-benzodiazepine hypnotics in the elderly: are all agents the same? CNS Drugs 2007;21(5):389–405.

55. McCrae CS, Ross A, Stripling A, et al. Eszopiclone for late-life insomnia. Clin Interv Aging 2007;2(3):313–26.

56. Reynolds CFI, Buysse DJ, Miller MD, et al. Paroxetine treatment of primary insomnia in older adults. Am J Geriatr Psychiatry 2006;14(9):803–7.

57. Edinger JD, Sampson WS. A primary care friendly cognitive behavioral insomnia therapy. Sleep 2003; 26(2):177–82.

58. McCrae CS, McGovern R, Lukefahr R, et al. Research evaluating brief behavioral sleep treatments for rural elderly (RESTORE): a preliminary examination of effectiveness. Am J Geriatr Psychiatry 2007;15(11):979–82.

59. McCurry SM, Logsdon RG, Teri L, et al. Evidence-based psychological treatments for insomnia in older adults. Psychol Aging 2007;22(1):18–27.

60. Lichstein KL. Relaxation. In: Lichstein KL, Morin CM, Lichstein KL, et al, editors. Treatment of late-life insomnia. Thousand Oaks (CA): Sage Publications, Inc; 2000. p. 185–206.

61. Bootzin RR. A stimulus control treatment for insomnia. Proc Am Psychol Assoc 1972;395–6.

62. Bootzin RR, Epstein DR. Stimulus control. In: Lichstein KL, Morin CM, Lichstein KL, et al, editors. Treatment of late-life insomnia. Thousand Oaks (CA): Sage Publications, Inc; 2000. p. 167–84.

63. Davies R, Lacks P, Storandt M, et al. Countercontrol treatment of sleep-maintenance insomnia in relation to age. Psychol Aging 1986;1(3):233–8.

64. Pallesen S, Nordhus IH, Kvale G, et al. Behavioral treatment of insomnia in older adults: an open clinical trial comparing two interventions. Behav Res Ther 2003;41(1):31–48.

65. Puder R, Lacks P, Bertelson AD, et al. Short-term stimulus control treatment of insomnia in older adults. Behav Ther 1983;14(3):424–9.

66. Friedman L, Bliwise DL, Yesavage JA, et al. A preliminary study comparing sleep restriction and relaxation treatments for insomnia in older adults. J Gerontol 1991;46(1):P1–8.

67. Lichstein KL, Riedel BW, Wilson NM, et al. Relaxation and sleep compression for late-life insomnia: a placebo-controlled trial. J Consult Clin Psychol 2001;69(2):227–39.

68. Riedel BW, Lichstein KL, Dwyer WO. Sleep compression and sleep education for older insomniacs: self-help versus therapist guidance. Psychol Aging 1995;10(1):54–63.

69. Germain A, Moul DE, Franzen PL, et al. Effects of a brief behavioral treatment for late-life insomnia: preliminary findings. J Clin Sleep Med 2006;2(4):403–6.

70. Morin CM, Colecchi C, Stone J, et al. Behavioral and pharmacological therapies for late-life insomnia: a randomized controlled trial. JAMA 1999;281(11):991–9.

71. McCrae CS, Dautovich N, Dzierzewski JM. Short-term and group treatment approaches. New York: Informa Healthcare; In press.

72. Morin CM, Kowatch RA, Barry T, et al. Cognitive-behavior therapy for late-life insomnia. J Consult Clin Psychol 1993;61(1):137–46.

73. Arent SM, Landers DM, Etnier JL. The effects of exercise on mood in older adults: a meta-analytic review. J Aging Phys Act 2000;8(4):407–30.

74. Colcombe S, Kramer AF. Fitness effects on the cognitive function of older adults: a meta-analytic study. Psychol Sci 2003;14(2):125–30.

75. Breen L, Stewart CE, Onambélé GL. Functional benefits of combined resistance training with nutritional interventions in older adults: a review. Geriatr Gerontol Int 2007;7(4):326–40.

76. King AC, Oman RF, Brassington GS, et al. Moderate-intensity exercise and self-rated quality of sleep in older adults. a randomized controlled trial. JAMA 1997;277(1):32–7.

77. King AC, Pruitt LA, Woo S, et al. Effects of moderate-intensity exercise on polysomnographic and subjective sleep quality in older adults with mild to moderate sleep complaints. J Gerontol A Biol Sci Med Sci 2008;63(9):997–1004.

78. McCurry SM, Reynolds CF, Ancoli-Israel S, et al. Treatment of sleep disturbance in Alzheimer's disease. Sleep Med Rev 2000;4(6):603–28.

79. McCurry SM, Gibbons LE, Logsdon RG, et al. Nighttime insomnia treatment and education for Alzheimer's disease: a randomized, controlled trial. J Am Geriatr Soc 2005;53(5):793–802.

80. McCurry SM, Logsdon RG, Teri L, et al. Sleep disturbances in caregivers of persons with dementia: contributing factors and treatment implications. Sleep Med Rev 2007;11(2):143–53.

81. Rybarczyk B, Lopez M, Schelble K, et al. Home-based video CBT for comorbid geriatric insomnia: a pilot study using secondary data analyses. Behav Sleep Med 2005;3(3):158–75.

82. Soeffing JP, Lichstein KL, Nau SD, et al. Psychological treatment of insomnia in hypnotic-dependant older adults. Sleep Med 2008;9(2):165–71.

83. Baillargeon L, Landreville P, Verreault R, et al. Discontinuation of benzodiazepines among older insomniac adults treated with cognitive-behavioural therapy combined with gradual tapering: a randomized trial. Can Med Assoc J 2003;169(10):1015–20.

84. Morin CM, Bastien CL, Guay B, et al. Randomized clinical trial of supervised tapering and cognitive behavior therapy to facilitate benzodiazepine discontinuation in older adults with chronic insomnia. Am J Psychiatry 2004;161(2):332–42.

Index

Note: Page numbers of article titles are in **boldface** type.

A

Accreditation Council for Graduate Medical Education (ACGME), physician trainees post-ACGME guidelines, 531
  mortality data, 532
  quality of life, 532
Actigraphy, in assessment of late-life insomnia, 597
Adaptation, physiologic and behavioral, to sleep loss, by physicians, 533–534
Adherence, treatment, to continuous positive airway pressure in obstructive sleep apnea, **473–485**
  adherence factors, 474–475
    disease severity and improvements in disease variables, 474
    patient-reported barriers, 474–475
    potential social factors, 475
    psychological and personality factors, 475
  mechanical interventions, 477–479
    humidification, 478
    mask types, 477
    PAP delivery modes, 478–479
    titration methods, 479
  nonadherence statistics, 473–474
  psychoeducational approaches, 479–480
    cognitive behavioral therapy, 480
    motivational enhancement therapy for CPAP, 480
    psychoeducation, 480
    self-management program, 479
    systematic densensitization, 479
  theoretical approach, 475–477
    health belief model, 475–476
    social cognitive theory and transtheoretical model, 476–477
    Wallston's health locus of control and social learning theory, 476
Advanced sleep phase disorder, 500–501
Age, effect on sleep deprivation in physicians, 533
Alzheimer's disease, insomnia in caregivers of persons with, **519–526**
Apnea. See Obstructive sleep apnea.
Ascending reticular activating system, in control of sleep and wakefulness, 551–553
Attentional processes, in chronic insomnia, 542–544
Attributional processes, in chronic insomnia, 544–545
Autoadjusting positive airway pressure, 478

B

Bandura, social cognitive theory and transtheoretical model, 476–477
Basal ganglia, role in sleep-wake regulation and dysregulation, 550–551
Behavioral adaptation, to sleep loss, by physicians, 533–534
Behavioral sleep medicine, 473–604
  chronic insomnia, cognitive mechanisms, **541–548**
    hypnotic discontinuation in, **583–592**
    neurobiologic mechanisms, **549–558**
  circadian rhythm disorders, **495–505**
  comorbid insomnia, **571–582**
  insomnia in caregivers of persons with dementia, **519–526**
  late-life insomnia, **593–604**
  nightmares in adults, **507–517**
  obstructive sleep apnea, **473–485**
  physicians and sleep deprivation, **527–540**
  primary insomnia, **559–569**
  restless legs syndrome and periodic sleep movement disorder, **487–494**
Benzodiazepines, management of hypnotic-dependent insomnia related to, **583–592**
Bi-level positive airway pressure, 478
Brain, neurobiologic structures involved in sleep-wake regulation, 549–551
Burnout, related to sleep deprivation in physicians, 534

C

C-flex positive airway pressure, 478–479
Cancer, comorbid insomnia and, 577–578
Caregivers, of persons with dementia, insomnia in, **519–526**
  cross-sectional correlates of sleep disturbances in, 520
  identifying dyads at greatest risk, 520–522
  treatment of, 522–524, 601
Chronic insomnia. See Insomnia, chronic.
Chronic pain. See Pain, chronic.
Circadian rhythm disorders, **495–505**
  advanced sleep phase disorder, 500–501
  delayed sleep phase disorder, 499–500
  effect of light on circadian system, 495–496
  endogenous and exogenous melatonin, 496

doi:10.1016/S1556-407X(09)00114-3
1556-407X/09/$ – see front matter

sleep.theclinics.com

United States Postal Service

Statement of Ownership, Management, and Circulation
(All Periodicals Publications Except Requestor Publications)

1. Publication Title	2. Publication Number	3. Filing Date
Sleep Medicine Clinics of North America	0 2 5 - 0 5 3	9/15/09

4. Issue Frequency	5. Number of Issues Published Annually	6. Annual Subscription Price
Mar, Jun, Sep, Dec	4	$150.00

7. Complete Mailing Address of Known Office of Publication (Not printer) (Street, city, county, state, and ZIP+4®)

Elsevier Inc.
360 Park Avenue South
New York, NY 10010-1710

Contact Person
Stephen Bushing

Telephone (Include area code)
215-239-3688

8. Complete Mailing Address of Headquarters or General Business Office of Publisher (Not printer)

Elsevier Inc. 360 Park Avenue South, New York, NY 10010-1710

9. Full Names and Complete Mailing Addresses of Publisher, Editor, and Managing Editor (Do not leave blank)

Publisher (Name and complete mailing address)

John Schrefer , Elsevier, Inc., 1600 John F. Kennedy Blvd. Suite 1800, Philadelphia, PA 19103-2899

Editor (Name and complete mailing address)

Sarah Barth, Elsevier, Inc., 1600 John F. Kennedy Blvd. Suite 1800, Philadelphia, PA 19103-2899

Managing Editor (Name and complete mailing address)

Catherine Bewick, Elsevier, Inc., 1600 John F. Kennedy Blvd. Suite 1800, Philadelphia, PA 19103-2899

10. Owner (Do not leave blank. If the publication is owned by a corporation, give the name and address of the corporation immediately followed by the names and addresses of all stockholders owning or holding 1 percent or more of the total amount of stock. If not owned by a corporation, give the names and addresses of the individual owners. If owned by a partnership or other unincorporated firm, give its name and address as well as those of each individual owner. If the publication is published by a nonprofit organization, give its name and address.)

Full Name	Complete Mailing Address
Wholly owned subsidiary of	4520 East-West Highway
Reed/Elsevier, US holdings	Bethesda, MD 20814

11. Known Bondholders, Mortgagees, and Other Security Holders Owning or Holding 1 Percent or More of Total Amount of Bonds, Mortgages, or Other Securities. If none, check box ☐ None

Full Name	Complete Mailing Address
N/A	

12. Tax Status (For completion by nonprofit organizations authorized to mail at nonprofit rates) (Check one)
The purpose, function, and nonprofit status of this organization and the exempt status for federal income tax purposes:
☐ Has Not Changed During Preceding 12 Months
☐ Has Changed During Preceding 12 Months (Publisher must submit explanation of change with this statement)

PS Form 3526, September 2007 (Page 1 of 3 (Instructions Page 3)) PSN 7530-01-000-9931 PRIVACY NOTICE: See our Privacy policy in www.usps.com

---

13. Publication Title	14. Issue Date for Circulation Data Below
Sleep Medicine Clinics of North America	September 2009

15. Extent and Nature of Circulation

			Average No. Copies Each Issue During Preceding 12 Months	No. Copies of Single Issue Published Nearest to Filing Date
a. Total Number of Copies (Net press run)			1151	1105
b. Paid Circulation (By Mail and Outside the Mail)	(1)	Mailed Outside-County Paid Subscriptions Stated on PS Form 3541. (Include paid distribution above nominal rate, advertiser's proof copies, and exchange copies)	535	521
	(2)	Mailed In-County Paid Subscriptions Stated on PS Form 3541 (Include paid distribution above nominal rate, advertiser's proof copies, and exchange copies)		
	(3)	Paid Distribution Outside the Mails Including Sales Through Dealers and Carriers, Street Vendors, Counter Sales, and Other Paid Distribution Outside USPS®	46	50
	(4)	Paid Distribution by Other Classes Mailed Through the USPS (e.g. First-Class Mail®)		
c. Total Paid Distribution (Sum of 15b (1), (2), (3), and (4))		▶	581	571
d. Free or Nominal Rate Distribution (By Mail and Outside the Mail)	(1)	Free or Nominal Rate Outside-County Copies Included on PS Form 3541	67	65
	(2)	Free or Nominal Rate In-County Copies Included on PS Form 3541		
	(3)	Free or Nominal Rate Copies Mailed at Other Classes Through the USPS (e.g. First-Class Mail)		
	(4)	Free or Nominal Rate Distribution Outside the Mail (Carriers or other means)		
e. Total Free or Nominal Rate Distribution (Sum of 15d (1), (2), (3) and (4))		▶	67	65
f. Total Distribution (Sum of 15c and 15e)		▶	648	636
g. Copies not Distributed (See instructions to publishers #4 (page #3))		▶	503	469
h. Total (Sum of 15f and g)		▶	1151	1105
i. Percent Paid (15c divided by 15f times 100)			89.66%	89.78%

16. Publication of Statement of Ownership
☐ If the publication is a general publication, publication of this statement is required. Will be printed in the December 2009 issue of this publication. ☐ Publication not required.

17. Signature and Title of Editor, Publisher, Business Manager, or Owner

[signature] Stephen R. Bushing

Stephen R. Bushing – Subscription Services Coordinator

Date September 15, 2009

I certify that all information furnished on this form is true and complete. I understand that anyone who furnishes false or misleading information on this form or who omits material or information requested on the form may be subject to criminal sanctions (including fines and imprisonment) and/or civil sanctions (including civil penalties).

PS Form 3526, September 2007 (Page 2 of 3)

Printed and bound by CPI Group (UK) Ltd, Croydon, CR0 4YY

03/10/2024

01040354-0013